Seminars in Addiction
Psychiatry

College Seminars Series

For details of available and forthcoming books in the College Seminars Series please visit: www.cambridge.org/series/college-seminars-series.

Seminars in Addiction Psychiatry

Second edition

Edited by
Ed Day

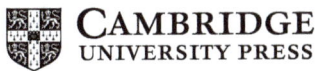

CAMBRIDGE
UNIVERSITY PRESS

University Printing House, Cambridge CB2 8BS, United Kingdom

One Liberty Plaza, 20th Floor, New York, NY 10006, USA

477 Williamstown Road, Port Melbourne, VIC 3207, Australia

314–321, 3rd Floor, Plot 3, Splendor Forum, Jasola District Centre,
New Delhi – 110025, India

103 Penang Road, #05–06/07, Visioncrest Commercial, Singapore 238467

Cambridge University Press is part of the University of Cambridge.

It furthers the University's mission by disseminating knowledge in the pursuit of
education, learning, and research at the highest international levels of excellence.

www.cambridge.org
Information on this title: www.cambridge.org/9781911623182
DOI: 10.1017/9781911623199

© The Royal College of Psychiatrists 2021

First published 1994, as Seminars in Alcohol and Drug Misuse by The Royal College of Psychiatrists
This second edition published by Cambridge University Press 2021

A catalogue record for this publication is available from the British Library.

Library of Congress Cataloging-in-Publication Data
Names: Day, Ed, editor.
Title: Seminars in addiction psychiatry / edited by Ed Day.
Description: Cambridge, United Kingdom ; New York, NY : Cambridge University Press, 2021. | Series:
College seminars series | Includes index.
Identifiers: LCCN 2021024704 (print) | LCCN 2021024705 (ebook) | ISBN 9781911623182 (paperback) |
ISBN 9781911623199 (ebook)
Subjects: LCSH: Substance abuse. | Compulsive behavior. | BISAC: PSYCHOLOGY / Mental Health
Classification: LCC RC564 .S455 2021 (print) | LCC RC564 (ebook) | DDC 362.29–dc23
LC record available at https://lccn.loc.gov/2021024704
LC ebook record available at https://lccn.loc.gov/2021024705

ISBN 978-1-911-62318-2 Paperback

Contents

Contributors

Dima Abdulrahim
NEPTUNE Project Principal Researcher & Program Manager, Central North West London NHS Foundation Trust

Alexandra Abry
Senior Clinical Research Coordinator, Recovery Research Institute, Center for Addiction Medicine, Massachusetts General Hospital, and Harvard Medical School, 151 Merrimac Street, 6th Floor, Boston, MA 02114.

Brandon G. Bergman
Assistant Professor of Psychology, Harvard Medical School, Recovery Research Institute, Center for Addiction Medicine, Massachusetts General Hospital, and Harvard Medical School, 151 Merrimac Street, 6th Floor, Boston, MA 02114.

Paul Bogowicz
CT3 in Psychiatry, Universal Crisis Team Northumberland/North Tyneside, Cumbria, Northumberland, Tyne and Wear NHS Foundation Trust, St George's Park, Morpeth NE61 2NU

Owen Bowden-Jones
Consultant in Addiction Psychiatry, Central North West London NHS Foundation Trust, Club Drug Clinic, 69 Warwick Road, Earls Court London SW5 9HB

Alex Copello
Professor of Addictions and Consultant Clinical Psychologist, Institute for Mental Health, School of Psychology, 52 Pritchatts Road, Edgbaston, Birmingham B152TT

Ed Day
Clinical Reader in Addiction Psychiatry, Institute for Mental Health, School of Psychology, University of Birmingham & Consultant in Addiction Psychiatry, Solihull Integrated Addiction Service, Institute for Mental Health, School of Psychology, 52 Pritchatts Road, Edgbaston, Birmingham B152TT

Emily Finch
Consultant in Addiction Psychiatry, Southwark, Central Acute and Addictions Directorate, South London and Maudsley NHS Foundation Trust, Marina House, 63-65 Denmark Hill, London SE5 8RS

Eilish Gilvarry
Professor and Consultant in Addiction Psychiatry, Newcastle Treatment and Recovery (NTaR), Plummer Court, Carliol Place, Newcastle NE1 6UR

Jennifer Harris
Consultant Clinical Psychologist, Wiltshire Psychological Service, Avon and Wiltshire NHS Mental Health Partnership NHS Trust

Andrea Hearn
Consultant in Addiction Psychiatry, Newcastle Treatment and Recovery (NTaR), Plummer Court, Carliol Place, Newcastle NE1 6UR

Rob Hill
Consultant Clinical Psychologist and Honorary Visiting Research Fellow, South London and the Maudsley NHS Foundation Trust, 63–65 Denmark Hill, London SE5 8RZ and the Institute of Psychiatry, Psychology & Neuroscience, King's College London

Nicola J. Kalk
Consultant Psychiatrist in Addictions and Visiting Clinical Lecturer, South London and the Maudsley NHS Foundation Trust & King's College London

Eileen Kaner
Professor of Primary Care & Public Health Research, Population Health Sciences Institute, Faculty of Medical Sciences, Newcastle University, Baddiley-Clark Building, Richardson Road, Newcastle upon Tyne NE2 4AX

Michael Kelleher
Consultant Addictions Psychiatrist and Clinical Lead for Lambeth Addictions, Lambeth Addictions Consortium, 12–14 Brighton Terrace, Brixton, London SW9 8DG

John F. Kelly
Elizabeth R. Spallin Professor of Psychiatry in the Field of Addiction Medicine at Harvard Medical School, Recovery Research Institute, Center for Addiction Medicine, Massachusetts General Hospital, and Harvard Medical School, 151 Merrimac Street, 6th Floor, Boston, MA 02114.

Fergus Law
Honorary Senior Clinical Lecturer, Faculty of Health Sciences, University of Bristol, Tyndall Avenue, Bristol BS8 1TH

Ann McNeill
Professor of Tobacco Addiction, National Addictions Centre, Institute of Psychiatry, Psychology & Neuroscience, King's College London, 4 Windsor Walk, Denmark Hill, London SE58BB

Luke Mitcheson

James Morris
Programme Manager, Alcohol and Drugs, Treatment and Recovery Team, Public Health England

David Pang
Consultant in Addiction Psychiatry, CGL Central & West Hub, 255 Hospital Street, Birmingham, West Midlands B19 2YF

Mark Pucci
Consultant in Acute Medicine, Clinical Pharmacology and Therapeutics, Queen Elizabeth Hospital, University Hospitals Birmingham NHS Foundation Trust

Duncan Raistrick
Consultant Addiction Psychiatrist & Visiting Senior Lecturer, The University of Leeds

Debbie Robson
Senior Research Fellow, National Addictions Centre, Institute of Psychiatry, Psychology & Neuroscience, King's College London, 4 Windsor Walk, Denmark Hill, London SE58BB

Emma Rourke
GP Registrar, Gloucestershire Hospitals NHS Foundation Trust, Great Western Road, Gloucester GL1 3NN

Mary Thornton
Core Trainee 3 and Honorary Clinical Research Fellow, South London and the Maudsley NHS Foundation Trust & King's College London

Gillian Tober
Consultant Addiction Psychologist & Visiting Sebior Lecturer, The University of Leeds

Preface

As a psychiatry trainee in the late 1990s I looked to the *College Seminars Series* as a vital source of information, both to pass college membership exams but also to go beyond the facts that standard textbooks provided. Here was a series written by people who were applying textbook knowledge at the 'coalface' of clinical practice. Reflecting my growing interest in the field, I found *Seminars in Alcohol and Drug Misuse* especially useful. I was particularly fascinated by the opening chapter, which outlined the evolution of the concept of dependence. Rereading that chapter when considering this book I was surprised to see reference to DSM-III-R, which reminded me that the last edition of the book was published in 1994. This new edition retains the core structure of the first edition, with revised and updated versions of each of the original book's 11 chapters written by new authors. In Chapter 1, the new edition reflects the changes in the diagnostic landscape that have occurred in the intervening quarter century. While ICD-11 has simplified the concept of dependence, DSM-5 has abandoned it altogether, leaving us with a potentially confusing difference in various parts of the world. Chapter 1 sets the scene for the book by reviewing the diagnostic issues that we consider when we think of 'addiction', and reviewing the historical path to our present understanding of this term.

The core work of the specialist addiction psychiatrist remains the treatment of heroin, cocaine (Chapters 2 and 3) and alcohol dependence (Chapters 5, 6 and 7). These topics are explored over the five chapters, covering epidemiology, aetiology, prevention and treatment. The prevalence of drug use has ebbed and flowed since the first edition, and our understanding of the aetiology of addiction has expanded. Large-scale epidemiological analysis has promoted a concept of risk and protective factors for developing a drug use disorder. Huge advances in the understanding of the neurobiology of addiction are reflected in both Chapters 2 and 6. Prevention and treatment strategies have also moved forwards, with the development since 1994 of a significant evidence base for take-home naloxone, opioid agonist treatment with buprenorphine and recovery-orientated systems of care. Prescription medication addiction has also increased in significance, with new drugs such as the gabapentinoids now meriting consideration (Chapter 4).

Psychological approaches remain the mainstay of treatment, and the developments in this area are captured in Chapter 8. Motivational interviewing has become an important strategy in the field, and it is a skill that all healthcare professionals should be able to use. Comorbidity of addiction and mental illness remains as common and as problematic as it did 25 years ago, and Chapter 9 covers the latest policy responses to the issue in the UK. Physical health problems resulting from drug or alcohol use are still as potentially serious as they were, but advances in medical knowledge mean that there is more hope of effective treatment (e.g. hepatitis C infection), as summarised in Chapter 10. The period from 2001 to 2008 saw rapid development of both evidence base and treatment services in the UK, only for much of the latter to wither away in the following decade. This is reflected in the chapter on treatment service provision (Chapter 11), reminding us that addiction remains a stigmatised issue and that its treatment is subject to political ideology.

This book includes four new chapters not present in the first edition, three covering long-standing issues and one a completely new one. Nicotine has long been the most prevalent substance of dependence around the world, and one of the largest causes of morbidity and mortality. The systematic application of evidence-based strategies across the public health and treatment world has reduced the impact of tobacco dependence (at least in the wealthier countries), and in many ways represents a model of the application of science to reduce a health burden. Chapter 12 provides a practical summary of this evidence, as well as exploring how it can be applied in psychiatric settings. Novel psychoactive substances (so-called legal highs) were not an issue in 1994, but a combination of globalisation and the ubiquity of the Internet meant that they came to prominence in the early twenty-first century. Chapter 13 summarises the current state of knowledge in this rapidly evolving area. Families have always felt the impact of psychoactive substance use by a loved one, but this has not always been acknowledged in the provision of treatment services. Chapter 14 highlights groundbreaking work from the UK in this area, with a focus on two pragmatic interventions that support and involve family and social network members. Finally, the term 'recovery' did not appear at all in the index of the first edition, and mutual self-help groups received very little attention. Chapter 15 rectifies this deficit, describing the evolution of the 12-Step Fellowships alongside four other mutual help organisations.

I hope this book will provide both the interested trainee and their consultant supervisor with a synthesis of the latest evidence and its application in policy and practice. My only regret is that there was not space to consider the next frontier of addiction science, that of behavioural addictions. Much is known about gambling, and it has been included for the first time in DSM-5. However, my teenage children and their generation have never known a world without the Internet, and an understanding of the mechanism of reward has underpinned many of the applications that run on today's smartphones. I anticipate that the next edition of this book will consider several of these behavioural addictions, and the title will reflect this change.

Ed Day
Birmingham, UK
April 2021

Historical and Conceptual Approaches to Addiction

Ed Day and James Morris

The Evolution of a Term: What Is 'Addiction'?

At the start of the twenty-first century, 'addiction' is said to be a 'disease' in most Western industrialised countries [1], and in the USA the National Institute on Drug Abuse (NIDA) refers to it as a 'brain disease'. However, when reading about the problems presented by drugs and alcohol you will encounter a range of terms ('addict', 'alcoholic', 'alcohol misuse', 'drug abuse', 'substance dependence') which seem to overlap and sometimes contradict each other. As is common with a lot of medical terminology, the meaning of many of these words has changed over time as they have started to be used out of their original context, and this can be a barrier to effective communication about the subject. Furthermore, the disease concept of addiction is not the only explanation of the problem, and some have argued that addiction is 'a set of ideas which have a history and a cultural location' [2].

The definition of addiction provided by the current edition of the Oxford English Dictionary is 'the state or condition of being dedicated or devoted to a thing, esp. an activity or occupation; adherence or attachment, esp. of an immoderate or compulsive kind' [3]. To the contemporary reader this feels familiar: the idea that human beings have a tendency to become so involved in a habit or pursuit that their involvement seems excessive to another observer. However, the word 'addiction' is derived from a Latin term used to denote a court sentence compelling one human being to follow the orders of another. This concept of slavery captures the essence of the modern-day scientific understanding of addiction – that is, that a pursuit or habit has moved beyond voluntary control to become a type of psychological slavery [4]. This can be illustrated by using the example of alcohol.

There is good evidence that alcohol has been produced by humankind for thousands of years, and there have been very few major civilisations that haven't learnt to harness the fermentation process to produce this psychoactive substance. Indeed, the enzyme alcohol dehydrogenase, which exists specifically to break down alcohol, demonstrates the human race's long-standing evolutionary relationship with ethanol. Drunkenness is a recurring theme in Greek mythology, and the worship of Dionysius or Bacchus (the wine god) was common in Mediterranean people. As religious beliefs came to be the organising principle of many societies, alcohol was often reserved for use in religious ceremonies, with wine and beer used as offerings to deities. It took on a key symbolic role in Christianity, which came to equate red wine with the blood of Christ in Holy Communion. Religions also began to control the excesses associated with alcohol. Islam chose total prohibition in AD 700, and Protestant sects in northern Europe (and later North America) saw abstinence as funda-mental. Attempts by religious groups to control excess led to what has been called the 'moral model' of addiction, whereby drunkenness is equated with 'sin'. Self-directed change was demanded of the sinner, and failure to conform was met with either intensified prayer or punishment.

However, fast-forward to the eighteenth century in Britain and, despite this 'moral model' of understanding, alcohol had become an integral part of the fabric of social life. The public house was the centre of many activities, including many public and private ceremonies. Business and trade were conducted in pubs, and wages were often paid there. However, alcohol could still be linked to social problems, as highlighted by the 'gin craze' of the 1730s and 1740s. This is best illustrated in two satirical prints produced by the artist Hogarth in 1751 in support of regulation of the production of gin, which was fast becoming the scourge of the poor. The first picture is set in the St Giles area of London in a street named Gin Lane, where people look thin and diseased, the pawnbroker is doing an excellent trade and buildings are falling into disrepair. Most shocking of all, a woman in the foreground is throwing away her baby in favour of the demon drink. In contrast, in Beer Street all is well. People are well fed and prosperous, the pawnbroker has closed down and new buildings are springing up.

The Disease of Addiction

Gin epidemics aside, Hogarth's prints illustrate that 'drink' such as beer was largely considered good for you in the eighteenth century. However, doctors in Georgian England were clear that heavy alcohol consumption was often responsible for ill health and disease. In the first part of the nineteenth century, two physicians simultaneously raised the idea that the habit of drunkenness was 'a disease of the mind'. Thomas Trotter was a ship's surgeon whose MD thesis at the University of Edinburgh in 1804 was entitled *An Essay, Medical, Philosophical, and Chemical on Drunkenness, and Its Effects on the Human Body*. Meanwhile, on the other side of the Atlantic the more celebrated *Inquiry into the Effects of Ardent Spirits upon the Human Body and Mind* by Benjamin Rush was published in 1816. However, it wasn't until 1849 that another physician, Magnus Huss, first used the term 'alcoholism' to describe a disease relating to excessive consumption of alcohol.

Although the emerging medical profession had begun to label and classify the effects of alcohol, it was change in wider society that started to make alcohol consumption a 'problem'. Levine argues that the idea of addiction emerged at a specific point in history and in a specific cultural context [5]. In early nineteenth-century America it was well recognised that certain people liked to drink alcohol and their drinking was often habitual. However, this was not given more significance than a 'preference' or a 'habit'. As the century wore on and the Industrial Revolution took shape, increasing personal mobility allowed people to move great distances to look for work. Extended family ties were often put under strain by this process, and social support networks became weaker. The fortunes of the nuclear family became more dependent on the self-control of the father/husband as the main earner. The maturing industrialised economies of the Western world required more disciplined workers, and intoxication and drunkenness were not compatible with arriving at work on time and working with machinery.

The emerging educated middle class in Victorian society devoted itself to moral causes to improve the health and well-being of the working poor, and one example was the Temperance movement. This philanthropic lobby group formed a strong alliance with the Church to act as a vehicle for polite society's increasing concern about personal self-control, particularly for adult males. Temperance campaigners preached mass abstinence, touring the countryside presenting accounts of drunken degradation and eternal salvation through taking a pledge to remain abstinent. Groups such as the Society for the Study and Cure of Inebriety, founded in 1884 in London (and now known as the Society for the Study of Addiction), came together to provide a place for Temperance reformers, physicians and public health doctors to discuss the problem of excessive alcohol consumption.

The 'medical model' of addiction was born, and with it came the first attempts at treatment. This usually involved secluding the inebriate in a large building in the country-side, and there was great enthusiasm for a variety of physical treatments. However, a strong moral element remained part of the medical model, and here we see the first attempts at demarcation of 'case' from 'non-case'. The term 'alcoholism' was applied to a 'worthy' sick person, one who had a progressive disease that required help, as opposed to an unworthy 'drunk' who was not interested in reform. Intense public alarm over excessive drinking led to a gradual change in the meaning of alcoholism. The term 'addiction', which the Temperance movement used interchangeably with 'alcoholism', had a narrow, moralised and medicalised meaning. Addiction was limited to drinkers, was always morally reprehen-sible and referred to a progressive disease; this became the dominant image of addiction in the nineteenth and early twentieth centuries in Western society [4].

In 1919 the Temperance movement was successful in driving through the Eighteenth Amendment to the US Constitution, banning the 'production, sale, and transportation of intoxicating liquors for beverage purposes'. Although this did succeed in reducing con-sumption and alcohol-related health problems, it also precipitated nationwide gangsterism and was repealed in 1933. Temperance ideas lost their appeal, but in 1935 the founders of Alcoholics Anonymous (AA) proposed a new approach that drew on medical, psychological and religious ideas. AA ideology has it that most people can drink socially without any problems. However, some people have a unique biological vulnerability to alcohol, whereby alcohol triggers an uncontrollable need for more alcohol. If an alcoholic continues to drink they will succumb gradually to a disease that can only result in either insanity or death.

A definition of 'alcoholism' was formulated into scholarly language in the 1950s by E. M. Jellinek, who used the concept set out by the fellowship of AA – that is, loss of control was the 'pathognomonic symptom of alcoholism'. Step one of the 12 Steps of AA emphasises loss of control of drinking, but also of one's life because of drinking. The user is failing to stop or regulate use despite the problems it is causing, and the recurrent problems them-selves have become part of the condition. By the mid-twentieth century, the meaning of 'addiction' had gradually expanded in scope, and the term had come to encompass all socially unacceptable uses of alcohol or drugs [4]. It was no longer limited to the 'over-whelming involvement' that was the essential component of addiction for the Temperance movement, but had taken on a less precise definition. As illicit psychoactive drugs became more available in the mid-twentieth century, so any use of a prohibited substance might be called 'addiction'. Furthermore, the application of science in the study of addiction has led to a recognition that problems that do not involve drugs or alcohol are similar, and can also be called 'addiction'. For example, gambling habits have the same psychological dynamics, can be overwhelming and dangerous, can be treated with the same therapies and can even have the same underlying neurochemistry.

As already mentioned, Room and others argue that the cultural framing of the concept of addiction is important [2]. Modern definitions of dependence (described later in this chapter) place a lot of importance on the concept of 'losing control' of consumption. Individual self-control and the expectation that an individual will take responsibility for their own life make sense in cultures where individuation and individualism are taken for granted. However, they make less sense in cultures where social control is more an external than an internalised matter and where individual goals and functioning are less important than the collective interests of the family and community. Furthermore, some of the definitions set out in the dependence syndrome (and enshrined in the diagnostic systems described in the next section of this chapter) are culture-specific. Neglect of alternative activities in favour of drinking is only a problem in the context of a culture attuned to the clock, where time is viewed as a commodity [2]. There is an assumption that desirable activities are an alternative to drinking, whereas in some cultural contexts most leisure activities involve drinking.

Reinarman challenges the idea of 'addiction-as-a-disease', arguing that 'the ubiquity of the disease concept of addiction obscures the fact that it did not emerge from the accretion of scientific discoveries' [1]. Rather than a discrete disease entity with a distinct aetiology, it may be best thought of as a concept that arose from a range of historical and cultural conditions, through a variety of actors and institutions. For most of the nineteenth century it was widely believed that alcohol was inherently addicting and therefore anyone who drank it would become addicted. We know that most drinkers and drug users do not become addicted, so the pharmacological properties of the psychoactive substances cannot be the primary cause of addiction-as-disease. More recently, the brain is cited as the organ in which addiction-as-disease is said to reside. However, although research confirms that there is a biological component, there is no specific locus of addiction-as-disease. Zinberg demonstrated that 'loss of control' was not the inevitable outcome of regular use but rather contingent on social and psychological variables [6]. Fingarette argued that heavy drinking was not technically a disease, and could just as easily be seen as a 'way of life' [7]. Davies employed attribution theory to show that people choose to interpret habitual drug taking as an addictive disease that is beyond the control of the user not because this interpretation best fits the observable facts, but because it is a view that serves useful purposes for users themselves and society in general. It functions as an excuse for bad behaviour, a means of absolving blame, an explanation of otherwise 'irrational' behaviour and as legitimation for punishment and/or treatment [8].

Severe addiction is now thought to involve not just a destructive habit, but a kind of slavery – 'the loss of a soul'. When people become severely addicted they not only change what they do, but who they are. However, this process can exist on a continuum of severity. Mild forms may be less than fully overwhelming, perhaps because they are short-lived, linked to a specific situation or episodic. Thus, there has been a move back towards the broader original OED definition, but the story has not gone full circle. What about overwhelming involvements that are socially acceptable? The lives of Martin Luther King and Mother Teresa show what can be achieved when a person becomes totally absorbed in, and devoted to, a cause to the exclusion of their own well-being [4]. Is this still addiction?

Terminology in Clinical Practice: Classification and Diagnosis

Various schools of knowledge have been applied to the issue of addiction. Epidemiologists or public health specialists describe levels and patterns of use and the harms that are associated with this; neuroscientists have described the key neurobiological changes and pathways; behavioural psychologists are interested in the learning processes of addiction and how they are influenced by the sociocultural environment; peer-led organisations such as AA and Narcotics Anonymous (NA) have adopted a model that sits somewhere between religion and medicine. Clinicians in contrast have described the key symptoms and psychopathology, and have developed classificatory systems to aid provision of treatment [9].

Classificatory approaches may utilise one of three strategies: categorical, ordinal or continuous. Categorical classification involves an assessment of the presence or absence of a given attribute, or the selection of the category best suited to a given individual among a number of options. This is the process of diagnosis, which is the bedrock of medicine. In contrast, a second approach is to provide a quantitative assessment of a specific individual attribute along a continuum of intensity, frequency or severity. Examples include blood pressure, symptom severity, quality of life or personality traits. Finally, ordinal classification provides a practical compromise between the two approaches. This uses a finite, ordered set of categories such as 'unaffected, mild, moderate or severe' to refine the diagnostic system. A 'cut point' can be used with any continuous scale to indicate a threshold for membership in a category. For example, when using the AUDIT screening tool for alcohol problems, a value greater than 8 is often used to define the presence of an alcohol use disorder [10]. In practice, quantitative thresholds are also embedded in most categorical diagnoses (e.g. DSM-5).

William Osler is famed for establishing many of the principles that still guide medical education and practice today, and in particular that diagnosis is based on detailed observation of signs, careful eliciting of the patient's symptoms and relevant investigations to confirm the presence of a pathological process [11]. Ideally, valid medical diagnoses are underpinned by an understanding of the disease process based on a specific cause (aetiology) and on a specific pathway to illness (pathogenesis). Most signs and symptoms can be the result of several different pathological processes, and the assessor has to sort through the possibilities and select the most likely cause.

The science of diagnosis, or 'nosology', implies that diagnostic categories are based on empirical data, but often they are not. The categories used in psychiatric diagnosis are based on observation of signs and symptoms rather than on pathological processes, and clinicians usually rely completely on subjective experiences reported by patients. Psychiatric diagnoses, with few exceptions, are *syndromes* rather than diseases, and the lack of clear disease categories has led to the use of the more general term 'disorder'. The definition of a psychiatric disorder in ICD-10 is: 'a clinically recognizable set of symptoms or behaviour associated in most cases with distress and with interference with personal functions' [12]. Despite these limitations, diagnosis performs a number of important functions: it validates the patient's suffering, confirming that something is indeed wrong; aids communication between professional and patient, and between professionals; helps to guide treatment; informs prognosis; and provides researchers with a tool for conducting investigations and for developing theoretical models of disease.

A good example of some of these issues comes from the US/UK Diagnostic Project of the late 1960s, where psychiatrists in New York and London were given detailed vignettes of cases and asked to make a diagnosis [13]. Although the vignettes were the same, psychiatrists in New York diagnosed schizophrenia twice as frequently as their counterparts in London, largely because they used a broad concept of the diagnosis that was psychodynamic in origin. Standardisation of diagnosis through rules of application or 'operational definitions' was required. An important change in psychiatric nosology therefore occurred in 1980 with the publication of the third edition of the *Diagnostic and Statistical Manual* (DSM-III). In the absence of knowledge about aetiology, its basic principle was to classify psychopathology in terms of signs and symptoms. Although it was anticipated that the system could change with research breakthroughs, it has been fairly stable during the past few decades. Unfortunately, diagnoses that were initially considered provisional have become set in stone over time. Although diagnoses based on the manual should not necessarily lead to any specific mode of treatment, it has been impossible to resist the linkage.

Alcohol and drug use provide an example of the difficulty in establishing a boundary between normality and disorder. In Western cultures the majority of people drink alcohol, and excess intake from time to time is far from unusual among otherwise 'low-risk' drinkers. There has been much debate about how problematic or unhealthy alcohol use should be conceptualised and classified [9]: an epidemiological approach using the mean daily or weekly consumption where the risk of harm is related to the amount or pattern of use, or a diagnostic approach that distinguishes an 'addict' from a 'non-addict'.

The Population Perspective

Use of any individual psychoactive substance occurs across a spectrum. At one end are people who do not use the substance at all. Others will use it occasionally and without problems, but as use increases in frequency and quantity so physical, psychological and social problems become more likely to develop. At the other extreme are people with severe dependence. The numbers at each stage of the spectrum will depend on the substance and the population under consideration, but these issues are easier to consider when applied to a (mostly) socially sanctioned substance such as alcohol.

'Low-Risk' Drinking

People may abstain from drinking alcohol for a variety of reasons (religious or cultural beliefs, health reasons, recovery from previously problematic use). However, assuming that an individual does drink alcohol, how much is too much? In order to answer this question there must be a standard way of quantifying the amount used. Although the WHO has described a 'standard drink' as containing 10 g of pure alcohol, there is a lack of worldwide consensus as to the amount of alcohol in a standard alcoholic drink. The USA defines a 'standard drink' as containing 14 g of pure alcohol, but a 'unit' of alcohol in the UK is classified as 8 g of pure alcohol, and a standard drink in other countries may contain as many as 20 g [14].

In the mid-1990s, 'low-risk' drinking was defined in the UK as being fewer than 21 units of alcohol per week for men and fewer than 14 units per week for women. Drinking alcohol at levels above this was considered to put the individual at risk of health-related harms, based on a review of the available epidemiological data. Consumption of 22–50 units per week for men and 15–35 units per week for women was labelled 'hazardous' drinking, and more than 50 units per week for men and more than 35 units per week for women was 'harmful' drinking. A further review of the evidence that focused on the risk of cancer led to a revising of this guidance in 2016, and both men and women are now advised not to drink more than 14 units/week on a regular basis, and to spread this evenly over three days with alcohol-free days [15]. Similar principles are followed around the world, but with some variations [14].

Hazardous Drinking

Hazardous drinking refers to consumption of more than the recommended low-risk weekly levels in the absence of any harm, a situation that is very common in most industrialised countries. The US National Longitudinal Alcohol Epidemiologic Survey calculated that a third of drinkers never exceed moderate alcohol consumption, a third do so occasionally and the rest do so habitually [16]. UK data shows that between 18 per cent (Wales) and 26 per cent (Scotland) of drinkers consumed more than 14 units in a week in 2016 (see Chapter 5). Defining and identifying 'hazardous' drinkers is important from a public health perspective, as interventions to help reduce (but not necessarily stop) drinking may have large national benefits. Alcohol Brief Interventions (ABI) have therefore been targeted at hazardous drinkers as a group, where more intensive treatment interventions are not typically required but simple advice from general health or social care practitioners can result in meaningful reductions. As such, NICE has recommended that ABIs be delivered opportunistically across a range of health and social care settings, although there have been questions about the extent and quality of their delivery in key setting such as Primary Care [17].

Binge Drinking

The UK government's Alcohol Strategy defines 'binge' drinking as exceeding 8 units (men) or 6 units (women) of alcohol on their heaviest drinking day in the week before interview. Binge drinking is not represented in diagnostic criteria because it is not specific to any level of consumption. In 2018 the proportion of adults reporting binge drinking on at least one day in the previous week was 12 per cent for women and 19 per cent for men [18]. However, binge drinking is not usually considered useful from a research or policy perspective since frequency of the drinking may vary widely, as indeed do drinkers' own ideas about what qualifies as 'binge' drinking. Nonetheless, heavy episodic drinking is associated with a range of harms, particularly acute harms such as accidents, injuries or effects on functioning.

The Diagnostic Perspective

Harmful Use

Harmful Use is a diagnostic category used in the International Classification of Diseases, tenth revision (ICD-10, see Table 1.1). It refers to a pattern of psychoactive substance use that is causing damage to health, which may be physical (as in cases of hepatitis from the

Table 1.1 ICD-10 criteria for harmful use [12]

Harmful use
A. There must be clear evidence that the substance use was responsible for (or substantially contributed to) physical or psychological harm, including impaired judgement or dysfunctional behaviour, which may lead to disability or have adverse consequences for interpersonal relationships.
B. The nature of the harm should be clearly identifiable (and specified).
C. The pattern of use has persisted for at least 1 month or has occurred repeatedly within a 12-month period.
D. The disorder does not meet the criteria for any other mental or behavioural disorder related to the same drug in the same time period (except for acute intoxication, F10.0).

self-administration of injected psychoactive substances) or mental (e.g. episodes of depressive disorder secondary to heavy consumption of alcohol). However, the boundary between 'normal' or hazardous use and a diagnosis of harmful use is often not clear.

Dependence

Although nearly 40 classification systems are recognised between the first use of the term 'alcoholismus' by Magnus Huss in 1849 and 1941, the process of trying to standardise diagnostic systems for alcoholism really began in the 1940s [19]. Early versions of both the DSM and the ICD classifications clustered alcoholism with personality disorders and neuroses. Separate criteria for alcohol abuse and dependence first appeared in ICD-9 and DSM-III in the 1980s. The modern conception of the alcohol dependence syndrome was first articulated by Edwards and Gross in 1976 and has seven elements which 'exist in degree', thus giving the syndrome a range of severity [20]. The description was intended to clarify the clinical picture of alcoholism and stimulate discussion and research that would lead to better diagnostic criteria. The authors were attempting to separate dependence, which was seen as being biologically driven, from alcohol abuse/harmful use – that is, drink-related disabilities such as cirrhosis, loss of job and car crashes [19]. As Stockwell has pointed out, 'a person may, for example, develop cirrhosis, lose his job, crash his car, or break up his marriage through his drinking without suffering from the dependence syndrome' [21].

The experience of being dependent is influenced by characteristics of the individual, and by their environment and culture. The exact nature of the presentation will also depend on the psychoactive substance in question (tolerance and withdrawal may appear within a matter of weeks with opioids, but take years to develop with alcohol). The character of dependence may also change over time. Criteria based on the dependence syndrome first appeared in DSM-III-R in 1987. The ICD-10 criteria for diagnosing dependence are shown in Table 1.2, and the DSM-IV criteria were very similar.

The Core Elements of Alcohol Dependence

Narrowing of repertoire: The type and form of alcohol consumed is usually influenced by the people around the drinker and their emotional state. A non-dependent pattern of drinking may typically involve a glass of cold beer on a warm day, wine with a meal or cocktails while celebrating at a party. Once dependence develops, the main goal – albeit perhaps not consciously – is to increase the blood alcohol level rather than enjoying a specific type of alcoholic drink, and cost and strength may be more influential on the drinking behaviour. Once dependence becomes severe, the individual may need to drink simply to avoid potentially fatal withdrawal effects – for example, they may need to top up every few hours in order to feel normal and to function.

Salience of drinking: The non-dependent drinker is able to weigh up the importance of the choice to drink, and to judge whether other internal or external factors are more important than consuming alcohol. In contrast, for the dependent drinker the views of others about their level of consumption become less important, and the consequences less relevant. Ultimately, drinking becomes more important than family, work, hobbies or other life goals. The extent of this change in priorities gives a diagnostic clue as to the severity of dependence.

Increased tolerance to alcohol: The heavy drinker may observe that they can 'drink others under the table', and may be able to sustain a high blood alcohol content without appearing

Table 1.2 ICD-10 criteria for dependence [12]

Dependence

Three or more of the following manifestations should have occurred together for at least 1 month or, if persisting for periods of less than 1 month, should have occurred together repeatedly within a 12-month period:

(1) a strong desire or sense of compulsion to take the substance;

(2) impaired capacity to control substance-taking behaviour in terms of its onset, termination, or levels of use, as evidenced by: the substance being often taken in larger amounts or over a longer period than intended; or by a persistent desire or unsuccessful efforts to reduce or control substance use;

(3) a physiological withdrawal state (see F1x.3 and F1x.4) when substance use is reduced or ceased, as evidenced by the characteristic withdrawal syndrome for the substance, or by use of the same (or closely related) substance with the intention of relieving or avoiding withdrawal symptoms;

(4) evidence of tolerance to the effects of the substance, such that there is a need for significantly increased amounts of the substance to achieve intoxication or the desired effect, or a markedly diminished effect with continued use of the same amount of the substance;

(5) preoccupation with substance use, as manifested by important alternative pleasures or interests being given up or reduced because of substance use; or a great deal of time being spent in activities necessary to obtain, take, or recover from the effects of the substance;

(6) persistent substance use despite clear evidence of harmful consequences (see F1x.1), as evidenced by continued use when the individual is actually aware, or may be expected to be aware, of the nature and extent of harm.

intoxicated. Steady levels of alcohol in the blood mean that the brain compensates by various homeostatic processes, and a greater level of alcohol is required to have the same subjective effect. This tolerance may also apply to sedative drugs such as benzodiazepines (known as 'cross-tolerance'), a fact that is exploited in the process of medically assisted withdrawal. The rate of development of tolerance varies considerably between individuals, and it may start to fade in the later stages of dependence.

Withdrawal symptoms: As dependence increases, so does the frequency and severity of withdrawal symptoms. Mild symptoms may begin to appear at any time of the day when blood alcohol levels begin to fall, but when dependence is severe and well established the individual experiences severe symptoms on waking (drenched in sweat, feeling very nauseous and a tremor so bad that it is hard to raise a glass to the lips). Many different symptoms are associated with alcohol withdrawal, some physiological (tremor, nausea, sweating, hyperacusis, tinnitus, muscle cramps), some psychological (mood disturbance, sleep disturbance, hallucinations) and some potentially very severe (seizures, delirium tremens).

Relief or avoidance of withdrawal symptoms by drinking: Alcohol withdrawal symptoms are unpleasant, and drinking more alcohol is a quick and effective way of alleviating them. In mild dependence the first drink can wait until lunchtime, but the severely dependent drinker often keeps alcohol by the bed to ensure it is readily available on waking.

Subjective awareness of compulsion to drink: 'Normal' drinking is characterised by a perception that the drinker can decide when to start, but more importantly, when to stop and how much to drink. In dependent drinkers, control is variably or intermittently impaired, and it becomes very hard to resist an alcoholic drink if it is available. Furthermore, once drinking starts it becomes extremely difficult to stop. The concept of 'craving' for a drink is often invoked, a sensation that is often strongly influenced by cues in the internal or external environment.

Reinstatement after abstinence: When a dependent drinker stops drinking for a period of time (weeks, months or even years), there may come a point when they decide to try alcohol again, usually with the intention of not repeating the mistakes of the past. Mildly dependent drinkers may manage to control their drinking with few problems, but the severely dependent often return to previous high levels of consumption within a matter of days.

Changes in DSM-5

Alcohol dependence has six diagnostic criteria in ICD-10, and in DSM-IV there are seven, with both systems requiring three to be present in the past 12 months for a diagnosis. Witkiewitz and colleagues have shown that the psychometric performance of both sets of criteria is very good, representing a unidimensional disorder across various studies and populations [22]. Reviewing his dependence syndrome ten years on, Griffith Edwards proposed two core elements for the alcohol dependence syndrome [1]: withdrawal and its attendant behaviour, including the subjective need for alcohol, salience and increased tolerance [2]; impaired control/loss of control [23]. In order to simplify things for clinical practice, the draft ICD-11 has proposed reducing the diagnostic guidelines for dependence from six to three, any two of which need to be present in order to make the diagnosis [9]:

(1) *impaired control over substance use* – that is, onset, level, circumstances or termination of use, often accompanied by a subjective sensation of urge or craving to use the substance.

(2) *substance use becomes an increasing priority in life*, such that its use takes precedence over other interests, daily activities, responsibilities or health or personal care. Substance use often continues despite the occurrence of problems.

(3) *physiological features* (i.e. neuroadaptation to the substance), as shown by (i) tolerance, (ii) withdrawal symptoms following cessation or reduction in use or (iii) repeated use of the substance to prevent or alleviate withdrawal symptoms.

The dependence syndrome appears to be a real entity, but not all the elements are equally consistent in psychometric terms and some may be redundant. Epidemiological data suggest the total of 11 criteria that make up the DSM-IV diagnoses of alcohol abuse [4] or dependence [7] represent a single dimension of alcohol problems along a continuum of severity, and so alcohol abuse is not an early stage of dependence. In DSM-5, alcohol abuse and dependence have been removed completely, and replaced by a broader disorder called Alcohol Use Disorder. This effectively merges DSM-IV alcohol abuse and DSM-IV alcohol dependence [9]. It includes the seven criteria used to diagnose dependence plus three of the four for abuse, adding in craving to bring it in to line with ICD. Reasons cited for this change [24] were:

- Confusion among health professionals about the use of the term 'dependence' (confused with 'physiological dependence').
- DSM-IV dependence had excellent psychometric properties, but abuse did not. Its natural history was not that of a unitary disorder.

Table 1.3 DSM-5 criteria for Alcohol Use Disorder [26]

Alcohol Use Disorder

1. Alcohol taken in larger amounts or over a longer period than was intended
2. Persistent desire or unsuccessful attempts to cut down or control alcohol use
3. Great deal of time is spent in activities necessary to obtain alcohol, use alcohol, or recover from its effects
4. Craving, or a strong desire or urge to use alcohol
5. Recurrent alcohol use resulting in a failure to fulfil major role obligations at work, school, or home
6. Continued alcohol use despite having persistent or recurrent social or interpersonal problems caused or exacerbated by the effects of alcohol
7. Important social, occupational, or recreational activities are given up or reduced because of alcohol use.
8. Recurrent alcohol use in situations in which it is physically hazardous
9. Alcohol use is continued despite knowledge of a persistent or recurrent physical or psychological problem that is likely to have been caused or exacerbated by alcohol
10. Tolerance, as defined by either:
    - a need for markedly increased amounts of alcohol to achieve intoxication or desired effect
    - a markedly diminished effect with continued use of the same amount of alcohol
11. Withdrawal, as manifested by either of the following:
    - characteristic alcohol withdrawal syndrome for alcohol
    - alcohol (or a closely related substance) taken to relieve or avoid withdrawal symptoms

- Some individuals (known as 'diagnostic orphans') met two of the seven criteria for dependence but also failed to meet the threshold for abuse.
- Item Response Theory analyses show that most of the DSM-IV dependence and abuse criteria fall on a continuum, with overlaps of abuse and dependence items

The 11 criteria for AUD provide a continuum of severity along which the frequency of a harmful pattern of drinking can be mapped. Addiction is now identified on a dimensional scoring procedure based on severity – that is, the number of criteria present (mild AUD if two or three criteria, moderate if four or five, severe if six or more). This means that patients can be diagnosed if they meet only two criteria, and although this approach is consistent with the DSM-5 manual's overall philosophy of including subclinical phenomena, critics have argued that this will pathologise too many people. Epidemiological survey work in Australia suggests that use of the DSM-5 criteria (see Table 1.3) could increase the prevalence in substance use disorders as a whole, but a North American study found only a 10 per cent increase [25].

A Case for Advancing a Continuum Model?

Changes such as those made in the DSM-5, alongside wider efforts to identify and engage hazardous or harmful drinkers, may represent a significant shift away from the historically dominant disease model of 'alcoholism'. However, some argue that further work is still needed to recognise the broad spectrum of use and harms in a wider range of contexts [27], while others highlight that the disease model remains widely endorsed but carries a number of under-recognised costs [28]. Increasingly, arguments for a more explicit recognition of a continuum model have been made on the grounds of the individual implications for those who experience alcohol problems [29].

Alcohol-related problems remain a highly stigmatised issue, and as such it has been suggested that the disease model's claimed stigma-alleviating benefits have failed to materialise [30]. Reviews of differences in the causal attributions of mental health and substance use problems suggest that disease model beliefs do indeed seem to carry some potential for blame alleviation (i.e. the person is not to blame if they have a disease). However, these benefits are likely to be offset by other stigma-related attitudes and beliefs such as more desire for social distance (i.e. unwillingness to interact with someone) or stereotypes about perceived dangerousness. Indeed, a fundamental component of stigma and associated discrimination is the perception of perceived difference between groups, which may be reinforced by categorisations which imply fundamental differences such as between 'alcoholics' and 'normal' drinkers. Other potential costs associated with a disease model have been explored, particularly in the context of treatment and recovery. Disease-model-aligned beliefs have been associated with poorer treatment outcomes, lower personal agency and self-efficacy and lower help-seeking [31]. This has led to calls to explore the 'positive implication of continuum beliefs' to alleviate the stigma of mental health and substance use disorders [32].

However, while continuum beliefs may hold promise in the context of experimental studies [29], a practical question relates to how a shift in problem framing will be received at the population level. There is currently limited understanding about the extent to which the public may endorse continuum-type beliefs about alcohol problems, and how these may interact with stigmatised attitudes towards the issue. One German study found just 27 per cent of people agreed with alcohol problems as a continuum [32], while disease-model-associated views appear to be endorsed by closer to half of people within Western populations [33] and have therefore been argued to remain the 'dominant conceptual paradigm' for understanding addiction. Furthermore, efforts to educate the public or reach hazardous drinking populations may have been hampered by a failure to connect with people's personal experiences of alcohol use [34]. For instance, the CMO's revised recommended drinking guidelines appear to have had little if any impact on drinking behaviours, in part because people tend to feel they 'know their own limits', or believe that meeting their responsibilities means that their drinking cannot be considered problematic [35]. One mechanism which may have potential for success may be the use of personal stories or 'narratives' that implicitly emphasise the continuum nature of alcohol problems. For instance, stories that tell a range of experiences of problems beyond stereotypes such as those who hit 'rock-bottom', or that highlight how many people 'recover' through moderating their drinking. Epidemiological data show most people recover from alcohol problems, particularly those lower in problem severity, through 'natural recovery', with many people simply 'maturing out' of problems with age and accrual of more responsibilities [36].

In short, alcohol problems and their causes are complex and influenced by a range of factors ranging from biogenetic, psychological and sociocultural. Any attempts at simplistic categorisation or labelling run the risk of overlooking such attributional complexity and interactions with individual-level variability. As such, further shifts towards models of alcohol use and problems more fundamentally aligned with a continuum model may go some way to better reflecting this complexity, and in turn mitigating some of the pitfalls presented by past categorisations.

References

1   Reinarman C. Addiction as accomplishment: The discursive construction of disease. *Addiction Research and Theory.* 2005; **13** (4): 307–20.

2   Room R. The cultural framing of addiction. *Janus Head.* 2003; **6** (2): 221–34.

3   Oxford English Dictionary. "addiction, n.": Oxford University Press; 2020.

4   Alexander B. *The Globalisation of Addiction: A Study in Poverty of the Spirit.* Oxford: Oxford University Press; 2008.

5   Levine H. G. The discovery of addiction: Changing conceptions of habitual drunkenness in America. *Journal of Studies on Alcohol.* 1978; **39** (1): 143–74.

6   Zinberg N. E., Harding W. M., Winkeller M. A study of social regulatory mechanisms in controlled illicit drug users. *Journal of Drug Issues.* 1977; **7** (2): 117–33.

7   Fingarette H. *Heavy Drinking: The Myth of Alcoholism as a Disease.* Berkeley, CA: University of California Press; 1988.

8   Davies J. B. *The Myth of Addiction.* 2nd ed. Amsterdam: Harwood Academic Publishers; 1997.

9   Saunders J. B., Peacock A., Degenhardt L. Alcohol use disorders in the draft ICD-11, and how they compare with DSM-5. *Current Addiction Reports.* 2018; **5** (2): 257–64.

10 Babor T. F., Higgins-Biddle J. C., Saunders J. B., Monteiro M. G. *AUDIT: The Alcohol Use Disorder Identification Test – Guidelines for Use in Primary Health Care.* Geneva: World Health Organization; 2001.

11 Paris J. *The Intelligent Clinician's Guide to the DSM-5.* New York: Oxford University Press; 2013.

12 World Health Organization. *The ICD-10 Classification of Mental and Behavioural Disorders.* Geneva: WHO; 1992.

13 Cooper J. E., Kendell R. E., Gurland B. J. *Psychiatric Diagnosis in New York and London: A Comparative Study of Mental Hospital Patients.* New York: Oxford University Press; 1972.

14 Kalinowski A, Humphreys K. Governmental standard drink definitions and low-risk alcohol consumption guidelines in 37 countries. *Addiction.* 2016; **111** (7): 1293–8.

15 Department of Health. *UK Chief Medical Officers' Alcohol Guidelines Review: Summary of the Proposed New Guidelines.* London: DH; 2016.

16 Dawson D. A., Archer L. D., Grant B. F. Reducing alcohol-use disorders via decreased consumption: A comparison of population and high-risk strategies. *Drug and Alcohol Dependence.* 1996; **42** (1): 39–47.

17 O'Donnell A., Angus C., Hanratty B., Hamilton F. L., Petersen I., Kaner E. Impact of the introduction and withdrawal of financial incentives on the delivery of alcohol screening and brief advice in English primary health care: An interrupted time–series analysis. *Addiction.* 2020; **115** (1): 49–60.

18 National Statistics. Health Survey for England 2018: Adult health-related behaviours: NHS Digital; 2019 [updated 3/12/2019. Available from: https://digital.nhs.uk/data-and-information/publications/statistical/health-survey-for-england/2018].

19 Li T.-K., Hewitt B. G., Grant B. F. The alcohol dependence syndrome, 30 years later: A commentary. *Addiction.* 2007; **102** (10): 1522–30.

20 Edwards G., Gross M. M. Alcohol dependence: Provisional description of a clinical syndrome. *British Medical Journal.* 1976; **1**: 1058–61.

21 Stockwell T. The alcohol dependence syndrome: A legacy of continuing clinical and scientific importance. *Addiction.* 2015; **110** (S2): 8–11.

22 Witkiewitz K., Hallgren K. A., O'Sickey A. J., Roosa C. R., Maisto S. A. Reproducibility and differential item functioning of the alcohol dependence syndrome construct across four alcohol treatment studies: An integrative data analysis. *Drug and Alcohol Dependence.* 2016; **158**: 86–93.

23 Edwards G. The Alcohol Dependence Syndrome: A concept as stimulus to enquiry. *British Journal of Addiction.* 1986; **81**: 171–83.

24   Hasin D. S., O'Brien C. P., Auriacombe M., Borges G., Bucholz K., Budney A., et al. DSM-5 criteria for substance use disorders: Recommendations and rationale. *American Journal of Psychiatry*. 2013; **170**: 834–51.

25   Agrawal A., Heath A. C., Lynskey M. T. DSM-IV to DSM-5: The impact of proposed revisions on diagnosis of alcohol use disorders. *Addiction*. 2011; **106** (11): 1935–43.

26   American Psychiatric Association. *Diagnostic and Statistical Manual of Mental Disordxers: Fifth Edition* (DSM-5). Arlington, VA: American Psychiatric Publishing; 2013.

27   Rehm J., Marmet S., Anderson P., Gual A., Kraus L., Nutt D. J., et al. Defining substance use disorders: Do we really need more than heavy use? *Alcohol and Alcoholism*. 2013; **48** (6): 633–40.

28   Racine E., Bell E., Zizzo N., Green C. Public discourse on the biology of alcohol addiction: Implications for stigma, self-control, essentialism, and coercive policies in pregnancy. Neuroethics. 2015; **8** (2): 177–86.

29   Morris J., Albery I. P., Heather N., Moss A. C. Continuum beliefs are associated with higher problem recognition than binary beliefs among harmful drinkers without addiction experience. *Addictive Behaviors*. 2020; **105**: 106–292.

30   Pescosolido B. A., Martin J. K., Long J. S., Medina T. R., Phelan J. C., Link B. G. 'A disease like any other'? A decade of change in public reactions to schizophrenia, depression, and alcohol dependence. *American Journal of Psychiatry*. 2010; **167** (11): 1321–30.

31   Burnette J. L., Forsyth R. B., Desmarais S. L., Hoyt C. L. Mindsets of addiction: Implications for treatment intentions. *Journal of Social and Clinical Psychology*. 2019; **38** (5): 367–94.

32   Schomerus G., Matschinger H., Angermeyer M. C. Continuum beliefs and stigmatizing attitudes towards persons with schizophrenia, depression and alcohol dependence. *Psychiatry Research*. 2013; **209** (3): 665–9.

33   Tikkinen K. A. O., Leinonen J. S., Guyatt G. H., Ebrahim S., Järvinen T. L. N. What is a disease? Perspectives of the public, health professionals and legislators. *BMJ Open*. 2012; **2** (6): e001632.

34   Lovatt M., Eadie D., Meier P. S., Li J., Bauld L., Hastings G., et al. Lay epidemiology and the interpretation of low-risk drinking guidelines by adults in the United Kingdom. *Addiction*. 2015; **110** (12): 1912–9.

35   Parke H., Michalska M., Russell A., Moss A. C., Holdsworth C., Ling J., et al. Understanding drinking among midlife men in the United Kingdom: A systematic review of qualitative studies. *Addictive Behaviors Reports*. 2018; **8**: 85–94.

36   Dawson D. A., Grant B. F., Stinson F. S., Chou P. S. Estimating the effect of help-seeking on achieving recovery from alcohol dependence. *Addiction*. 2006; **101** (6): 824–34.

Chapter 2

Illicit Drug Use: Epidemiology, Aetiology and Prevention

Ed Day

Epidemiology of Drug Use

In their 2020 World Drug Report, the World Health Organization highlight that the global market for psychoactive drugs is expanding, fuelled by population growth along with increasing urbanisation and income [1]. This market has steadily increased in complexity over more than a century, driven by new technologies, new substances entering the market, increasing poly-drug use and a blurring of the boundary between legal and illegal markets. Drug use is on the rise both in terms of overall numbers of people using and percentage of the worldwide population. This increase is more rapid in developing countries, and is most prevalent in people of the lowest socioeconomic status. Cannabis is the most used illicit drug in the world (192 million people in the past year), but stimulant use is increasing faster (27 million reported amphetamine or prescription stimulant use). Illicit drug use is estimated to cause nearly 60,000 deaths/year worldwide, and is responsible for 42 million disability-adjusted life years (DALYs, which combine premature mortality as years of life lost [YLLs] and disability as years lived with disability [YLDs]). Opioid use accounts for half of the DALYs and a significant proportion of the deaths.

Sources of Data about Illicit Drug Use

Illicit drug use is difficult to monitor accurately, largely because of its illegal nature. However, the following list provides an example of the types of information available in England (Scotland, Wales and Northern Ireland have comparable data available elsewhere).

The Crime Survey for England & Wales:

The Crime Survey for England and Wales (CSEW, formally known as the British Crime Survey) is commissioned by the Home Office and based on a nationally representative household survey. Drug use estimates are produced from responses to a self-completion module of the full CSEW survey, which is completed at the end of the main face-to-face interview (which mainly covers questions on experiences of being the victim of crime and perceptions of crime-related issues). CSEW data are weighted to ensure that figures reflect the age and sex distribution of the population under study (adults aged 16 to 59 and 60 to 74, resident in households in England and Wales).

Deaths Related to Drug Misuse in England and Wales

The Office for National Statistics (ONS) produces annual statistics on the number of registered deaths that can be attributed to drug misuse. Deaths are included if the

15

underlying cause was drug poisoning and where a drug controlled under the Misuse of Drugs Act 1971 is mentioned on the death certificate: https://bit.ly/3fozBKG.

The Adult Psychiatric Morbidity Survey:

Information on drug dependence is available from the NHS Digital Adult Psychiatric Morbidity Survey: Survey of Mental Health and Wellbeing, England. This survey has been conducted every seven years since 1993, and the most recent version was carried out in 2014: https://bit.ly/3deDdfm.

Information about People Seeking Treatment for Drug Use Problems

Information on treatment for drug misuse is available from the National Drug Treatment Monitoring System (NDTMS), administered by Public Health England. All specialist treatment services in England report anonymised data about all clients receiving treatment from structured community-based or residential inpatient services: https://bit.ly/3fqDEpT.

The UK in Comparison with the Rest of Europe:

Comparisons of drug use prevalence across European countries are available from the European Drug Report: Trends and Developments, published by the European Monitoring Centre for Drugs and Drug Addiction (EMCDDA) every year (https://bit.ly/2PmuYWP).

The UK in Comparison with the Rest of the World:

The United Nations Office on Drugs and Crime (UNODC) publishes the World Drug Report each year, which provides a global overview of the extent of and trends in drug use, and its health consequences: https://wdr.unodc.org/wdr2020/index.html.

Waste Water Analysis

Waste water analysis is a new scientific discipline with the potential for monitoring real-time data on geographical and temporal trends in illicit drug use. Originally developed to monitor the environmental impact of liquid household waste, the method has since been adapted to estimate illicit drug consumption across whole cities. London and Bristol participate with 70 other cities in the Europe-wide annual waste water campaigns under-taken by the Sewage Analysis Core Group Europe (SCORE, see www.emcdda.europa.eu/topics/pods/waste-water-analysis_en). This study provides data based on the levels of illicit drugs and their metabolites found in sources of waste water across a whole city. The results point to a possible increase in cocaine use in Bristol since the initiation of the study (2014). Furthermore, higher levels of cocaine metabolites were detected at the weekends.

Seizures of Drugs in England and Wales:

The Home Office provides an annual statistical bulletin presenting data on seizures of all drugs controlled under the Misuse of Drugs Act 1971 made in England and Wales by the police and Border Force: https://bit.ly/3dpNeX8.

Drug Use in England

Statistics on Drug Misuse in England in 2019 reported that around 1 in 11 (9.4 per cent) of adults aged 16 to 59 had taken a drug in the last year [2], which equated to around 3.2 million people. The 2019 estimate was not significantly higher than the previous year

(9.0 per cent, in 2017/18), although there had been an upward trend since 2015/16 (8.3 per cent). However, the 2018/19 estimate still remained lower than the figure in 1996 (11.2 per cent), the year the time series began. Cannabis remained the most commonly used illicit drug, with powder cocaine second. Around 1 in 25 (3.7 per cent) adults aged 16 to 59 had taken a Class A drug in the last year (mainly heroin and crack cocaine), which equates to around 1.3 million people. This is similar to the 2017/18 estimate (3.5 per cent). Table 2.2 compares the 2017 results from England and Wales with findings from other European Union countries.

Estimating the Prevalence of Opiate and Crack Cocaine Use

Heroin and crack cocaine have a low prevalence of use relative to other drugs, but their health and social impact is much greater. In order to estimate the need for treatment services, two epidemiological and statistical techniques are used to estimate the size of the hidden drug-using population: the capture-recapture method (preferred method) and the multiple indicator method (alternative method) [3]. The capture-recapture method examines the overlap between four different sources of data on individual drug users that are available at the local level (treatment services, probation, police and prison). The overlap between data sources is determined by comparison of (anonymised) initials, date of birth and gender within each local area. The multiple indicator method models the relationship between all of the available capture-recapture estimates and readily available drug-indicator data, and then applies that relationship to the areas where capture-recapture estimates are not available to provide an estimate.

Using these methods it was estimated that there were 313,971 opiate and/or crack cocaine users (OCUs) aged 15 to 64 in England in 2016/17 (see Table 2.1) [3]. Within this group, 261,294 were estimated to use opiates and 180,748 crack cocaine, giving overall prevalence rates per thousand population of 8.85 for OCU, 7.37 for opiate use and 5.10 (95 per cent CI: 4.98 to 5.30) for crack cocaine use. This represented a statistically significant 4.4 per cent increase in OCUs in England when compared to 2014/15 (300,783 to 313,971).

Prevalence rates were highest in the 25 to 34 age group. However, the estimated number of OCUs in the 35 to 64 group increased by 12 per cent between 2014/15 and 2016/17, while the estimated number aged 25 to 34 decreased by 10 per cent. This rise in the older age group is due to an ageing subpopulation who started using heroin in the 1980s and early 1990s. The highest rates of for both OCU and opiate use were in the North East, North West and Yorkshire and Humber regions, with the largest rate of increase in the East of England. London had the highest estimated rate of crack cocaine use.

Table 2.1 Estimates for number of opiate and crack users in England in 2016/17

Drug	Estimate	95% confidence interval	Rate per 1000 population	95% confidence interval
Opiate and/or crack cocaine use (OCU)	313,971	309,242–327,196	8.85	8.72–9.23
Opiate use	261,294	259,018–271,403	7.37	7.30–7.65
Crack cocaine use	180,748	176,583–188,066	5.10	4.98–5.30

Table 2.2 Prevalence of drug use by adults in England and Wales compared with the ranges found in European countries (adapted from [6])

	Year	England & Wales data	European Union range	
			Min.	Max.
Cannabis				
Last year prevalence of use: young adults (15–34) (%)	2017	12.3	1.8	21.8
Last year prevalence of drug use: all adults (16–59) (%)	2017	7.2	0.9	11
All treatment entrants (%)	2017	24.2	1.0	62.9
First-time treatment entrants (%)	2017	45.3	2.3	74.4
Cocaine				
Last year prevalence of use: young adults (15–34) (%)	2017	4.7	0.1	4.7
Last year prevalence of drug use: all adults (16–59) (%)	2017	2.7	0.1	2.7
All treatment entrants (%)	2017	17.6	0.1	39.2
First-time treatment entrants (%)	2017	22.1	0	41.8
Amphetamines				
Last year prevalence of use: young adults (15–34) (%)	2017	1	0	3.9
Last year prevalence of drug use: all adults (16–59) (%)	2017	0.5	0	1.8
All treatment entrants (%)	2017	2.1	0	49.6
First-time treatment entrants (%)	2017	2.7	0	52.8
MDMA				
Last year prevalence of use: young adults (15–34) (%)	2017	3.3	0.2	7.1
Last year prevalence of drug use: all adults (16–59) (%)	2017	1.7	0.1	3.3
All treatment entrants (%)	2017	0.5	0	2.31
First-time treatment entrants (%)	2017	1.1	0	2.85
Opioids				
High-risk opioid use (rate/1,000)	2014–15	8.42	0.48	8.42
All treatment entrants (%)	2017	49.8	3.99	93.45
First-time treatment entrants (%)	2017	21.8	1.8	87.36
Injecting/death				
Injecting drug use (cases rate/1,000 population)	2004–11	3	0.1	10.0
Drug-induced deaths – all adults (cases/million population)	2016	73.6	2.4	129.8

Table 2.2 (cont.)

	Year	England & Wales data	European Union range	
			Min.	Max.
Health and social responses				
Syringes distributed through specialised programmes	n.a.	n.a.	245	11,907,416
Clients in substitution treatment	2017	149,420	209	178,665
Treatment demand				
All entrants	2017	118,342	179	118,342
First-time entrants	2017	37,577	48	37,577
All clients in treatment	2017	237,841	1 294	254,000

High-Risk Drug Use and Trends

The studies just mentioned can help to identify the extent of the more entrenched drug use problems, while data on first-time entrants to specialised drug treatment centres can inform an understanding of the nature and trends in high-risk drug use. In England, the National Drug Treatment Monitoring System (NDTMS) collects information on the provision of drug and alcohol treatment (see Figure 2.1). Reporting data is a requirement of any nationally funded provider, and around 1,000 treatment services report information each month in community, residential and prison settings. Overall, 279,793 individuals were in contact with drug and alcohol treatment services in 2016/17, a slight (3 per cent) decrease from the previous year [4]. Around 25 per cent of people treated for heroin use reported using by injection, but increased rates of crack and amphetamine injection have caused more concern, alongside the emergence of injection of new psychoactive substances (NPS).

Heroin is the most commonly reported primary substance among those seeking treatment for drug use problems. However, there has been a long-term reduction in first-time patients seeking treatment for heroin use. Among patients receiving their first episode of treatment, cannabis is the most commonly reported substance followed by cocaine. Studies in certain populations (homeless people, people in prison) indicate that use of synthetic cannabinoid receptor agonists is high among some groups [4].

Prevalence in Mental Health Services

The majority of patients treated for drug and alcohol use disorders experience comorbid psychiatric disorder. In the best designed and implemented study of its type in the UK, 44 per cent of Community Mental Health Team patients were found to have used an illicit drug or were harmful users of alcohol, whereas 75 per cent of a sample of the population of a specialist drug/alcohol treatment service had at least one psychiatric disorder [5]. The authors estimated that the prevalence of severe depression and personality disorder was

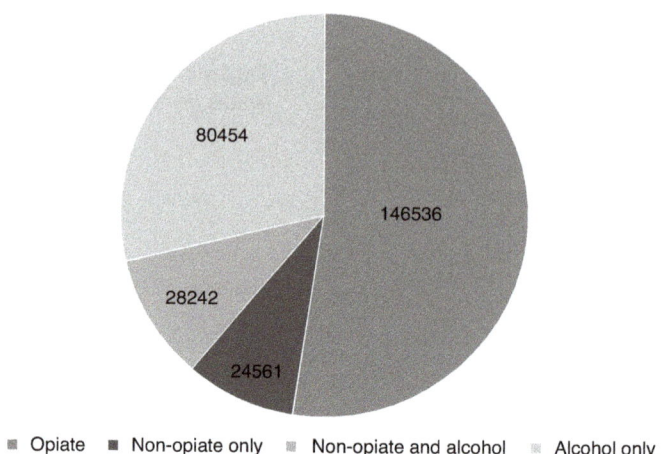

Figure 2.1 Number of people receiving treatment for drug or alcohol use disorders in England in 2016/17 according to the National Drug Treatment Monitoring Service [4]

consistent with other studies of comparable populations. However, the prevalence of psychosis (drug service patients, 8 per cent; alcohol service patients, 19 per cent) was significantly higher than previously reported and was 10 times (drug) and 24 times (alcohol) the prevalence rate for psychosis in the urban UK population (0.8 per cent).

Aetiology of Drug Use and Dependence

The description of the changing place of the concept of 'addiction' in society over the centuries in Chapter 1 illustrates three broad models of understanding the aetiology of drug dependence. Initially, many societies adopted a 'personal responsibility' model. Problems with alcohol or drugs were seen as a failure of self-control or a violation of moral or religious standards, and the solution was often punishment, repentance, and social sanctions. Underlying this was an assumption that drug use was a voluntary, chosen behaviour for which an individual was responsible. The Temperance movement in the nineteenth and early twentieth centuries placed the emphasis on the drug itself, a so-called 'agent' model. Anyone who was exposed to the drug was at risk because of its addictive properties and tendency to cause problems. Another example of an agent model is the more recent 'war on drugs' (see later in this chapter), which advocates physically ridding society of drugs by destroying the source and imprisoning the producers. Finally, a 'dispositional model' places the primary cause of addiction within the person, but sees the cause as constitutional and beyond the individual's control. This might also be called a 'disease model', and by arguing that the person is not responsible for having the condition, opens up an argument for treatment rather than punishment.

As White and Kurtz have pointed out, different cultures across time have viewed psychoactive substance problems and their resolution in various ways [7]:

- religious (sin and redemption)
- spiritual (hunger for meaning and personal transformation)

- criminal (amorality/immorality and reformation)
- disease (sickness and recovery)
- psychological (flawed thinking/coping and maturation)
- socio-cultural (historical trauma/oppression and liberation/cultural renewal)

Depending on which model of understanding is adopted, the solution may be the responsibility of priests, judges, physicians, psychologists, addiction counsellors or community activists. Drug use disorders are perhaps best understood as biopsychosocial problems in which genetic factors, adverse early life events and development, drug exposure, social norms and market availability all play a part in the progression of the disorder [8]. Not everyone tries or uses psychoactive substances, and not everyone that does becomes dependent on them. The likelihood of developing a substance use disorder is influenced by some factors that increase risk (risk factors) and others that decrease it (protective factors).

Risk and Protective Factors for Drug Use Disorders

Drug use is most likely to start in adolescence, and surveys of young people consistently show that the frequency of use begins to increase in mid-adolescence and peaks in early adulthood. Studies in many countries have reported a typical sequential order of drug initiation: tobacco (12–14 years), alcohol (13–14), cannabis (14–16), psychostimulants (17–19) and finally heroin (19–20). Starting earlier and using more frequently is associated with being more likely to progress to use of the next drug in the sequence [9]. This pattern has led to some drugs being labelled as 'gateway' drugs (particularly cannabis). However, not all countries show the same pattern of drug use, and varying patterns of initiation in different cultures suggest that a young person's entry into illicit drug use might be representative of a combination of social context, illicit drug availability and personal characteristics and social settings that facilitate or deter drug use [9].

This conclusion is supported by a systematic review of the social and contextual factors associated with the initiation of substance use [10] (see Table 2.3). Developmental *risk factors* independently increase the probability that an individual or group will engage in harmful patterns of drug use, and *protective factors* mediate or moderate the influence of risk factors. Knowledge of these factors has come from follow-up research studies and a range of intervention studies. The cumulative number of risk factors across the course of development can additively or exponentially impact on substance use and related harms, with evidence of the cascading effects of risk factors across development [11].

An Example: Risk Factors for Opioid Use Disorder

Drugs that occur later in the sequence of progression can produce the most significant problems. For example, once heroin use disorder is established, the dominant trajectory appears to be long-term, frequent use, with intermittent cycles of treatment, abstinence and relapse [12]. It follows that this population tends to experience the most risk factors, and Shane Darke has described these in detail in his book, *The Life of the Heroin User* [13]. The following paragraphs describe these risk factors as applied to heroin users in the categories used in Table 2.3.

Table 2.3 Risk and protective factors for adolescent and young adult substance use [10]

	Risk Factor	Protective Factor
Individual or peer factors	**Early initiation of substance use** Engaging in alcohol or drug use at a young age	**Social, emotional, behavioural, cognitive and moral competence** Interpersonal skills that help a young person integrate feelings, thinking and actions to achieve specific social and interpersonal goals
	Early and persistent problem behaviour Emotional distress, aggression, 'difficult' temperaments in adolescents	**Self-efficacy** Belief that a person can modify, control or abstain from substance use
	Rebelliousness High tolerance for deviance and rebellious activities	**Spirituality** Belief in a higher being, or involvement in spiritual practices or religious activities
	Favourable attitudes to substance use Positive feelings towards alcohol or drug use, low perception of risk	**Resilience** Capacity for adapting to change and stressful events in healthy and flexible ways
	Peer substance use Friends and peers who engage in alcohol or drug use	
	Genetic predictors Genetic susceptibility to alcohol or drug use	
Family	**Family management problems** Parents' failure to set clear expectations for behaviour, failure to supervise and monitor children, or excessively severe, harsh or inconsistent punishment	**Bonding** Attachment and commitment to, and positive communication with, family (and school and wider community)
	Family conflict Conflict between parents or between parents and children (including abuse or neglect)	**Marriage or committed relationship** Living with partner who does not misuse alcohol or drugs
	Parental attitudes to drugs Parents have positive attitudes to drugs or approve of drug use	**Recognition for positive behaviour** Parents (and teachers or other community members) provide recognition for effort and achievements to motivate individuals to engage in positive behaviours

Table 2.3 (cont.)

	Risk Factor	Protective Factor
	Family history of substance use Persistent, progressive, and generalised substance use, and substance use disorders by family members	**Healthy beliefs and standards for behaviour** Family (and school/community) norms that communicate clear and consistent expectations about not misusing drugs
School	**Academic failure beginning in primary school** Poor grades in school	
	Lack of commitment to school Role of student not considered meaningful and rewarding	
Community	**High availability of substances**	**Opportunities for positive social involvement** Developmentally appropriate opportunities to be involved with community (or family or school)
	Community norms favourable to substance use Reinforcement of norms that drug use is acceptable for young people	
	Low neighbourhood attachment	
	Community disorganisation High population density, lack of natural surveillance of public places, physical deterioration, high rates of adult crime	
	Low parental socioeconomic status Measured through a combination of education, income, and occupation	
	Transitions and mobility High rates of mobility within or between communities	

Individual/peer factors: Childhood abuse is highly prevalent in heroin users, with 33–50 per cent reporting physical abuse, 33–50 per cent reporting sexual abuse (women more than men) and more than 50 per cent reporting emotional abuse or neglect. Multiple forms of abuse are common. Major depression is seen in at least 25 per cent of adult heroin users entering treatment, 33–50 per cent have anxiety disorders and 50 per cent or more have post-traumatic stress disorder. Much of the serious morbidity seen in adulthood has origins in childhood behavioural and emotional problems, and poor outcomes are more common in children whose psychopathology was not treated. Childhood ADHD prevalence rates range from 10 to 80 per cent, and 40 to 80 per cent meet the diagnostic criteria for childhood conduct disorder. The latter independently predicts the persistence of substance use into adulthood, but longitudinal research suggests the transactional process between early onset psychopathological risk and environmental adversity establishes a trajectory involving substance dependence.

Parental/family factors: Studies consistently show that 33–50 per cent of heroin users had at least one substance-dependent parent, compared with an estimate of 2 per cent in the general population. Violence in the family home of heroin users is common, both between parents and upon the child, with high rates of psychopathology among the parents. At least a third of heroin users report parental separation or absence during childhood. A history of childhood trauma is associated with an earlier age of first intoxication and more extensive poly-drug use.

Community factors: An important risk factor for drug use disorder is the availability of illicit or prescribed drugs. Countries that have higher rates of prescribing of opioid drugs (e.g. in Western Europe, North America and Australia) have greater rates of non-medical use and opioid overdose deaths. The USA and Canada have seen an epidemic of opioid prescribing turn in to a public health emergency that is still ongoing. There were nearly 47,000 deaths from opioid overdose in 2018, 32 per cent of which involved prescription opioids [14]. Risk factors have been shown to differ between countries. An assessment of the initiation and progression to illicit drug dependence in 17 countries showed that earlier onset of drug use, using more types of illicit drugs and having already developed externalising or internalising disorders predicted the development of dependence in drug users [15]

An impoverished social environment is associated with higher rates of initiation into tobacco, alcohol and illicit drug use, and the development of substance dependence. Social disadvantage tends to produce a cluster of risk factors for drug use: high rates of crime, delinquency and substance availability, limited educational opportunities, low rates of completion of basic schooling, low levels of employment, high rates of imprisonment and high levels of stress on individuals and families. In addition, children from lower socioeconomic background families are more likely to experience childhood abuse and neglect, depression and to have parents who smoke and use alcohol and/or illicit drugs. Prolonged unemployment is the norm among cohorts of adult heroin users, and prolonged unemployment perpetuates the cycle of social disadvantage for the children of heroin users.

The Brain Disease Model of Addiction

A wide range of neurobiological research over the past 40 years has characterised drug addiction as a chronic, relapsing disease that results from the prolonged effects of drugs on the brain. By the end of the twentieth century it was understood that although each drug of abuse had some unique mechanisms of action, virtually all of them had direct or indirect effects on the mesolimbic reward pathway deep in the brain. Activation of this system appeared to be the common element in what kept users taking drugs [16]. Initial work using animal models was synthesised into the theory that chronic drug use 'flicked a neurochemical switch' in the brain, making it very difficult for people addicted to drugs to stop using them. Researchers at NIDA have since done a huge number of neuroimaging studies on people with drug addiction and they have elaborated on this theory to explain how chronic drug use hijacks the brain's reward systems.

Consuming food or having sex causes the release of dopamine within the basal ganglia and produces feelings of pleasure, which in turn motivates individuals to continue to engage in these activities and ensures the survival of the species. In the face of danger, activation of the brain's stress systems within the extended amygdala drives 'flight or fight' responses, also critical for survival. These basic survival systems are 'hijacked' by addictive substances. A repeating three-stage cycle of drug use disorder has been hypothesised, based on conceptual frameworks from animal models, human brain imaging studies and social psychology:

- **binge/intoxication**, where an individual consumes a psychoactive substance and experiences its rewarding or pleasurable effects
- **withdrawal/negative affect**, where an individual experiences a negative emotional state in the absence of the substance
- **preoccupation/anticipation**, where the individual seeks substances again after a period of abstinence

The cycle may occur over weeks or months, or several times per day. The speed of progress and the intensity of each stage vary between individuals, but the cycle tends to intensify over time. The following section summarises the brief description of this model in chapter 2 of the US Surgeon General's 2016 *Report on Alcohol, Drugs and Health* [17]. The interested reader can find more detailed versions in the work of George Koob and colleagues [18, 19], and the model is summarised in Figure 2.2.

Binge/Intoxication Stage

The **basal ganglia** (BG) have a role in coordinating body movements, learning routine behaviours and forming habits. Two subregions of the BG are particularly associated with the development of addiction:

(i) **nucleus accumbens** – involved in motivation and experiencing reward
(ii) **dorsal striatum** – involved in habit formation and other routine behaviours

The BG control the rewarding/pleasurable effects of substance use and the formation of habitual substance taking. Initial substance use may involve an element of impulsivity. If the experience is pleasurable, this feeling positively reinforces the substance use, making the individual more likely to take the substance again. Addictive substances produce feelings of pleasure, and brain-imaging studies in humans show activity in the nucleus accumbens and activation of dopamine and opioid signalling systems. At the same time, the individual learns to associate the stimuli present while using (people, places, moods, paraphernalia) with the rewarding effects of the substance. Over time, these stimuli can activate the dopamine system on their own and trigger powerful urges to take the drug (**incentive salience**). These urges can persist after the rewarding effects of the substance have reduced, and exposure to people, places, moods or things can serve as 'triggers' (**cues**) that promote substance seeking. This explains why addicted individuals who are trying to maintain abstinence are at increased risk of relapse if they continue to have contact with people they previously used drugs with or the places where they used them. The situation is compounded by habit formation. The release of dopamine, activation of the brain opioid systems and release of glutamate can trigger changes in the dorsal striatum, changes which serve to strengthen drug-seeking and drug-taking habits as addiction progresses.

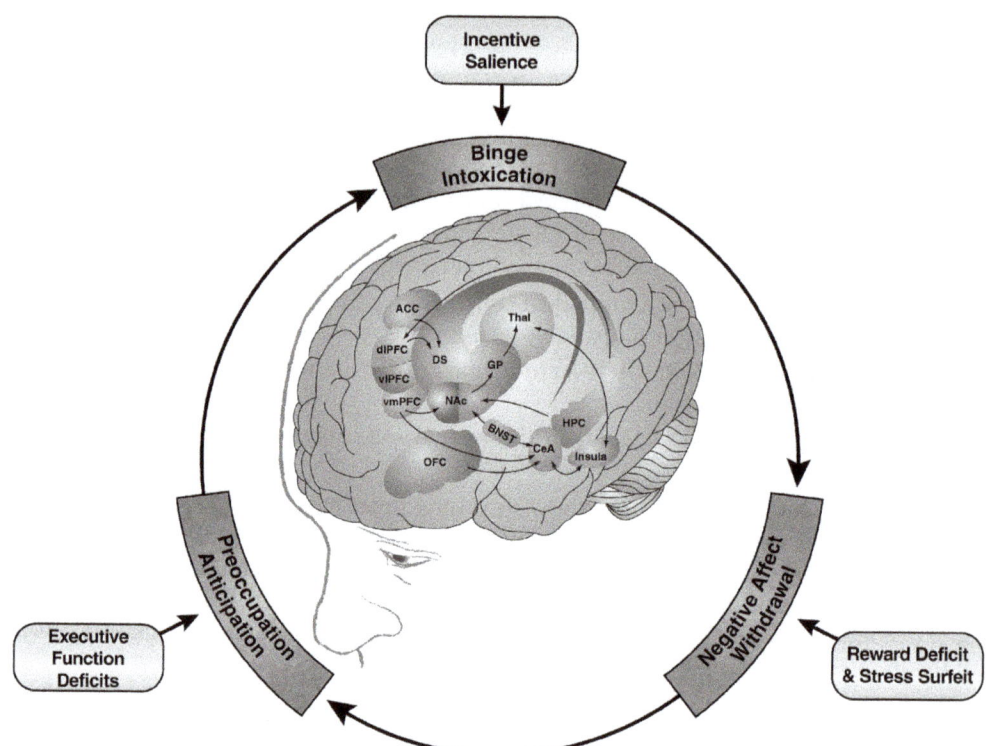

Figure 2.2 Conceptual framework for the neurobiological basis of addiction
ACC, anterior cingulate cortex; BNST, bed nucleus of the stria terminalis; CeA, central nucleus of the amygdala; DS, dorsal striatum; dlPFC, dorsolateral prefrontal cortex; GP, globus pallidus; HPC, hippocampus; NAC, nucleus accumbens; OFC, orbitofrontal cortex; Thal, thalamus; vlPFC, ventrolateral prefrontal cortex; vmPFC, ventromedial prefrontal cortex.
Reproduced with permission from Koob and Schulkin 2019 [18]

The reward induced by drugs such as opioids, cocaine or amphetamine leads to the association of the reward with drug-associated stimuli such as smells, visual cues or specific contexts – for example, sitting inside a drug using friend's car. This triggers drug craving (conditioned reinforcement/incentive salience). Conditioned responses trigger the 'expectation of reward' (i.e. learned associations) in environments where the drug has been experienced.

Withdrawal/Negative Affect Stage

The extended **amygdala** is located beneath the BG. Its role is to regulate the brain's reactions to stress, including 'flight or fight' reactions and negative emotions such as anxiety and irritability. It interacts with the hypothalamus, which in turn has an indirect role in controlling reactions to stress through the pituitary gland. The amygdala is involved in the feelings of unease, anxiety and irritability that typically accompany substance withdrawal.

At first, substance use may generate pleasure, but it may also relieve negative feelings such as stress, anxiety or low mood. This temporary relief from negative feelings is also rewarding (**negative reinforcement**), thus increasing the chance that the individual will use the substance again. Both positive and negative reinforcement can also be driven by other environmental and social stimuli – for example, peer approval can be a positive reinforcement, or using drugs with others can provide relief from social isolation (negative reinforcement). Repeated use of a substance tends to reduce its reinforcing effects (**tolerance**), and this may lead to more frequent use or use in greater quantities in order to achieve the original effect. Eventually, in the absence of the substance the individual may experience negative emotions such as stress, anxiety or depression, or feel physically ill (**withdrawal**). Further substance use will then relieve these withdrawal symptoms.

Symptoms of withdrawal may occur with all addictive substances, but vary in intensity and duration. Negative affect is often prominent due to both reduced activation of the reward circuitry of the basal ganglia and activation of the brain's stress systems in the extended amygdala. The overall reduction in the sensitivity of the brain's reward system in addiction, especially the circuits involving dopamine, means that people who develop a substance use disorder fail to get the same level of satisfaction from once-pleasurable activities. This explains the steady increase in substance use as the individual attempts to recreate the pleasurable feelings previously provided by the reward system.

Another motivation for substance seeking among people with substance use disorder is to suppress overactive brain stress systems that produce negative emotions/feelings. The three neurotransmitters corticotropin-releasing factor (CRF), norepinephrine and dynorphin play a key role in the negative feelings associated with withdrawal and in substance use triggered by stress. The desire to overcome negative feelings of withdrawal can be a strong motivator for continued drug use, strengthened by negative reinforcement. This promotes a vicious cycle – taking drugs to lessen withdrawal symptoms during abstinence causes those symptoms to be worse next time.

Preoccupation/Anticipation Stage

Use of an addictive substance gradually becomes an ingrained behaviour, and impulsivity turns into compulsivity. The primary drivers of repeated use shift from positive reinforcement (pleasure) to negative reinforcement (relief), and the individual is using the drug to escape low feelings rather than to get 'high'. Compulsion and the sense of loss of control over use are key features of addiction (see Chapter 1). In this stage an individual seeks drugs after a period of abstinence (which might only be a period of hours). The addicted person becomes preoccupied by using drugs (**craving**), a process that involves the prefrontal cortex.

The **prefrontal cortex** (PFC) is responsible for the brain's 'executive function' – that is, organising thoughts and activities, prioritising tasks, managing time, making decisions and regulating actions, emotions, and impulses. This includes exerting control over substance taking in the presence of triggers such as cues or stressful experiences. The functions of the PFC can be split into a '**Go system**' and an opposing '**Stop system**'. The Go system helps to make decisions where either significant attention is required, or planning to achieve goals. When substance-seeking behaviour is triggered by environmental cues (incentive salience), the Go circuits are activated and the nucleus accumbens creates a powerful urge to use the substance through release of glutamate. The Go system engages habit-response systems in the dorsal striatum, thus contributing to impulsivity. Habitual responding can occur automatically and subconsciously, and the individual may not be aware that they are engaging in such behaviours.

The Stop system inhibits Go system activity through control of the dorsal striatum and nucleus accumbens, and by controlling habit responses it plays a role in inhibiting incentive salience. Lower activity in the Stop component of the PFC is also associated with increased activity of the stress circuitry of the extended amygdala, and this drives substance-taking behaviour and relapse. Executive function deficits parallel changes in the prefrontal cortex and suggest decreased activity in the Stop system and greater reactivity of the Go system in response to substance-related stimuli. A smaller volume of the PFC in abstinent but previously addicted individuals predicts a shorter time to relapse.

Why Do Only Some People Become Addicted?

Why do some people become addicted when exposed to drugs whereas others do not? There are many ways in which genetic and environmental factors may lead to variation in vulnerability to addiction in general, and addiction to specific drugs in particular. Genetics must play an important role given that the heritability of addictive disorders has been estimated at around 30–50 per cent. Prolonged low mood, stress responsiveness and trait anxiety are important in predisposing to addiction impulsivity. Reward sensitivity and reduced capacity to learn from punishment also appear to be important.

Substance use disorders are inherited as common, complex diseases that show no obvious pattern of Mendelian transmission [20]. Environmental interactions are crucial, but the origin of the complexity is not well understood. It is clear from the description just given that a variety of pathways are involved in becoming addicted, and each must involve numerous genes with potential functional variants. It is therefore reasonable to imagine that addictions are polygenic, with vulnerability arising from the simultaneous impact of functional variations at several genes. However, MZ:DZ twin concordance ratios show no clear polygenic pattern in the inheritance of addiction. In most cases, the MZ:DZ ratios converge to 2:1, which is consistent with alleles of individual effect, and the genetic heterogeneity model (see [20] for a more detailed explanation). The relative importance of polygenicity versus heterogeneity has implications for the potential diagnostic use of genetic markers and for strategies to identify gene effects.

For example, the risk of developing the opioid use disorder has a significant genetic component according to twin and family studies [21]. Identification of the genetic variants underlying this inherited risk has focused on two different methods: candidate gene studies and genome-wide association studies (GWAS). The most studied candidate genes have included the mu-opioid receptor (OPRM1), the delta-opioid receptor (OPRD1), the dopamine D2 receptor (DRD2) and brain-derived neurotrophic factor (BDNF). Variants in these genes have been associated with relatively small, but reproducible, effects on the risk of developing opioid use disorder [21]. The genetic associations identified so far explain only a small portion of the risk of dependence.

Challenges to the Brain Disease Model of Addiction

At the heart of President Richard Nixon's War on Drugs in the early 1970s was the belief that taking drugs inevitably causes addiction. However, two important studies challenged this belief. At around the same time, almost half (45 per cent) of Army-enlisted men fighting in Vietnam reported trying opioids, either in the form of heroin or opium. These drugs were cheap and of high purity, and could be used by non-injecting methods (e.g. mixing with tobacco and smoked) that appealed to a majority of soldiers. One in five soldiers interviewed claimed that while in Vietnam they had felt addicted to opioids, and almost all had used them heavily for a considerable time and suffered the classic symptoms of withdrawal for at least a few days. Almost 11 per cent of Army-enlisted men tested positive at departure from Vietnam, meaning that about 1,400 recently or still addicted enlisted soldiers were arriving in the USA per month. This caused concern that treatment services in the USA would be overrun by drug-addicted Army veterans, and Professor Lee Robins was asked to conduct an evaluation of their outcomes.

Much to everyone's surprise, she found that in the first year after return only 5 per cent of those addicted in Vietnam remained so on their return home. Even veterans still on narcotics at departure from Vietnam were doing very well eight to twelve months after return. The curve showing the likelihood of any use, heavy use and addiction for veterans was the mirror image of that for treated civilians [22]. Even when followed up three years later, only 12 per cent of those addicted in Vietnam had been addicted at any time in the period since return, and for those re-addicted the addiction had usually been very brief.

A second challenge came from animal research. Drugs 'hijacking' the brain had been demonstrated using the Skinner box, a cage equipped to utilise reward or punishment to condition a rat's behaviour. When a surgically implanted catheter was linked to a supply of heroin or cocaine that the animal self-administered by pressing a lever, rats became slaves to the drug, repeatedly pressing a lever to obtain further doses to the exclusion of eating or drinking. However, Bruce Alexander and his co-researchers noticed that the rat had few alternative sources of pleasure to compete with the drugs. They built a Rat Park, an enclosure 200 times the size of a standard cage that was filled with a wide range of alternative interests and activities, including up to 20 other rats of both sexes. They then set up an experiment whereby rats in Rat Park and control animals in standard laboratory cages had access to two water bottles, one filled with plain water and the other with morphine-laced water. When offered a choice, the occupants of Rat Park overwhelmingly preferred plain water to morphine [23]. Furthermore, when rats were given nothing but morphine-laced water for eight consecutive weeks until they were physically dependent on the drug, the animals in Rat Park still switched to plain water more often than the caged rats did when given the opportunity to do so (thus putting themselves into opiate withdrawal). This effect is also shown in experiments with cocaine users, who respond less for cocaine when there are alternative reinforcers available [24]

This research shows that the environment has a key role in the development of dependence on drugs, and that use does not equate to dependence. It is well established that more than 90 per cent of people can use even the most potent drugs with little long-term impact. For example, findings from research investigating the impact of recreational methamphetamine use on human cognition challenges the belief that it causes severe cognitive deficits [25]. The data on acute effects show that methamphetamine improves cognitive performance in selected domains – for example, visuospatial perception, attention and inhibition.

When long-term effects on cognitive performance and brain-imaging measures are considered, only a minority of measures show statistically significant differences between methamphetamine users and control participants. Furthermore, cognitive functioning overwhelmingly falls within the normal range when compared against normative data, thereby limiting the potential clinical significance of these findings. In spite of these observations, there is a general trend to interpret any cognitive and/or brain difference(s) as a clinically significant abnormality. Carl Hart argues that this interpretation has bolstered support for the 'war on drugs' and draconian drug policies, and led to disproportionately high rates of incarceration of Black people and countless Black deaths [26].

Psychological Models of Addiction

Robert West and Jamie Brown have reviewed and synthesised the wide range of psychological models that aim to explain addiction in their book, *Theory of Addiction* [27]. Their approach also uses observations drawn from the brain disease model described in this chapter. The following account represents a brief summary of some of their thinking that forms a prelude to their new integrated theory, the PRIME theory of addiction (see chapters 7 and 8 of *Theory of Addiction*).

Addiction as Reflective Choice

West and Brown start with what they consider to be the simplest 'common sense' approach to the problem. The *Rational Choice* theory argues that addiction arises from a reasoned decision to engage in an activity that is based on weighing up its costs and benefits, and assumes that the individual is well informed about the possible consequences and is always consistent in trying to maximise these benefits/minimise costs. This cost-benefit analysis may favour an increase in frequency, intensity or dose if the individual gets less of a reward from each instance (e.g. pharmacological tolerance), or if abnormal functioning or unpleasant symptoms occur with abstinence. This theory also explains why the individual gives up the activity when the benefits of stopping it are judged to be greater than the costs. If it were the whole story, it would be relatively easy to reduce the prevalence of an addiction just by making it more expensive in financial terms, or in personal terms (e.g. making it illegal or stigmatising it).

Addiction as Irrational Choice

Unfortunately, the numbers of people attending treatment services (and the need for this book) suggest that genuine attempts to restrain use fail. There are large numbers of cases where addicted people show every sign of wanting to stop permanently but still resume the activity soon afterwards. Rational Choice theory requires the decision-maker to be unbiased in their beliefs, but unfortunately irrationality in decision making is common. Many people with substance use disorder are biased in their beliefs about their activity, and they often underestimate the costs and overestimate the benefits. Furthermore, this theory does not take account of emotions, which often win out over rational thought, and ignores *Cognitive Bias* theories. The latter suggest that people in the throes of addiction pay closer attention to information relating to their preferred behaviour than non-addicts.

Addiction, Compulsion and Self-Control

Choice involves conscious consideration of alternatives, but most human behaviour occurs in response to stimuli, or follows pre-made plans. One thing often leads to another and the extent of deliberation varies from situation to situation. A model purely based on rational choices presumes that the individual makes the best choice at the time, even though they may regret it later. However, people with substance use disorder usually describe a difficult process of trying to exercise restraint that it is often unsuccessful. 'Self-control' involves consciously prioritising what we should or should not do over what we feel an urge to do. In relapse to drug use after a period of abstinence people rarely decide to engage in the behaviour as a positive step, but instead describe a sense of failure to exert control followed by regret. Addiction may result when the desire to engage in an activity is abnormally strong or the ability to resist the desire is abnormally weak or both. The journey from normal to addictive behaviour may therefore be explained by a number of processes: changes to the individual's circumstances, development of habituation or sensitisation to the rewarding effects of the activity, onset of unpleasant symptoms during abstinence or a progressive reduction in the person's ability to exercise restraint.

Addiction, Instrumental Learning and Habit

The association between the level of reward provided by a substance and the level of addiction is complex, and the level of addiction is more closely related to dose than reward. Likewise, there is only a weak association between severity of withdrawal symptoms measured prior to relapse and likelihood of relapse. Urge to use and relapse cannot be fully explained by the perceived rewards or the discomfort that would be relieved.

Habits are behaviour patterns that become routine through repetition, and they occur without conscious intent (i.e. they are at least partly 'automatic'). Much of human behaviour is shaped by rewards and punishments without making any conscious choices or weighing up preferences – that is, *instrumental* or *operant learning*. Once a behaviour has been rewarded in some way, it is more likely to occur when the conditions that preceded it are repeated. Connections are made between the conditions that preceded the behaviour (cues), the behaviour itself (the response) and the reward (the 'positive reinforcer'). At times, taking a psychoactive substance leads to an increase in dopamine in the nucleus accumbens which causes the activity to be repeated if the stimulus is encountered again. As this process is not influenced by beliefs about what is good or bad, it can conflict with the individual's conscious choices, and a strong impulse to smoke crack cocaine may override conscious choices not to engage in this activity. This explains why degree of addiction can be dissociated from enjoyment or conscious feelings. The subjective manifestation is the sensation of an *urge* or *compulsion* if attention is drawn to it (because it conflicts with conscious wishes that drive attempts to abstain), but when attention is not drawn to it the behaviour is simply automatic. The process by which the link between the cue and the response weakens over time is gradual and rarely complete, and so although relapse rates are highest soon after instigating abstinence they rarely drop away completely.

Operant learning may also explain why people vary in their susceptibility to addiction. Differences in the dopamine receptor levels will influence the level of reinforcement provided by psychoactive substances, and at least some of these differences are inherited. Such differences may also underpin behavioural traits that increase or decrease the likelihood of developing addiction – for example, impulsivity or antisocial behaviour.

Unfortunately, operant learning and its neurobiological underpinnings discussed earlier cannot explain all the features of addiction, which goes far beyond simple cue-response behaviour. The action chain that leads the opiate-dependent individual to their drug needs to be flexible in order to cope with changing situations (means of obtaining money, finding supply etc). This could be described as 'foraging' behaviour, whereby the individual will use whatever mental and physical resources they have at their disposal to achieve the goal of obtaining and using the chosen drug. This is not easily explained in cue-response terms. Most human behaviour is guided by plans at some level, as we look ahead and work out how to reach our desired goals. Furthermore, much of our life is governed by routines, which cannot be said to be habits as they involve many different behaviours and usually involve conscious acts of will. Routines are plans that are triggered automatically by certain conditions as a result of repetition.

Addiction therefore needs more than a simple theory of choice and more than operant conditioning. West and Brown provide their own integration of these various theories in the form of the PRIME theory of addiction, and the interested reader should explore their book *Theory of Addiction* to find out more. Clinical applications of some of these theoretical concepts will be explored in Chapter 8 of this volume. Robert West's summary of the various theories of addiction, both individual- and population-level is presented in Table 2.4.

Prevention of Illicit Drug Use Disorder

Consideration of the risk/protective factors for initiation and continuation of illicit drug use just outlined suggests that adolescence and early adulthood is the best time of life in which to intervene to prevent drug use. Research evidence suggest that programmes designed to prevent, delay or reduce the use of illicit drugs and drug-related problems are more effective with younger people than at later periods in life. Indeed, workplace prevention programmes have been found to have little effect on illicit drug use.

Rudolf Moos has highlighted four related theories that have been applied to identify key social processes that protect individuals against the initiation and development of substance use problems and facilitate their resolution [29, 30]:

- *Social control theory*: Strong bonds with family, friends, school, work, religion and the wider community motivate people to engage in responsible behaviour and avoid substance use, mainly through monitoring, supervision and the highlighting of acceptable goals. Families that lack cohesion and structure, friends who encourage problematic behaviours and lack of supervision and structure at school or work may all contribute to weak bonds, leading to individuals being less likely to follow 'normal' behaviour and more likely to misuse substances.
- *Behavioural economics or behavioural choice theory*: Rewards provided by activities other than substance use can protect people from exposure to drugs and drug-using opportunities, and form part of a strategy to break addictive patterns of use [31]. The choice of one rewarding behaviour (e.g. drug use) depends on access to other competing rewards (e.g. education, work, physical activity, leisure pursuits).

Table 2.4 West's classification of theories of addiction [28]

INDIVIDUAL-LEVEL MODELS

Addiction arises out of either pre-existing or acquired characteristics of individuals that combine with a given set of environmental circumstances to produce powerful motivations to engage in harmful patterns of behaviour.

Automatic processing theories

Addictive behaviours are acquired through mechanisms that shape behaviours without the need for conscious decisions or intentions and/or influence our capacity for self-regulation.

Learning theories

Addiction involves learning associations between cues, responses and powerful positive or negative reinforcers.

- Operant learning theory (operant conditioning)
- Classic (Pavlovian) conditioning theory
- Incentive-sensitisation theory
- Behavioural momentum and inertia theory

Drive theories

Addiction involves the development of powerful drives underpinned by homeostatic mechanisms.

- The 'disease' model of addiction
- Serotonin theory of nicotine addiction
- Control systems dynamical model of smoking urges

Inhibition dysfunction theories

Addiction involves impairment of the mechanisms needed to control impulses.

- Dysfunction of inhibitory brain circuitry
- Orbitofrontal gyrus dysfunction in cocaine addiction

Imitation theories

Addiction has its origins in the imitation of behaviour patterns and assimilation of ideas and identities.

- Social learning theory
- Automatic imitation

Reflective choice theories

'Rational' choice theories

Addicts choose to engage in the addictive behaviour, and recovery involves choosing not to engage in it. The choice may be rational or biased, but always involves a comparison of the costs and benefits.

Addiction involves making a rational (in the sense that preferences are decided using reason and analysis and then acted upon) choice that favours the benefits of the addictive behaviour over the costs.

- Subjective expected utility theory
- Multi-attribute utility theory
- Prospect theory
- Theory of planned behaviour
- Protection motivation theory
- Theory of rational addiction
- Positive & negative expectancy theories

Table 2.4 (cont.)

Theory category	Description	Theories
'Biased' choice theories	*Addiction arises at least in part from the influence of emotional and other biases on the process by which options to engage or not engage in addictive behaviours are compared.*	• Unstable preference theory • Temporal discounting theory • Cognitive bias models • The affect heuristic • Gateway theory • Conflict theory
Positive reward theories	*Addiction arises out of the pleasure and satisfaction caused by the activity. The greater the pleasure and satisfaction, the greater the risk of addiction.*	• Failure of habituation to positive reward • Body image theory of steroid addiction • Weight control theory of tobacco smoking
Acquired need theories	*Addiction involves the development of physiological or psychological needs, as a result of engaging in the addictive behaviour, which are then met by the addictive behaviour.*	• Drug withdrawal theory • Opponent-process theory
Pre-existing need theories	*Addiction involves engaging in behaviours that meet important pre-existing needs.*	• Self-medication theory • Attachment theory • Affect regulation theory
Identity theories	*Addiction arises from, and is at least partly maintained, by aspects of one's self-identity (how one views oneself).*	• Identity theory • Prototype willingness model • Self-affirmation theory • Self-identity model of recovery
Self-regulation theories	*Addiction involves a failure of an individual's strategies, skills and capacity for self-control to counter the immediate impulses and desires underlying the addictive behaviour. This failure can be linked to 'ego depletion'.*	• Cognitive control theory • Executive dysfunction theory • Self-regulation theory • Self-determination theory • Implementation intentions
Goal-focused theories	*Addiction arises out of pleasure seeking or avoidance of distress or discomfort or, at least in part, out of identification with others engaging in the addictive behaviour.* *Prevention and promotion of recovery involves limiting access to the sources of these goals, reducing their reward value, meeting the needs in other ways or boosting the impact of conflicting goals.*	
Integrative theories	*Addiction involves a combination of mechanisms in which environmental factors and internal states and traits interact to generate conscious and non-conscious motivations based on seeking pleasure or satisfaction or avoiding discomfort.*	

Broader integrative theories

Addiction involves a range of processes depending on the behaviour, population, context and individual. Social and environmental factors interact with pre-existing dispositions to trigger initiation of the behaviour. An interactive process then leads to changes in the personal environment and personal dispositions to increase the strength of motivation to engage in the behaviour relative to competing behaviours.

- The pathways model of pathological gambling
- Externalising & internalising pathways to addiction
- Excessive appetites theory
- PRIME theory

Biological theories

Addiction is primarily a 'brain disease' in which neural pathways of executive function become disordered and particular motivational processes become amplified as a result of an interaction between behaviours (usually drugs) and their effects in the brain.

- Neural circuitry in addiction
- Individual differences in neural circuitry
- Expectancy-reward theory

Process-of-change theories

Addiction involves a wide range of processes for different behaviours, populations, contexts and individuals. Social and environmental factors interact with different pre-existing dispositions to trigger initiation of the behaviour and this leads, through an interactive process, to changes in the personal environment and personal dispositions to increase the strength of motivation to engage in the behaviour relative to competing behaviours.

- Cognitive-dissonance theory
- Elaboration likelihood theory
- Transtheoretical model
- Acceptance and commitment theory
- Relapse prevention

Table 2.4 (cont.)

POPULATION-LEVEL MODELS
Addiction can be understood in terms of the interplay between population-level parameters.

Social network theories
The rates of transition into and out of addiction on the part of individuals within a group are a function of the social connections between individuals who are and are not promoters of addiction, and the nature of these connections.

- **Diffusion theory**
- **Social contagion theory**
- **Actor-network theory**

Economic models
The prevalence, incidence and/or rate of addictive behaviours in populations can be predicted by functions from economic theory, including current and future financial and other costs relating to the behaviour and/or competing/alternative behaviours.

- **Price elasticity**
- **Cross-elasticity models**

Communication/marketing models
The development of and recovery from addiction is influenced by the persuasive communications and marketing activities of those promoting or seeking to combat the behaviours concerned.

- **Contemporary marketing theory**

Organisational systems models
Addictive behaviours can be understood in terms of systems of mutually interacting components at a societal level (e.g. government, tobacco industry, public). The effects of innovation introduced into the system can be nullified by compensatory changes in another or can propagate through the system or even be amplified.

- **Tobacco use management system**
- **Systems approach to healthcare delivery**

- *Social learning theory*: Role models provide positive norms and expectations, and observation of family members or friends who use drugs may lead to imitation and social reinforcement of drug-taking behaviour.
- *Stress and coping theory*: Those who lack self-confidence and coping skills may use drugs to avoid problematic situations or to escape from stressful life circumstances that lead to distress and alienation.

Early prevention programmes highlighted the dangers of drug use in a didactic style. However, as cannabis use became more widespread, people became more familiar with the positive outcomes of the drug and no longer accepted the idea that use invariably led to serious harm. Simply providing objective information about drugs could increase levels of knowledge but it rarely changed actual drug use. Therefore, later approaches began to attempt to influence risk factors for drug use. As low self-esteem could leave young people vulnerable to drugs, so prevention initiatives started to focus on trying to improve self-esteem. Likewise, as young people were often influenced by peer pressure, 'resistance training' facilitated students to 'say no' without losing face. Over time, the 'resistance skills' idea has become a more general 'social influences' approach (i.e. consideration of social and psychological factors in the onset of drug use), including norm setting (objective information to persuade young people that use of alcohol and drugs is the exception not the norm) and broader theories of impacting antisocial behaviour, criminal activity, health and well-being.

The Institute of Medicine in the USA has described three categories of prevention interventions [32]. *Universal* interventions are designed for everyone in a given population, irrespective of risk (e.g. all children of a certain age). They attempt to reduce specific problems by both reducing a range of risk factors and promoting protective factors. *Selective* interventions are for subgroups known to be at risk for a particular problem, and where the balance of risks versus benefits and costs of prevention indicate that universal approaches are not favourable. Finally *indicated* interventions are targeted at individuals already identified as being at increased risk – for example, individuals already using substances but not yet exhibiting problems. Examples of drug prevention strategies illustrating different forms (columns) and functions (rows) for preventive interventions are given in Table 2.5 [33, p126]).

Prevention in Schools

School-based drug prevention curricula that deliver didactic information about drugs and their effects have no effect on drug use compared to normal classroom activities. A more sophisticated approach is to pay attention to:

- social competence: teach generic personal and social self-management skills, such as goal-setting, problem-solving and decision-making and cognitive skills to resist media and interpersonal influences, enhance self-esteem, cope with stress and anxiety, increase assertiveness and interact with others.
- social influence: normative education methods and anti-drug resistance training that aims to correct overestimates of the drug use rates of other adolescents and adults, recognising high-risk situations, increasing awareness of media, peer and family influences and teaching refusal skills.

Table 2.5 Examples of drug prevention illustrating different forms (columns) and functions (rows) for preventive interventions (from [33, p126])

	Universal	Selective	Indicated
Environmental	Legislation to prohibit drug use	Targeted enforcement and actions to deal with drug dealing in high risk areas	Electronic tags to restrict the movement of an individual
Developmental	Primary school classroom behaviour management strategies	Home visiting programmes with vulnerable pregnant women	Individual counselling programmes for adolescent males with impulse control problems
Informational	Mass media campaigns to raise awareness of the dangers of drug use	Informational interventions targeted at young males in deprived areas with strong gang cultures	Normative feedback interventions for individuals who screen positive for substance misuse

When these components are added to information-giving strategies, there is evidence that they can prevent cannabis and other drug use at 12-month follow-up [33]. Programmes that change the classroom/school environment are more effective than those that try to change individual behaviour. Here the focus is on improving discipline and school climate, and strengthening teachers' classroom-management skills, which in turn improve child on-task behaviour and prosocial development. The use of mandatory random student drug testing has led to lower rates of self-reported drug use, but this approach lacks clear evidence of effectiveness.

Prevention via Families and Communities

These programmes are based on social learning and social development models that stress the importance of protective factors (e.g. parents spending time with children) and risk factors (e.g. drug-using peers). There is some evidence that parent training (using cognitive behavioural therapy), family skills training and structured family therapy can prevent illicit drug use in low-risk and high-risk young people [34], although merely providing education to parents is not effective. Other interventions are based on theories of community organisation and participation, and are usually multicomponent interventions comprising environmental, developmental, informational approaches targeting schools, families, peers and the wider community to try to shape drug use norms. Significant effects have not been detected in multicomponent community interventions [35].

Mass media campaigns are another common approach, and often have a sound theoretical underpinning such as aiming to present positive role models who reject substance use. They may be capable of raising awareness of the negative consequences of use, and can work indirectly – for example, by messages targeted at parents (encouraging them to spend more time with their children). However, they are often competing with powerful opposing influences such as a pro-drug club culture or pro-drug music, and there is also evidence that such campaigns may even increase use.

Overall Evidence of Effectiveness

Some prevention programmes (see Table 2.5) do work, but the effects are not large and the evidence is limited. Interventions with a developmental orientation are more likely to be effective. There is less evidence for selective and indicated prevention interventions targeted at those at higher risk. One positive example is the UK-based Preventure programme [36]. In this developmental prevention intervention, school children aged 13 to 15 were screened on four personality dimensions associated with problematic substance use: anxiety-sensitivity, hopelessness, impulsivity and sensation seeking. Those scoring one standard deviation above the school mean on any of these were invited to participate in two 90-minute group workshops focusing on developing adaptive coping skills for their personality profile. This approach produced evidence of impact on alcohol use [37], but mixed results for drugs. Universal programmes are most effective for young people who have not already initiated drug use, and may have little or no impact on those who are at most risk because they have already started to use drugs. This begs the question: should universal programmes be delivered earlier (i.e. before drug use has been initiated)?

There are significant methodological issues with this research evidence base (difficulty in achieving blinding, unknown validity of self-report measures, frequent use of cluster designs weakening statistical power) [33]. Therefore marginal results do not provide a high level of confidence. There is also an issue of whether a delay in drug use has a long-term impact – it is very difficult to measure with certainty the extent to which less substance use in the teenage years translates into reduced drug dependence, blood-borne virus infection or overdose deaths years later.

Summary

In reality, the pathway to problematic patterns of drug use and their ultimate resolution involves a mixture of interacting risk and protective factors. For example, being the child of a person with substance use disorder may mean a genetic liability to addiction, less supervision as a child, more access to drugs from an earlier age, positive modelling of drug-taking behaviour, an increased risk of neglect or abuse and poverty. Living in a neighbourhood with increased rates of drug dealing and crime, on a low income, may lead to a restricted range of opportunities for reward, and psychoactive substance can provide regular and reliable rewards. Neurobiological, psychological and social theories of addiction help us to conceptualise these risks in order to develop more effective interventions at an individual, family or community level.

References

1 United Nations Office on Drugs and Crime. World Drug Report. United Nations publication, Sales No. E.20.XI.6; 2020.

2 NHS Digital. Statistics on Drugs Misuse, England, 2019: Health and Social Care Information Centre; 2019 [updated November 2019. Available from: https://bit.ly/2O90MxL.]

3 Hay G., Rael dos Santos A., Reed H., Hope V. Estimates of the Prevalence of Opiate Use and/ or Crack Cocaine Use, 2016/17: Sweep 13 report. Liverpool John Moores University: Public Health Institute; 2019.

4 Public Health England. *Adult substance misuse statistics from the National Drug Treatment Monitoring System (NDTMS): 1 April 2016 to 31 March 2017*. London: PHE; 2017.

5 Weaver T., Madden P., Charles V., Timso G. S., Renton A., Tyrer P. et al. Comorbidity of substance misuse and mental illness in community mental health

and substance misuse services. *British Journal of Psychiatry*. 2003; **183**: 304–13.

6 European Monitoring Centre for Drugs and Drug Addiction. United Kingdom: Country Drug Report 2019. Luxembourg: : Publications Office of the European Union; 2019.

7 White W., Kurtz E. *Recovery – Linking Addiction Treatment and Communities of Recovery: A Primer for Addiction Counselors and Recovery Coaches*. Pittsburgh, PA: Institute for Research, Education and Training in Addictions (IRETA); 2006.

8 Strang J., Volkow N. D., Degenhardt L., Hickman M., Johnson K., Koob G. F. et al. Opioid use disorder. *Nature Reviews Disease Primers*. 2020; **6**(1): 3.

9 Degenhardt L., Stockings E., Patton G., Hall W. D., Lynskey M. The increasing global health priority of substance use in young people. *The Lancet Psychiatry*. 2016; **3** (3): 251–64.

10 Stone A. L., Becker L. G., Huber A. M., Catalano R. F. Review of risk and protective factors of substance use and problem use in emerging adulthood. *Addict Behaviour*. 2012; **37** (7): 747–75.

11 Toumbourou J. W., Catalano R. F. predicting developmentally harmful substance use. In: Stockwell T., Gruenewald P. J., Toumbourou J. W., Loxley W., eds.. *Preventing Harmful Substance Use*. Chichester: John Wiley & Sons; 2005. p. 53–65.

12 Hser Y.-I., Longshore D., Anglin M. D. The life course perspective on drug use: A conceptual framework for understanding drug use trajectories. *Evaluation Review*. 2007; **31**: 515–46.

13 Darke S. *The Life of the Heroin User: Typical Beginnings, Trajectories and Outcomes*. Cambridge: Cambridge University Press; 2011.

14 Wilson N., Kariisa M., Seth P., Smith H., Davis N. L. Drug and opioid-involved overdose deaths – United States, 2017–2018. *Morbidity and Mortality Weekly Report*. 2020; **69** (290–7).

15 Degenhardt L., Dierker L., Chiu W. T., Medina-Mora M. E., Neumark Y., Sampson N. et al. Evaluating the drug use 'gateway' theory using cross-national data: Consistency and associations of the order of initiation of drug use among participants in the WHO World Mental Health Surveys. *Drug and Alcohol Dependence*. 2010; **108** (1): 84–97.

16 Leshner A. I. Addiction is a brain disease, and it matters. 1997; **278** (5335): 45–7.

17 US Department of Health and Human Services (HHS): Office of the Surgeon General. *Facing Addiction in America: The Surgeon General's Report on Alcohol, Drugs, and Health*. Washington, DC: HHS; 2016.

18 Koob G. F., Schulkin J. Addiction and stress: An allostatic view. *Neuroscience and Biobehavioral Reviews*. 2019; **106**: 245–62.

19 Koob G. F., Volkow N. D. Neurocircuitry of addiction. *Neuropsychopharmacology Reviews*. 2010; **35**: 217–38.

20 Goldman D., Oroszi G., Ducci F. The genetics of addictions: Uncovering the genes. *Nature Genetics*. 2005; **6**: 521–32.

21 Crist R. C., Reiner B. C., Berrettini W. H. A review of opioid addiction genetics. *Current Opinion in Psychology*. 2019; **27**: 31–5.

22 Robins L. N. Vietnam veterans' rapid recovery from heroin addiction: a fluke or normal expectation? *Addiction*. 1993; **88**: 1041–54.

23 Alexander B. K., Beyerstein B. L., Hadaway P. F., Coambs R. A. Effect of early and later colony housing on oral ingestion of morphine in rats. *Pharmacology, Biochemistry and Behavior*. 1981; **15**: 571–6.

24 Hart C. L., Haney M., Foltin R. W., Fischman M. W. Alternative reinforcers differentially modify cocaine self-administration by humans. *Behavioural Pharmacology*. 2000; **11** (1): 87–91.

25 Hart C. L., Marvin C. B., Silver R., Smith E. E. Is cognitive functioning impaired in methamphetamine users? A critical review. *Neuropsychopharmacology*. 2012; **37**(3): 586–608.

26 Hart C. L. Exaggerating harmful drug effects on the brain is killing black people. *Neuron*. 2020; **107** (2): 215–18.

27 West R., Brown J. *Theory of Addiction*. 2nd ed. Chichester: Wiley Blackwell; 2013.

28 West R. *Models of Addiction*. Lisbon: EMCDDA; 2013.

29 Moos R. H. Theory-based processes that promote the remission of substance use disorders. *Clinical Psychology Review*. 2007; **27**: 537–51.

30 Moos R. H. Theory-based active ingredients of effective treatments for substance use disorders. *Drug and Alcohol Dependence*. 2007; **88** (2–3): 109–21.

31 Meyers R. J., Miller W. R. *A Community Reinforcement Approach to Addiction Treatment*. New York: Cambridge University Press; 2001.

32 National Research Council and Institute of Medicine. *Preventing Mental, Emotional, and Behavioral Disorders Among Young People: Progress and Possibilities*. Washington (DC): National Academies Press; 2009.

33 Babor T. F., Caulkins J., Fischer B., Foxcroft D., Humphreys K., Medina-Mora M. E. et al. *Drug Policy and the Public Good*. Oxford: Oxford University Press; 2018.

34 Kumpfer K. L., Alvarado R., Whiteside H. O. Family-based interventions for substance use and misuse prevention. *Substance Use and Misuse*. 2003; **38** (11–13): 1759–87.

35 Stockings E., Hall W. D., Lynskey M., Morley K. I., Reavley N., Strang J. et al. Prevention, early intervention, harm reduction, and treatment of substance use in young people. *The Lancet Psychiatry*. 2016; **3** (3): 280–96.

36 Conrod P. J., Castellanos-Ryan N., Strang J. Brief, Personality-targeted coping skills interventions and survival as a non-drug user over a 2-year period during adolescence. *Archives of General Psychiatry*. 2010; **67** (1): 85–93.

37 Conrod P. J., O'Leary-Barrett M., Newton N., Topper L., Castellanos-Ryan N., Mackie C. et al. Effectiveness of a selective, personality-targeted prevention program for adolescent alcohol use and misuse: A cluster randomized controlled trial. *JAMA Psychiatry*. 2013; **70** (3): 334–42.

Chapter

3

Illicit Drug Use: Clinical Features and Treatment

Ed Day

The Scope of Psychoactive Drug Use

Humans have extracted, prepared and used psychoactive substances for thousands of years: examples include Peruvian hill farmers chewing coca leaves for their stimulant effects, the use of opium in medical poultices in ancient Greece or the use of mescaline from the peyote cactus in the religious ceremonies of the indigenous people of Mexico. The last hundred years have seen the development of a sophisticated industry to develop drugs as medicines, alongside a concerted drive by the wealthiest countries to prohibit the use of many psychoactive substances. In the UK, a number of waves of illicit heroin use have occurred since the 1980s, but by the end of the second decade of the twenty-first century use of heroin is falling. However, it is important to see this in the wider historical context, as use of psychoactive drugs has increased every decade since the Second World War. More importantly, people's first introduction to drugs occurs at a younger age, and this is significant because earlier use is associated with an increased risk of developing significant problems.

As the overall trend moves upwards, use of different substances comes and goes. New drugs appear and rapidly gain prominence (MDMA or 'ecstasy' in the 1980s and 1990s), old drugs appear in new forms (the current 'epidemic' of prescribed opiates in the USA) and some populations start to use drugs in new ways (men who have sex with men, MSM). Psychoactive drug use is rarely out of the news, often provoking strong or contradictory political responses. Cannabis use perhaps demonstrates this variability best in its transition from exotic substance from the East, to the cause of 'reefer madness', to medicinal product for the twenty-first century. Technology has often played a part in the story of humanity's interaction with psychoactive substances, and nowhere is this more obvious than with the emergence of the World Wide Web, coinciding with advances in chemistry to lead to the production of the 'novel psychoactive substances' (NPS) such as synthetic cannabinoids.

Illicit drug use has much in common with use of mainstream substances such as alcohol, but also a number of significant differences. The illegality of use adds new problems such as the risk of legal sanctions, and is also associated with increased levels of stigma and a need to keep the activity covert. All healthcare professionals should be aware of them and be able to take a basic history and signpost the individual towards help and support. The medical perspective on this issue is just one of many, and effective responses to people who struggle with the use of psychoactive substances incorporate a wide range of interpersonal, familial, community and societal strategies. Such is the nature of drug use, any textbook chapter hoping to provide an up-to-date account of how to manage these issues is doomed to be out of date within a relatively short time. Therefore this chapter will focus on broad principles of practice. Specific guidance can be found from Government (e.g. the Orange Book [1]) or national/international bodies (e.g. National Institute for Health and Care Excellence [NICE], https://bit.ly/39vYUqf; European Monitoring Centre for Drugs and Drug Addiction [EMCDDA], www.emcdda.europa.eu/topics/treatment; World Health Organization, www.who.int/health-topics/drugs-psychoactive).

Components of the Assessment Process

The process of assessment follows a similar pattern to that of any mental health disorder, with certain key exceptions or new areas of emphasis. Comprehensive assessment is essential to identify treatment needs and start the process of developing the goals of treatment with the patient. Assessment of risk and the development of a plan to mitigate this is also important. The following broad areas should be covered [1]:

- Confirm that the patient is taking psychoactive substances based on history taking (including information from past clinical records), examination and objective drug testing. It is important to assess the degree of problem use or dependence (see Chapter 1), including the types of psychoactive drugs used (see the next section) and routes of administration (including any injecting). Use of legal substances such as alcohol, tobacco and prescribed medication must also be considered.
- Physical and mental health problems, including current or previous physical complications of drug use (see Chapter 10).
- Current or previous psychological problems, such as personality issues, self-harm, history of abuse or trauma, depression, anxiety and severe psychiatric comorbidity. Any past episodes of treatment should be recorded.
- Social problems including problems in personal relationships (including domestic violence and abuse), family, housing and living arrangements, education, employment, benefits and financial problems. Safeguarding considerations mean it is important to enquire about childcare issues, including parenting, pregnancy and child protection.
- Criminal involvement, offending and other legal issues, including arrests, fines, outstanding charges and warrants, probation, imprisonment, violent offences.
- Explore the patient's personal, family, social and other strengths. An assessment of the social network can be particularly helpful in developing the goals of treatment [2], as can establishing the details of past successes and difficulties in achieving stability or in making improvements.

The final component of the assessment is to understand the patient's motivation for change and their preferred treatment options. Table 3.1 details the essential information required in order to commence substitute medication or other prescribing for dependence.

Substance Use

Screening for illicit drug use is important in any setting and requires a little skill, as people will not often volunteer this information unprompted. The range of psychoactive substances potentially available to use is increasing rapidly (see Chapter 13), and understanding the range of substances used and their effects is helped by adopting the six broad categories used in Mark Adley's 'Drugs Wheel' (www.thedrugswheel.com):

Stimulants: e.g. amphetamine, cocaine, mephedrone, khat

Opioids: e.g. heroin, methadone, buprenorphine, codeine

Table 3.1 Recommended information to be collected prior to prescribing replacement opiates, such as methadone and buprenorphine (adapted from Orange Guidelines [1])

Ideally, the following should be carried out before the initial prescribing appointment:

- Confirmation of the patient's identity through identification check.
- Check the patient's name against any regional prescribing database to prevent double prescribing.
- Check whether the patient is registered with a GP, and if not help them to find one.
- Urine drug screen for opioids, cocaine, amphetamine, and benzodiazepines (see below).
- Consider a pregnancy test if this is a possibility.

Do not start the prescription without evidence of:

- Daily use of heroin or other opioid drugs confirmed on urine drug screen.
- Psychological dependence from patient or informant history – that is, inability to stop after several attempts.
- History or objective evidence of physical withdrawal symptoms (sneezing, runny eyes and nose, yawning, leg, back and joint aches, abdominal cramps, diarrhoea, nausea and vomiting, restlessness, insomnia, anxiety, irritability, sweating, flushing, hot and cold shivers, dilated pupils, piloerection).

Other important elements of the initial history are:

- Details of current physical health problems (e.g. hypertension, diabetes, epilepsy, tuberculosis, HIV, hepatitis B or C infection, asthma).
- Current medication.
- Known allergies.

A physical examination, baseline blood tests (full blood count [FBC], liver function tests [LFTs]) and infectious diseases screen (hepatitis B and C, HIV) are desirable. If the patient is suspected of having hepatitis, LFTs are essential, particularly if buprenorphine is being considered. A baseline electrocardiogram (ECG) is useful if methadone is being considered, or if other medications that prolong the QTc interval are prescribed.

Depressants: e.g. benzodiazepines, gabapentin, pregabalin

Cannabinoids: e.g. cannabis, 'Spice', 'Mamba'

Psychedelics: e.g. LSD, mescaline, psilocybin

Empathogens: e.g. MDMA (ecstasy), MDA, PMA

It is useful to have an awareness of the names that people use for each substance (street names, which tend to vary regionally), and more importantly a feel for capturing quantity, frequency and route of use.

- *Frequency* of use is the most important variable, and this can most easily be assessed by asking about the number of days on which the drug was used in the past week. Daily use of drugs like heroin suggests physical dependence, whereas powder cocaine may only be used at weekends.
- The *quantity* is difficult to gauge, as the purity of illicit substances is variable. However, enquiring about the amount of money spent per day or week is helpful for understanding both the potential impact of the substance use on the individual's life, and their likely level of dependence.

- *Route of use* is important, as some routes are more harmful than others. Injecting carries a high risk of accidental overdose, transmission of blood-borne viruses and physical trauma or associated problems such as deep vein thrombosis. Smoking is increasingly associated with respiratory problems such as chronic obstructive pulmonary disease, and snorting may cause local trauma such as perforation of the nasal septum with cocaine use.

There is often concern about how truthful a history of illicit drug use is. In reality, this may vary as a function of how well the patient is known to the assessor and what the implications of the assessment are. Patients may exaggerate use to obtain a prescription, but minimise it if there are implications such as child protection issues.

Objective Tests for Psychoactive Drugs

Objective testing can be used for initial assessment of drug use, confirming or challenging the patient's self-report and allowing an assessment of use of a range of substances. Although testing does not confirm dependence or tolerance and should be used alongside other methods of assessment, it is essential before prescribing methadone or buprenorphine. Objective tests can also be used to confirm that a patient is taking prescribed medication, and monitor progress towards a mutually agreed goal such as abstinence (important as part of some psychosocial interventions, e.g. contingency management).

Such is the technology available today in the best clinical toxicology laboratories that in theory it is possible to screen for any substance (known or unknown). However, in reality the range is limited by the test medium used, the time since last use and the frequency of drug use. Testing for illicit drugs only ever forms part of the assessment process, and the results must always be interpreted as part of a larger picture by someone with an understanding of the process being used. Staff performing tests should be competent in taking samples and in interpreting the results.

A variety of biological samples are available (urine, saliva, hair, blood) using different testing methods. The sensitivity and varying 'window of detection' of different drug tests can result in false negatives or false positives. Inconsistent or unexpected results should always be interpreted in the light of other clinical information and should not be treated as definitive in themselves.

- *Urine* is the most versatile biological fluid for testing. Collection of a reasonable-sized sample is physically non-invasive, and drugs are present in relatively high concentrations. As urine contains predominantly drug metabolites it is possible to get a picture of drug use over the past three to five days.
- *Oral fluid* is even easier to collect, and direct observation of the process makes it harder to switch or adulterate samples. However, the smaller sample size and lower concentration of drugs within it can present technical problems, and the detection window for oral fluid testing of 24–48 hours means that only very recent drug use can be detected.
- *Hair* testing is poor at detecting very recent use and cannot distinguish sporadic from continual use, but can increase the detection window to several weeks to months. The process of hair collection, preparation and analysis is much more technically demanding, which increases its cost and limits its availability.

Two testing formats are available for urine and oral fluid: 'instant', point of care screening tests and confirmatory laboratory tests. Screening tests have the advantage of being quick, cheap and easy to complete, but there is a real risk of false positive or false negative results.

They use an immunoassay system, and should not be relied upon when important decisions depend on the results – for example, criminal or child protection cases. A confirmatory test may be reserved for samples that have produced a positive result on a screening test. Testing laboratories use either gas or liquid chromatography coupled to mass spectrometry (GC/MS or LC/MS), methods that detect drugs and their metabolites with greater accuracy than screening tests but are usually slower and more expensive.

Drug-testing results form part of the larger assessment picture, and can support the need for prescribing interventions. Once specialist treatment is under way, random intermittent drug screening is probably the most practical and cost-effective option for providing reliable information about an individual's recent drug use. As a therapeutic alliance with the patient develops, many patients will admit to continued drug use without the need for repeat testing, although it may still be needed to assess compliance with medication. Drug testing can be used as part of a specific intervention using contingency management principles, when the testing regimen should be determined in line with the principles of that intervention.

Collection procedures should aim to ensure the integrity of specimens. The time of sample collection should always be noted along with reported consumption of relevant prescribed and illicit drugs over the previous few days. Urine samples can be deliberately diluted by drinking lots of fluid beforehand, adulterated by adding substances to them (e.g. bleach, methadone) or merely substituted for someone else's sample. Direct observation of the patient giving the urine sample can reduce this, but is seldom used for obvious reasons. However, various strategies help to limit false results (removing coats and bags before entering the toilet, checking the colour and temperature of the sample after voiding, checking the dilution in the lab). As urine mainly contains metabolised drug products, spotting substances added to the urine is usually straightforward in a lab, but may be problematic in near patient ('instant') tests. Where serious consequences might follow a positive (or negative) test, procedures should be more rigorous and might include a stricter 'chain of custody' procedure with more security of the specimen collection site and secure packaging for delivery to the testing site.

General Health Assessment

Health problems may be directly linked to drug taking, a complication of a drug-using lifestyle or an incidental comorbid finding. Table 3.2 outlines the important elements of physical assessment.

Possible healthcare interventions initiated in a specialist drug treatment service include information and advice about, and immunisation against, hepatitis B (and possibly A); advice and testing for blood-borne virus infections, with referral for treatment if required; general health information; treatment of direct complications of injecting, including deep vein thrombosis and abscesses; safer injecting advice and provision of injecting parapher-nalia; advice about contraception and safer sex, referral to sexual health service; information about local NHS dental services or direct referral to special care dental services if appropriate.

Principles of Treatment

Use of psychoactive substances is common, and not always problematic. However, when the harmful consequences of use start to outweigh the benefits, attempts are often made to cut

Table 3.2 Components of the comprehensive assessment of the physical health of an illicit drug user (adapted from the Orange Guidelines [1])

History

- Presenting symptoms of a physical health concern
- Past medical history including operations, injuries and periods in hospital
- For women, relevant contraception history and cervical screening, menstrual and pregnancy history
- Sexual health and sexually transmitted infections history (including any partners with HIV or hepatitis C)
- Current oral health problems and recent dental attendance
- Current problems with respiratory or cardiac health
- Current prescribed and non-prescribed medication including over the counter medicines
- Cigarette, cannabis and alcohol consumption
- Any allergies or sensitivities

Physical examination

- Assessment of injection sites in all limbs and inguinal areas, particularly if injecting (or injected in the past)
- General assessment of respiratory, cardiovascular and other body systems, paying attention to any symptoms offered and complaints described (which can lead to a basic medical examination of body system or signposting the patient to their GP for this)
- Measurement of weight and blood pressure – baseline measurements can be useful in monitoring progress and may be needed in cases where there are concerns

Special examinations

- Electrocardiogram (ECG)
- Chest X-Ray
- Pulmonary function tests such as peak flow and FEV/FVC
- Detailed examination of gastrointestinal system, including dentition and liver
- Pregnancy test
- Testing for HIV, hepatitis C (including PCR testing for the presence of HCV RNA) and hepatitis B infection
- Other blood tests to assess liver function, thyroid function, renal function and haematological indices
- Neurological examination (indications = loss of sensation, organic causes of confusion, forgetfulness, convulsions, blackouts)
- Urine testing for markers of conditions such as diabetes and infection

down or stop use. If these attempts are unsuccessful, the individual may seek help from a professional healthcare agency. Use of psychoactive drugs can begin in response to physical health problems such as pain, and use of such drugs commonly leads to a variety of physical health problems (see Chapter 10). Mental health problems are also strongly associated with psychoactive substance use, and may precede or follow use. The illicit nature of the substance used means that financial problems often follow, and their effects may compound this by causing the individual to lose their job. Most drugs used in this way are illegal, and so merely using the drug may lead to fines, imprisonment and associated stigma. Therefore it is not surprising that the helping response required to overcome these problems is complex and multifaceted, and may need to continue for many years. As described in Chapter 1, the nature of psychoactive substance dependence is such that once the problem is established it is very hard to stop, and drug dependence is best considered as a chronic, relapsing illness. Therefore the framework for providing healthcare should adopt a chronic care rather than an acute care model [3].

A debate has raged in drug treatment and policy fields over several decades about the best strategy to adopt when faced with helping people with drug use disorders. This debate, like many issues relating to psychoactive drug use, is often presented in a polarised manner, with 'harm reduction' strategies at one end, and abstinence-based 'recovery' at the other. In reality, such polarised thinking is very unhelpful, and the ideal treatment system would include both elements in equal measure. As professionally led treatment services for alcohol and drug problems developed in the twentieth century, they increasingly adopted an 'acute care' model, driven by insurance companies in the USA. This model sees drug addiction as an acute problem like appendicitis. A severe episode results in a hospital admission directed by medical procedures (detoxification), followed by a short (days to weeks) period of recovery and rehabilitation and discharge (cured). Sadly the nature of dependence is that two-thirds will have lapsed or relapsed within 12 months. Such is the stigma and shame surrounding the issue, people are then reluctant to return to the original treatment provider, allowing significant problems to mount up.

This chapter will consider four broad medical strategies:

(1) harm reduction
(2) medically assisted withdrawal (sometimes known as detoxification)
(3) Opioid Assisted Treatment (OAT; sometimes known as Maintenance Treatment or Opioid Substitution Treatment, OST)
(4) relapse prevention

Figure 3.1 shows how these may be sequenced within the wider biopsychosocial treatment model described in the following sections.

Harm Reduction

Although dependence on psychoactive substances is a chronic condition, many (and probably a majority) of people can become abstinent in the long term. However, the process may take years, and during that time the stigmatised nature of illicit drug use often means that physical and social harms accumulate. Mortality rates in people dependent on heroin are considerably higher than among those who are not. Therefore, a simple all-or-none approach to treatment that requires abstinence as the only marker of success is doomed to failure for the majority.

A *harm reduction* strategy refers to policies, programmes and practices that aim to reduce the harms associated with the use of psychoactive substances in people unable or unwilling to stop. The defining feature of this approach is the focus on prevention of harm, rather than the prevention of drug use itself, and therefore meeting drug users 'where they're at'. The approach came to prominence in the 1980s in Europe when many countries were faced with an epidemic of HIV infection that was strongly linked to injecting drug use. The approach is nicely summed up in a quote from the Advisory Council on the Misuse of Drugs (ACMD) report, *AIDS and Drug Misuse: Part 1*, published in 1988 [4]:

The report's first conclusion is that HIV is a greater threat to public and individual health than drug misuse. The first goal of work with drug misusers must therefore be to prevent them from acquiring or transmitting the virus. In some cases this will be achieved through abstinence. In others, abstinence will not be achievable for the time being and efforts will have to focus on risk-reduction. Abstinence remains the ultimate goal but efforts to bring it about in individual cases must not jeopardize any reduction in HIV risk behaviour which has already been achieved.

Harm reduction complements approaches that seek to prevent or reduce the overall level of drug consumption. It is based on the recognition that many people throughout the world continue to use psychoactive drugs despite even the strongest efforts to prevent them. Access to good treatment is important for people with drug problems, but many people with drug problems are unable or unwilling to get treatment.

Key components of a harm reduction approach to illicit drug use include:

- information on the safe handling and disposal of injecting equipment
- access to blood-borne virus testing, vaccination and treatment services
- help to stop injecting drugs, including access to drug treatment (e.g. Opioid Agonist Treatment) and encouragement to switch to safer drug taking practices
- other health and welfare services, including condom provision
- provision of naloxone to prevent death from accidental opioid overdose

Needle and syringe programs (NSPs) provide needles, syringes and other injecting paraphernalia, and provide a safe place to return used equipment. A variety of multimedia materials are available to help people understand the potential harms of injecting, and to inject more safely (e.g. avoiding groin injecting, using better sterile technique). The rapid development of this approach in the UK in the 1980s was credited with averting widespread HIV infection.

A major threat to public health is the risk of spreading blood-borne viruses such as hepatitis B and C and HIV through the sharing of drug injecting paraphernalia. UK drug treatment services have provided a very successful *hepatitis B vaccination* programme, leading to very low levels of the disease. However, hepatitis C remains a major concern. New treatments provide a realistic expectation of cure from hepatitis C, but the challenge remains getting those at risk to access them.

Advice on safer injecting practices is incorporated into NSPs and other treatment services. The World Health Organization (WHO) describes information, education and communication approaches as an essential component of the response to BBV infection among injecting drug users. The same principles are also employed to address many other forms of drug-related harm, including respiratory and cardiac problems secondary to smoking crack cocaine. Provision of condoms and assessment, advice and treatment of sexually transmitted infections is important.

Advice on how to avoid and manage an overdose is now combined with provision of naloxone for people at risk of accidental overdose of opioid drugs. Naloxone is a full opioid antagonist and is an effective antidote in reversing the effects of heroin overdose. This is a standard and well established treatment procedure in emergency medicine settings, but recently the prescription of 'take home' naloxone to heroin users has been recommended in an attempt to reduce heroin overdose and death. This approach is gathering momentum as a public health and harm reduction intervention in the USA, Europe, Australia and the UK.

Between 40 and 70 per cent of injecting drug users have overdosed at least once in their drug using careers, and overdose is the most common cause of death in heroin addicts (see [5] for a detailed review). The majority of heroin overdoses occur with other people present, and the people most likely to be present as witnesses are other drug users. Administration of naloxone can reverse opioid-induced respiratory depression and so prevent death, hence the case for educating and distributing naloxone to drug users and their families in the hope that prompt provision of this antidote will save lives. Naloxone is ineffective orally and should be administered parenterally, and this requires some initial training (at the time of writing intranasal versions are starting to be used but are expensive). It has an excellent safety profile and is virtually devoid of any side effects. In the absence of opiates, it has no pharmacologic action (hence no potential for abuse) and doses of up to 90 mg are well tolerated.

Changes to UK legislation have increased access to naloxone for use in opioid overdose. Naloxone was reclassified by the UK Parliament in June 2005, meaning that it was added to the list of prescription-only medicines (POM) that anyone (not just healthcare professionals) can administer by injection for the purpose of saving a life (similar to epinephrine in an EpiPen). This means that naloxone can be given by any member of the public, including all drug service/hospital staff, to a person suspected of taking an opioid overdose. However, naloxone could only be prescribed directly to a named patient ('someone who uses, or has used, opiates and is at risk of overdose'), or supplied to an individual by means of a patient specific direction (PSD) or a patient group direction (PGD). New legislation in October 2015 outlined exemptions from the restriction on supply of a POM in the case of naloxone, meaning it could be supplied to individuals by drug services without prescription. Establishing intravenous access in overdose victims can be difficult, so patients are advised to administer naloxone intramuscularly. It is available in the UK in minijets or prefilled syringes (0.4 mg per 1 ml), and a needle should also be supplied with the prescription.

Prescribing naloxone to take home is not seen as a one-off event, but rather as a process that requires regular monitoring. A review should take place at least every three months, considering whether the supplied naloxone has been used, and if so the appropriateness, impact and experience of such use. Knowledge and understanding should be reassessed, and refresher training delivered if necessary. A new naloxone supply may be needed if the expiry date has been reached.

Opiates

Medically Assisted Withdrawal

Medically assisted withdrawal (MAW) is usually known as 'detoxification', and is defined by NICE as 'the process by which the effects of drugs are eliminated from dependent users in a safe and effective manner, such that withdrawal symptoms are eliminated' [6]. Opiate withdrawal symptoms present significantly less threat to life than severe alcohol withdrawal, and yet those that have experienced them will go to great lengths to avoid them, and many present to healthcare providers in crisis induced by withdrawal symptoms. Management of these symptoms should be an active process carried out after a joint decision between the patient and the healthcare professional, with continued treatment, support and monitoring. Outcomes are better when the individual is committed to a longer-term process of abstinence-based recovery after the medicated episode ends, rather than seeing detoxification as a cure to their problems. In fact, opiate withdrawal can increase the risk of mortality, as opiate tolerance disappears rapidly after abstinence is achieved [7].

Failed episodes of withdrawal also reduce self-efficacy, and preparation work is crucial in order to maximise the chances of success. The process is most likely to be successful if the individual is well engaged in treatment or mutual aid processes and actively addressing issues relating to drug use, including stabilising the amount used, resolving life problems, cutting links with other drug users and the development of strategies for relapse prevention. Actual attempts are better evidence than stated intentions, and the best marker of long-term success is the development of clear plans and social supports to sustain abstinence following detoxification, including a programme of activities or work to prevent boredom and ideas on how to replace the role of opioids.

Preparation

This is based on a dialogue between the prescriber, the keyworker, the patient and members of their social support network. Key issues to be addressed include determining readiness for withdrawal, discussing learning points from previous attempts to stop, coping strategies other than pharmacotherapy for dealing with withdrawal symptoms, identifying a support person and plan for the withdrawal period, identifying a post-withdrawal plan and assessment of risks such as accidental overdose post-withdrawal. Throughout the preparation phase patients should be encouraged to reduce their substance use, and a drug diary may be helpful. In all cases of complete withdrawal the prescription of relapse prevention medication should be considered and prepared for.

Risk Assessment

The setting for MAW will depend upon an assessment of the risks involved. An accurate interpretation of risk requires an understanding of the withdrawal syndromes of the substance(s) in question, any potential interactions with medications, and the physical and mental health of the patient. It is important to consider a history of seizures or delirium, high dosages (particularly with short-acting depressant drugs such as lorazepam) or polypharmacy, and pre-existing conditions, such as hypertension, ischaemic heart disease, significant liver or renal impairment, diabetes, mental illness including organic brain damage or pregnancy. Likewise, risks relating to the available levels of support and supervision will influence the treatment plan – for example, lack of a non-using support person and/or a person willing to supervise medicine, childcare difficulties or the distance to the treatment centre. Even with planned withdrawal episodes unexpected problems may arise and so careful monitoring of withdrawal symptoms is necessary using standardised scales – for example, the Short Opiate Withdrawal Scale (SOWS) and Clinical Opiate Withdrawal Scale (COWS). Monitoring throughout MAW may reveal either physical or mental illness previously masked by substance use and which may require referral to an appropriate specialist.

There are two broad MAW strategies that might be adopted:

(1) Stop the opioid drug abruptly and manage the withdrawal symptoms until they stop.

(2) Stabilise the situation using a long-acting opioid medication such as methadone or buprenorphine, and then taper this medication down to zero at a rate that the patient can cope with.

Abrupt Opiate Discontinuation and Symptomatic Relief

Opioid withdrawal can be associated with both psychological and physiological discomfort for the patient, and some discomfort is inevitable as signs and symptoms of withdrawal are rarely completely abolished. Making the patient aware of this prior to commencing MAW is helpful in reducing distress and discomfort [8].

Medications for reducing the discomfort of the opioid withdrawal syndrome are listed in Table 3.3.

Lofexidine is an alpha-2 agonist that reduces the adrenergic surge of the opioid withdrawal syndrome. It was initially developed as an antihypertensive, and so blood pressure should be measured regularly. It reduces the intensity of the opioid withdrawal syndrome

Table 3.3 Medications used to reduce the symptoms and signs of opiate withdrawal

Autonomic symptoms (sweating, tachycardia, myoclonus)	• Lofexidine 0.2 to 0.6 mg oral every 6 hours; hold dose if blood pressure <90/60 mmHg (0.4 mg 4 times daily is commonly used in the outpatient setting) *Recommend test dose (0.4 mg oral) with blood pressure check 1 hour post dose; obtain daily blood pressure checks; increasing dose requires additional blood pressure checks. Re-evaluate in 3 to 7 days; taper to stop; average duration 15 days.*
Anxiety, dysphoria, lacrimation, rhinorrhea	• Promazine 25 mg up to 6-hourly (and 50mg nocte) • Diphenhydramine 25 mg every 6 hours as needed • Small doses of benzodiazepines may be useful (e.g. diazepam 2-5mg up to 8-hourly), but has high addiction potential *Anxiety levels are an important feature of the opioid withdrawal syndrome. Providing good information prior to the detoxification can help to reduce this [8], and reassurance and other non-pharmacotherapeutic techniques are also useful.*
Myalgia	• NSAIDs (e.g. ibuprofen 400 three times daily) • Paracetamol 1g every 6 hours as needed • Topical medications like menthol/methylsalicylate cream
Sleep disturbance	• Zopiclone 7.5 mg orally at bedtime • Nitrazepam 10 mg orally at bedtime *Difficulty sleeping is common with opioid dependence, and medication will only help to a limited degree. Sedating antidepressants such as Mirtazapine or Trazadone may be useful, and carry less potential for physical dependence. However, they are not without side effects and are not licensed as hypnotics.*
Nausea	• Prochlorperazine 5 to 10 mg every 4 hours as needed • Promethazine 25 mg orally or rectally every 6 hours as needed • Ondansetron 4 mg every 6 hours as needed
Abdominal cramps	• Dicyclomine 20 mg every 6 to 8 hours as needed
Diarrhoea	• Loperamide 4 mg orally initially, then 2 mg with each loose stool, not to exceed 16 mg daily

and has the advantage of not being dependence forming. It is contraindicated in pregnancy and in patients with severe cardiovascular disease. It should be used with caution in patients taking medications that cause postural hypotension or prolong the QTc interval. This regimen is best suited to a day care setting, but could also be utilised in a community environment if reliable support from the patient's social network is available alongside review by a clinician in the patient's home.

Table 3.4 shows a sample lofexidine-dosing schedule. Patients may be started on the 'moderate severity' regimen, with modifications made according to the actual severity of opioid withdrawal symptoms that occur. Symptoms are monitored using objective rating scales (SOWS and/or COWS), and if the withdrawal symptoms are unexpectedly severe it may be necessary to move from the 'moderate' to the 'severe' regimen (or from the severe to the moderate regime if they are unexpectedly mild). Random urine drug screens are performed to test for opioid use. If the patient uses heroin or another opioid during the peak withdrawal period, then the peak dosing phase will typically need extending by two days. This is only appropriate for one-off heroin use, and is not for those who relapse to regular use who may be better served by discussing maintenance treatment options (see the next section). Blood pressure should be monitored daily (standing and sitting) for the first few days if possible. The next lofexidine dose should be omitted if the diastolic falls below 50 mmHg, if there is a postural drop of more than 20 mmHg, or if the patient reports feeling dizzy or unwell.

Stabilisation Followed by Taper from Buprenorphine or Methadone

NICE Clinical Guideline 52 (Opioid Detoxification) recommends that methadone or buprenorphine should be offered as the first-line treatment in opioid detoxification [9]. Furthermore, when deciding between these medications, healthcare professionals should take into account whether the patient is already receiving treatment with methadone or buprenorphine, as well as patient preference.

Buprenorphine has high service-user acceptability and has the benefit that it is straight-forward to convert to stabilisation or maintenance prescribing (if the MAW is unsuccessful) by continuing buprenorphine or switching to methadone. It has a high affinity for opioid receptors and is able to displace methadone and heroin while at the same time blocking withdrawal effects. Buprenorphine binds to the receptor long after elimination from blood, thus there is a mild protracted residual withdrawal; this is similar to, but of less severity than with, methadone. There should be evidence of withdrawal before commencing buprenor-phine otherwise withdrawal will be precipitated (see section Buprenorphine). The last dose of methadone should be at least 48 hours prior to commencement of a crossover regime.

Patients already stabilised on buprenorphine should receive a gradual reduction in dose, with the rate of reduction limited primarily by psychological preparedness of the individual not by withdrawal symptoms. As a general rule, reduce by up to 2 mg each time until 4 mg is reached, 0.4–0.8 mg each time until about 0.4 mg is reached, then halve the dose and then stop. Adjunctive medications are not typically needed, although a hypnotic maybe useful for the 10 day period around termination of the dose.

Patients not already stabilised on buprenorphine (i.e. using heroin) may benefit from a brief period of stabilisation followed by a reduction over a 10-day period. Stabilisation may occur over one to two days at between 8 and 16 mg/day, followed by a steady reduction to zero over the next eight days (e.g. 8–16–12–8–6–4–2–1.2–0.8–0.4–0).

Table 3.4 Lofexidine regimens used in managing mild, moderate and severe opiate withdrawal symptoms

Phase of withdrawal	Mild – moderate Opioid withdrawal	Severe opioid Withdrawal	Both regimes
	Regular lofexidine	Regular lofexidine	Prn lofexidine
Induction (to minimise the impact of hypotension)	*Day 1 – 0.2 mg qds*	*Day 1 – 0.2 mg qds* *Day 2 – 0.4 mg tds*	0.2 mg qds prn daily
Peak dosing (coincides with peak opioid withdrawal symptoms)	*Days 2–5 – 0.2 mg qds*	*Days 3–8 – 0.4 mg qds*	
Early reduction	*Day 6 – 0.2 mg tds* *Day 7 – 0.2 mg bd*	*Day 9 – 0.4 mg tds* *Day 10 – 0.2 mg qds* *Day 11 – 0.2 mg bd*	
Late reduction (to prevent any rebound effects from lofexidine)	*Days 8–10 – 0.2 mg od*	*Days 12–14 – 0.2 mg od*	None
Total prescribed tablets	56 [0.2 mg qds for 14 days]	112 [0.4 mg qds for 14 days]	

Methadone: Following stabilisation on methadone the dose can be reduced at a rate which will result in zero at around 12 weeks (usually a reduction of 5 mg every seven to fourteen days). Patients often prefer a faster reduction at the beginning although there is no research evidence to indicate the superiority of a linear or exponential dose reduction. What evidence there is suggests that a rate directed by the patient is most likely to be successful [10], and a period of reduction followed by stabilisation is most often successful. A significant number of patients supplement their methadone prescriptions when the dose falls below 20 mg daily and this holds true for either slow reduction or MAW regimens. Thus the regimen is best suited to more stable patients with positive alternatives to drug use that are well established.

Opioid Agonist Treatment (OAT)

The manifestations of heroin dependence are both medical and social – for example, unsafe injecting, criminal activity and family and relationship dysfunction. Treatment with a long-acting opioid agonist (sometimes called Opioid Substitution Treatment or 'maintenance' therapy) aims to manage these problems, allowing the patient to tackle other issues without having to deal with the daily cycle of intoxication and withdrawal. The aim of a prescription is to bring about stability in four domains: substance use, physical and psychological health, social functioning and offending. If an adequate dose of medication fails to bring about any improvements in these domains it should be reviewed, as there is the possibility that prescribing simply adds to, rather than reduces, the total amount of drug taken. OAT should only be used as part of a treatment package that includes a structured care-planning approach.

Methadone

There is a large evidence base for the use of methadone in managing the harms associated with illicit heroin use. Evidence from systematic reviews [11] and long-term cohort studies [12] demonstrates that methadone treatment can lead to reduced illicit heroin use, reduced crime and imprisonment, reduced injection-related risk behaviour, reduced HIV infection, reduced mortality and improved psychosocial well-being.

Methadone is a synthetic μ-opioid receptor agonist with similar activity to morphine. Its pharmacological profile makes it ideal for use as a maintenance drug: the oral route avoids the risks associated with injecting, its long half-life allows it to be taken as a single daily dose, and accumulation in the body means that steady state plasma levels are easily achieved after repeated administration. No serious adverse reactions or other organ damage have been associated with continued maintenance treatment extending more than 30 years in some patients. It has a high bioavailability when ingested orally, with 80–90 per cent absorbed through the gastrointestinal tract. Once absorbed into the bloodstream 90 per cent of the methadone is bound to blood proteins and after repeated administration accumulates in various tissues in the body, including the brain. At steady state the elimination half-life has been estimated to be 24–36 hours, but there is considerable individual variation (from 10 to 80 hours). In contrast, the half-life of morphine is about three hours, and so heroin users need to use the drug at least two to three times per day.

The liver is the main site of biotransformation of methadone (via CYP 3A4 enzymes, in particular), and it is eliminated in the form of metabolites resulting from biotransformation and by direct excretion of the drug itself in urine and faeces. In stabilised patients, methadone does not have the pronounced narcotic effects seen with shorter-acting opioids such as heroin. Some drugs influence the amount of methadone present in blood plasma by induction of microsomal liver enzyme activity, thus speeding up the elimination of methadone from the body – for example, rifampicin, phenytoin and some antiviral drugs used in the treatment of HIV infection. Other drugs, such as fluvoxamine, may have the opposite effect on methadone metabolism and increase plasma levels. Knowledge of these interactions allows the appropriate adjustment of methadone dose for effective treatment.

Research involving variable doses of methadone shows that the best results are achieved at doses above 60 mg/day, and although there is technically no upper limit provided the dose is increased cautiously, in practice doses over 150 mg are the exception. The 1 mg/1 ml solution used in routine practice has low potential for abuse by injection. Potential side effects are nausea and vomiting, constipation, drowsiness, respiratory depression and hypotension. Difficulty with micturition, dry mouth, sweating, headache, facial flushing or decreased libido are less commonly described.

Some medical conditions are relative contraindicators (e.g. head injury, elevated intra-cranial pressure, respiratory conditions including asthma, renal problems, acute abdomen, hepatic disease), but the risks should be balanced against the risk of overdose or blood-borne virus transmission when using street heroin. Patients should be advised to avoid the use of sedative or hypnotic drugs including benzodiazepines, alcohol and other opioids in conjunction with methadone. Many treatment services provide naloxone and training in how and when to use it to new inductees to methadone treatment. Alongside other drugs used in psychiatry, methadone has a dose-related effect in prolonging the QTc interval [13]. Patients with known heart or liver disease, electrolyte abnormalities, a known history of ECG abnormalities (particularly prolonged QTc interval) or taking medication known to inhibit the CYP3A4 system in the liver should therefore be monitored carefully.

Buprenorphine

Buprenorphine emerged as an alternative treatment option to methadone in the 1990s, a move largely driven by the desire to prescribe OAT in office-based psychiatry practice in the USA. It is both a partial μ-opioid receptor agonist and a k-opioid receptor antagonist, and its low intrinsic agonist activity gives a milder, less euphoric and less sedating effect than full opioid agonists such as heroin or methadone. It is taken sublingually, and has an onset of effect within one hour and peak effect within four hours. The maximum daily dose is 32 mg, but doses of 12 mg or more appear to produce blockade of the opioid receptors to the effect of heroin.

Buprenorphine has a number of differences in its mode of action to methadone. Its high affinity for μ-opioid receptors reduces the impact of additional 'on top' heroin or other opioid use by preventing receptor occupation. Furthermore, the high lipophilicity of buprenorphine combined with its affinity for μ-opioid receptors means that it has a prolonged duration of action at higher doses (48–72 hours), which potentially allows alternate-day and even three-days-a-week dispensing regimes. A monthly depot version of the drug has recently become available in the UK. Doses many times greater than normal therapeutic doses rarely result in clinically significant respiratory depression. However, the safety of buprenorphine is not clear when it is mixed with high doses of other sedative drugs such as alcohol or benzodiazepines. The sublingual tablets can be crushed to snort or inject, with significantly more potent effects on the user.

Patients should be cautioned about the possibility of 'precipitated' opiate withdrawal symptoms if buprenorphine is commenced within 12 hours of heroin or 72 hours of methadone use. Its high affinity for the opioid receptor may remove full agonists occupying brain receptors, and the resulting partial agonist effect will be experienced as opiate withdrawal. It follows that buprenorphine should be used with caution in people with recurrent acute or chronic pain conditions where opioid analgesia with a full opioid agonist is required. Patients should be advised to avoid the use of sedative or hypnotic drugs including benzodiazepines, alcohol and other opioids in conjunction with buprenorphine, although it would be expected to be safer than methadone. There is a small risk of toxic hepatitis, and baseline and repeat liver function tests are advised in those with known hepatitis C or other abnormal liver function. Evidence is emerging for its efficacy and safety in pregnancy and breast-feeding.

Buprenorphine-Naloxone

Buprenorphine is available with the opioid antagonist naloxone in a combined sublingual tablet (buprenorphine:naloxone in a 4:1 ratio). When taken sublingually as intended the naloxone has very low bioavailability and does not diminish the therapeutic effect of the buprenorphine. However, if injected the naloxone has high bioavailability and is liable to precipitate withdrawal in an opioid-dependent patient, therefore discouraging further misuse. If taken intranasally the effect of the naloxone appears to be variable. The combination tablet may provide the same therapeutic benefit while preventing or reducing the liability for misuse.

Assessment and Early Recovery Planning

The components of the optimum assessment for OAT are laid out in the UK Orange Guidelines [1]. Receiving a prescription at an early stage in the treatment process may be a key factor in engaging the person in treatment, but it is important to remember that other approaches may also be useful. In particular, starting a substitute prescription is likely to remove some of the drivers that led the individual to seek help in the first place, and so it is important to work intensively with the patient to continue the momentum towards recovery in the first three months of treatment. The service should present a positive, optimistic attitude at the point of initial assessment, emphasising the patient's strengths and existing 'recovery capital' and possible exits out of treatment [14]. An early meeting with someone in recovery can inspire hope, and all potential pharmacological, psychological and social options should be presented prior to the first meeting with a prescriber.

The usual minimum criteria for commencing OAT are opioid dependence by ICD-10 criteria *and* at least three months regular opioid use *or* high-risk behaviour *or* failed attempts at abstinence. An OAT prescription should never be commenced in a new patient that does not have an oral fluid/urine test positive for opioids (although be aware of the limitations and potential false positives associated with each type of testing). The assessment process should establish the initial aims of prescribing, agree a plan of care with the patient/ keyworker and set default conditions for stopping the prescription. The goal may be:

(1) *Short- or medium-term stabilisation:* Here an opioid prescription is a means of achieving stability in order to make lifestyle changes that will lead to abstinence. The aim is to provide enough opioid medication to replace the illicit drugs used and to completely

relieve/prevent withdrawal symptoms. It is useful to agree practical goals to be achieved and a rough timescale to achieve them. The ultimate aim will be to achieve abstinence from all opioid drugs by moving towards a withdrawal phase once stability has been reached. If MAW is unsuccessful, it may be necessary to switch to strategy 2.

(2) *Longer-term maintenance treatment*: This usually involves moving to doses above those required for stabilisation in order to extinguish opioid craving and block the reinforcing effects of illicit opioids. The key to optimising outcomes seems to be to focus on the goal of maintenance as acceptable in its own right, rather than treating it merely as a stepping stone to abstinence.

An extensive body of evidence shows that long-term higher dose (>60 mg/day) methadone-prescribing programmes produce better outcomes than short-term, low-dose programmes [11]. However, there are successes from short-term, low-dose programmes and a 'one size fits all' approach does not always apply. UK prescribing guidance recommends maintaining individuals on a daily dose of methadone between 60 mg and 120 mg [1]. Higher doses can reduce heroin and other opioid consumption, but caution needs to be observed if there is associated alcohol or other benzodiazepine dependence.

Methadone or Buprenorphine?

Methadone can be said to be the 'gold standard' for OAT that newer therapies are measured against. However, buprenorphine has emerged as an extremely useful alternative, and it is possible to weigh up the pros and cons of either medication.

Buprenorphine may be used instead of methadone in patients who:

- refuse methadone.
- are determined to withdraw from opioids and do not want long-term maintenance treatment.
- cannot tolerate methadone (e.g. too sedated, insufficiently clearheaded).
- may benefit from the 'blocking' effects of buprenorphine in order to stop 'on top' heroin use (and high doses of methadone are considered inappropriate).
- are at risk of overdose or suicide.
- are admitted to general medical/psychiatric hospitals and need an agonist agent, and where there is no guarantee that the prescription can be continued on discharge. Buprenorphine is preferred here as it is easier to reduce quickly and is probably safer. One exception to this rule is the need for full opioid agonists for pain relief.
- are vomiting their methadone (e.g. pregnant women who are suffering from morning sickness).

Relapse Prevention

Naltrexone

Naltrexone is an opioid antagonist that has a high affinity for opioid receptor sites, and therefore competitively displaces opioid agonists but has little intrinsic action of its own. Naltrexone hydrochloride is available as a 50 mg tablet which is rapidly absorbed (peak blood levels achieved after 60 minutes), and has a relatively short plasma half-life (four hours). It is primarily metabolised in the liver to a metabolite (6-β-naltrexol) which has a plasma half-life of about 10 hours, is excreted by the kidneys and is also an opioid antagonist. Despite both compounds having relatively short half-lives, the duration of naltrexone blockade is much longer (up to 72 hours).

Naltrexone is used to help to prevent a relapse back to opioid use following MAW. The patient knows that if they take the naltrexone tablets as prescribed, any use of heroin or other opioid drugs will have no effect. Therefore naltrexone can be seen as a form of protection against a sudden temptation to use opioids, although it will not stop cravings to use heroin or maintain motivation to remain abstinent. It is contra-indicated if there is physiological dependence on opioids (withdrawal is required before starting naltrexone), acute opioid withdrawal (there should be a drug-free interval before commencing naltrexone), chronic pain requiring opioid pain relief, acute hepatitis or liver failure (naltrexone can be hepatotoxic in high doses) or known adverse reactions to naltrexone.

It should be used with caution in women who are pregnant or breast feeding, patients concurrently dependent on multiple drugs or patients with impaired renal function. Side effects are reported by more than 10 per cent of users but tend to be mild and transient, and include insomnia, anxiety, nausea and vomiting, headache, loss of energy, abdominal pain and joint and muscle pain. The biggest problem is the increased risk of death from accidental overdose in patients who return to opioid use after being treated with naltrexone. The loss of tolerance produced by naltrexone means that a dose of heroin that the user had been accustomed to inject during their last period of addiction may now prove fatal. Furthermore, there is a serious risk of overdose if a patient who has taken naltrexone in the previous few days tries to take larger doses of heroin in order to overcome the blockade and achieve a pleasurable effect. Training to use take-home naloxone may be very useful in this group.

Published literature on relapse prevention shows that only a minority of opioid-dependent people seek naltrexone treatment, and there is a very high rate of drop out. However, a significant proportion of people remaining in naltrexone treatment for periods of three months or more remain abstinent from heroin.

Investigations to Consider before Commencing Naltrexone Treatment

- *Pregnancy test*: Patients should be advised of the potential risks of naltrexone during pregnancy.
- *Urinalysis*: If the patient has an opioid-positive sample, ensure that they have been opioid-free for the relevant number of days prior to starting naltrexone.
- *Liver function tests*: The margin of separation between a safe dose of naltrexone and the dose causing hepatic injury appears to be fivefold, but do not start naltrexone if the Alanine Transaminase (ALT) is greater than two times normal. Check the LFTs three to six monthly after starting treatment, discontinuing it if ALT rises to more than three times normal.

It may be useful to confirm that a person is no longer physically dependent on opioids by starting with a small dose of oral naltrexone (12.5 mg) and checking for opiate withdrawal symptoms, before starting the therapeutic dose of 50 mg/day. Various depot and implantable forms of naltrexone are available, but not yet licenced in the UK.

Integrating Medication with Psychosocial Interventions

Opioid dependence is a chronic disease with a prolonged, and commonly lifelong, course. There is little debate about the role of medication in the management of other chronic disorders (e.g. diabetes, epilepsy, asthma, hypertension, chronic obstructive pulmonary disease), and Vincent Dole, the original developer of methadone maintenance treatment, believed that the patient receiving OAT should therefore be viewed no differently than patients requiring daily doses of insulin, anti-convulsive medication or hypertensive medication [15]. However, as just described, over the course of the past 50 years opioid treatments have been conceptualised along a spectrum from acute care (heroin detoxification) to palliative care (long-term medication maintenance as a form of social pacification, e.g. control of crime and disease), with services often becoming polarised as either providing 'harm reduction' or 'abstinence-based' treatment.

More recently, the concept of Recovery-Orientated Methadone Maintenance (ROMM) has been articulated [14, 16]. In the words of William White, treatment systems 'follow a person-centred model of long-term recovery management whose primary goals are defined in terms of remission of primary and secondary substance use disorders, enhancement of personal/family health and functioning, and positive community reintegration. The ultimate aim of ROMM is an enhanced quality of life for each MM patient and his or her family, with larger social benefits viewed as flowing from this primary achievement' [16].

In summarising the evidence for the effectiveness of treatment systems, Dwayne Simpson has developed a coherent model that can be useful for thinking and talking about treatment as a process [17]. Findings from large-scale national evaluations of drug treatment services and clinical trials show that more time in treatment is related to better outcomes. Furthermore, outcome research suggests that reliable behavioural change only appears after about three months of treatment. Despite extensive efforts to understand which characteristics of patients entering the 'black box' of treatment predict the best results, no clear pattern has been established. However, when the treatment process is broken down into stages (similar to the well-known 'Stages of Change' of Prochaska and Diclemente [18]), some key markers of retention in treatment and subsequent outcomes emerge. For example, higher pre-treatment levels of patient motivation and readiness for treatment are related to better treatment results. Treatment progress can then be thought of in three stages:

(1) *Early engagement*: Patients entering treatment must participate (i.e. attending treatment sessions) and begin forming positive therapeutic relationships with the treatment staff. These indicators of early engagement are especially important in the first two months after treatment admission, and they are positively related to client motivation and treatment readiness.

(2) *Early recovery*: Indicators of early recovery such as behavioural change (i.e. substance use) and psychosocial change (i.e. addressing problems in housing, relationships) by month three are directly related to the level of early engagement shown by clients.

(3) *Retention/transition*: Favourable evidence on early recovery indicators predicts better retention in treatment.

It follows that different outcome measures are important at different stages of the journey, and that psychosocial interventions should be tailored to the relevant stage. There are many effective psychosocial interventions in the addictions field (see

Chapter 8), including motivational enhancement therapy (MET), cognitive behavioural treatment (CBT) and behaviourally oriented family counselling (BFC), 12-step facilitation treatment (TSF) and contingency management (CM) and community reinforcement approaches (CRA) [19]. Moos has identified four common elements that appear to underlie all such effective approaches, and these can be incorporated into a model of treatment:

(1) *Focus on engagement, structure and goal direction:* The quality of the relationship between patient and therapist has been consistently associated with treatment outcome. When a stronger therapeutic alliance is established, patients are more likely to actively explore problems, experience less distress and better mood, abstain from alcohol and drugs during treatment and achieve better long-term substance use outcomes. Following an underlying theory of treatment also tends to produce better treatment outcomes, as does greater clarity and organisation of treatment sessions and an emphasis on goal-directed work driven by the patient's personal milestones and objectives.

(2) *Set up opportunities to use rewards and rewarding activities:* Providing rewards for positive change works better than punishing negative actions in shaping future behaviour. The systematic reinforcement of desired behaviours is known as Contingency Management [20]. Initial work focused on using vouchers and prizes that were contingent on being abstinent from drugs (i.e. substance-free urine samples), but later work emphasised rewards for goal-directed activities that could have continuing benefits. For example, the Community Reinforcement Approach focuses more directly on changing individual life contexts to provide rewards for remaining substance-free and increase the likelihood of pleasurable activities [21]. One of the key determinants of long-term abstinence is the ability to find a (non-pharmacological) substitute for drugs.

(3) *Link to abstinence-oriented norms and models wherever possible:* People tend to evaluate and change their drug use with reference to prevailing social norms. Therefore, provision of normative feedback is an important ingredient of treatment, and linking patients to peers in recovery may provide this. The overall goal may be to help the patient change their social network from one populated mainly by drug users to one where positive support for change is provided by non-users.

(4) *Focus on building self-efficacy and coping skills:* There is evidence that patients' coping skills and self-efficacy improve during treatment and are associated with treatment outcome. Therefore, treatment may focus on building an individual's self-efficacy and skills to manage high-risk situations and life stressors, to resist the urge to return to substance use when under stress and to obtain rewards that can serve as alternatives to substance use.

These approaches have been summarised and packaged in a node-link map form [22], and are available from www.gov.uk/government/publications/routes-to-recovery-from-substance-addiction. The process of treatment may be seen as a journey from professionally delivered interventions to peer- and community-led strategies. Whereas the initial goal may be reduction of risks, as engagement builds there is a shift to behaviour change and adaptation of the patient's environment towards one that supports abstinence, citizenship and self-efficacy.

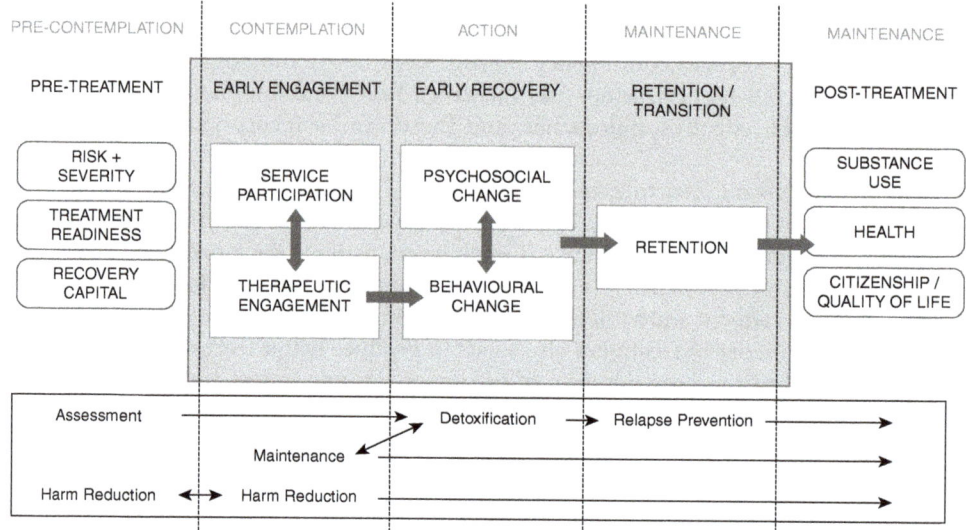

Figure 3.1 The 'black box' of treatment showing the stages that must be negotiated, with the relevant potential treatment strategies shown at the bottom

Stimulants

The most commonly used stimulant drugs are cocaine, amphetamine and methamphetamine, and they can be synthetic (amphetamines) or plant-derived (cocaine). Stimulant drugs are used to increase alertness, attention and energy, but also elevate blood pressure, heart rate and respiration. They include a range of drugs that have historically been used to treat conditions such as obesity, ADHD and depression, and like other prescription medication can be diverted for illegal use. They may be taken orally, snorted, smoked or injected.

Stopping regular use of stimulant drugs leads to fatigue, sleep problems and increased appetite. Although stimulant withdrawal does not produce a pronounced physical syndrome in the same way as opioids, the symptoms of stimulant use disorder include craving, failure to control use when attempted, continued use despite interference with major obligations or social function, use of larger amounts over time, development of tolerance and spending a great deal of time to obtain and use stimulants. Treatment of the withdrawal syndrome is entirely symptomatic. Much work exploring the therapeutic potential of drugs such as desipramine, bromocriptine and lithium has failed to yield positive results, and psychosocial strategies remain the mainstay of treatment. The therapeutic model already described in this chapter is useful, and a potential treatment structure is highlighted in Table 3.5.

Amphetamine and cocaine can both result in the development of a drug-induced psychosis, in which paranoia and persecutory delusions may occur in clear consciousness, alongside ideas of reference and auditory or visual hallucinations. Urinalysis may be helpful in establishing the use of stimulant drugs, and also in determining whether an individual has been abstinent in treatment. Symptomatic treatment and management is sufficient, and the condition will recover spontaneously over the course of a few days to weeks, and should not recur unless there are further episodes of high dose stimulant use.

Table 3.5 A psychosocial treatment plan for stimulant use (adapted from the Treatment for Stimulant Use Disorders Treatment Improvement Protocol (TIP) [23].

A psychosocial treatment program for stimulant use may last between 12 and 24 weeks, and be split into three stages:

1. *Treatment Initiation:*

    This early phase lasts 3–14 days, and is characterised by low mood, difficulty concentrating, poor memory, irritability, fatigue, craving for stimulant drugs, and paranoia.

    The main goals are *engagement* i.e. establish treatment attendance (multiple weekly visits in the first few weeks), discontinuing drugs and start urinalysis schedule (random testing every week), strongly encourage participation in self-help groups, assess psychiatric co-morbidity, and reduce stimulant 'withdrawal' symptoms (proper sleep and nutrition, exercise). The greatest risk of stimulant withdrawal is harm to self or others due to withdrawal-related dysphoria and depression. Continuing agitation and persistent inability to fall asleep can be treated symptomatically using diphenhydramine, sedating antidepressants (e.g. mirtazapine, trazadone), or low dose, short-duration benzodiazepine.

2. *Abstinence attainment period:*

    Establish structure and support, set short-term goals, with brief frequent sessions to reinforce short-term abstinence goal and build therapeutic alliance. Address secondary drug use, encourage the throwing out of all substance-related items, initiate avoidance strategies, provide education about cognitive impairment and forgetfulness, identify cues and triggers, develop an action plan for cues and triggers, enlist family participation + establish social support systems.

3. *Long-term abstinence support plan:*

    Teach functional analysis of stimulant use and examine types of circumstances, situations, thoughts, and feelings that increase likelihood of use. Examine positive immediate but short-term consequences and review negative and delayed consequences.

    Relapse Prevention techniques include education about the relapse process and how to interrupt it, identifying 'High Risk Situations' and relapse warning signs, developing coping and management skills, enhancing self-efficacy in dealing with potential relapse situations, counteracting euphoric recall and the desire to test control over use, developing a balanced lifestyle, responding safely to slips, and establishing behavioural accountability for slips and relapse using testing.

Cannabis

Cannabis is the most widely used illicit drug in the UK. The drug is usually smoked with a mixture of tobacco and dried leaves (marijuana) or resin (hash). There are various psychoactive components within cannabis, but the most active constituent is delta-9-tetrahydrocannabinol (often abbreviated to THC), but this is balanced by cannabidiol (CBD) which may have protective effects on the brain. As with all drugs, the effects of cannabis depend greatly on the circumstances of use, and particularly on the individual's expectations and previous experiences.

For most users, and for most episodes of use, there will be no serious untoward physical or psychiatric complications. However, short term adverse reactions do occur, including anxiety states and panic attacks, brought on by the drug in novice users, and may occur in the absence of any prior psychopathology. Short-term psychotic reactions may occur, although it remains unclear whether these reactions only occur within vulnerable individuals or in any drug user. Anxiety, depersonalisation and confusion are prominent features of the acute cannabis psychosis, and the condition is usually managed adequately with symptomatic relief and reassurance.

Chronic psychotic episodes have been described in association with cannabis use, but the evidence for this causal link between prior use of the drug and subsequent psychosis remains inconclusive. Use of cannabis can certainly act as a trigger to the recurrence of schizophrenia or manic depressive states, but the existence of a specific motivational syndrome is less clear. The extent to which cannabis interferes with motor performance is often overlooked. Studies of simulated driving/air pilot flying conditions demonstrate the extent to which cannabis interferes with estimations of time and distance, as well as impairment of attention and short-term memory. These effects may still be discernible 24–48 hours after last use of the drug. Cannabis is fat-soluble and is only slowly eliminated, so that urine tests after high dose cannabis use can remain positive for several weeks.

Treatment strategies are predominantly psychosocial, and may follow a similar structure to the one described in Table 3.5.

The Concept of Recovery

As the modern science of medicine has developed, the focus of much of its work has moved from cure to the management of chronic diseases which cannot yet be cured. In general health care, treatments that reduce the symptoms of a chronic disease to normal or 'subclinical' levels are said to produce remission. Serious substance use disorders are chronic conditions that can involve cycles of abstinence and relapse, possibly over several years following attempts to change. An episode of treatment that leads to abstinence cannot be said to be a cure. Instead, sustaining remission requires a personal programme of sustained recovery management. With a lesser degree of severity, remission may end a chapter in that person's life that never recurs. In more severe cases, remission requires broader change in behaviour, outlook and identity – a move from being immersed in the culture of addiction to the culture of recovery [24]. This change occurs over a period of time, and alters how an individual thinks about themselves and their lives. Such people describe themselves as being 'in recovery' [25].

Recovery is about the accrual of positive benefits, and requires the building of aspirations and hope from the individual, their family and those around them. It may be associated with various types of support and interventions or may occur without any formal external help: no 'one size fits all'. Recovery is a process, not a single event, and takes time to achieve and effort to maintain. It must be voluntarily sustained in order to be lasting, although it may sometimes be initiated or assisted by 'coerced' or 'mandated' interventions within the criminal justice system.

Recovery has three important elements [26]:

(1) A comfortable and sustained freedom from compulsion to use substances, although abstinence alone does not equate to recovery. For many people this will require abstinence from the problem substance or all substances, but for others it may mean abstinence supported by prescribed medication or consistently moderate use of some substances (e.g. the occasional alcoholic drink).

(2) Recovery maximises health and well-being, encompassing both good physical and mental health as far as they may be attained for a person.

(3) Recovery is about building a satisfying and meaningful life, as defined by the person themselves, and involves participation in the rights, roles and responsibilities of society. (Re-)entry into society and the improved self-identity that comes with a productive and meaningful role is important. For many people this is likely to include being able to participate fully in family life and be able to undertake work in a paid or voluntary capacity.

The diversity in pathways to recovery has sometimes led to debate about the value of some pathways over others. An unhelpful split occurred in the UK about 10 years ago where recovery became equated with abstinence, and was presented as being in opposition to 'harm reduction' approaches such as opioid agonist treatment [27]. This led to further divisions between professionals and people in recovery. In reality, a chronic disease often requires both intensive and extensive treatment to bring about remission, and the ideal system of care blends both professional treatment services and peer-led recovery support services in a seamless Recovery Oriented System of Care (ROSC).

Recovery Orientated Systems of Care (ROSC)

The ROSC model/framework was designed to support communities in the coordination of services supporting recovery from substance use disorders [28]. Professional treatment services and peer-led recovery support services (RSS) are organised into a framework that incorporates the whole health and social care system. The ROSC should be easy to navigate, transparent and responsive to the cultural diversity of the community in which they operate. Two prominent examples of the development of a ROSC have been described in the USA, one in a city (Philadelphia) [29] and the other in a state (Connecticut) [30].

Davidson and White describe the guiding principles [31]:

(1) Recovery looks different for different individuals.
(2) Matches should be made to where an individual is in their recovery process with appropriate interventions and resources.
(3) Recovery is a process along a continuum.
(4) Peer support, family support and involvement and spirituality are important components of any recovery process.

The ROSC framework avoids the polarised debate that often develops between harm reduction and abstinence-based approaches, and between 'experts by training' and 'experts by experience'. As Figure 3.2 shows, the best system contains both elements,

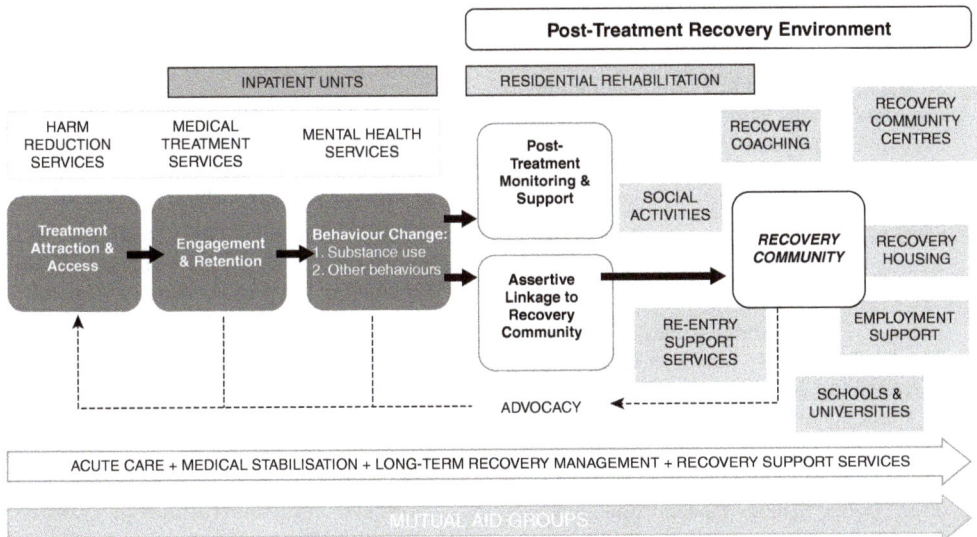

Figure 3.2 A schematic diagram showing a Recovery Orientated System of Care (ROSC). Services led by 'experts by training' are shown on the left, and those led by 'experts by experience' are on the right.

with a gradual transition towards self-care and peer-support as the process of recovery develops. The emphasis may be placed on each group of services delivering their component of the system to the highest level, with assertive linkage between professional and recovery support services and resources within the surrounding community.

Professional treatment of SUD is often conceptualised as an acute intervention, and if success rates are considered in terms of abstinence periods, treatment is successful in 20–60 per cent of the time [32]. However, when combined with long-term recovery support, outcomes improve dramatically [33]. It is estimated that approximately 10 per cent of the population of the USA is in remission from a substance use disorder of any severity [34, 35], but these data are not available in the UK.

References

1 Independent Expert Working Group. Clinical Guidelines on Drug Misuse and Dependence Update, 2017. Drug Misuse and Dependence: UK Guidelines on Clinical Management. Department of Health, 2017.

2 Day E. Building bridges to positive social identities: the social network diagram and opiate substitution treatment. In: *Addiction, Behavioural Change and Social Identity* (eds. S. A. Buckingham, D. Best). Routledge, 2017.

3 O'Brien C. P., McLellan A. T. Myths about the treatment of addiction. *The Lancet.* 1996; **347**: 237–40.

4 Advisory Council on the Misuse of Drugs. AIDS and Drug Misuse: Part 1. HMSO, 1988.

5 Strang J., McDonald R. Preventing Opioid Overdose Deaths With Take-Home Naloxone. European Monitoring Centre for Drugs and Drug Addiction, 2016.

6 National Collaborating Centre for Mental Health. Opiate Detoxification for Drug Misuse, 2007.

7 Strang J., McCambridge J., Best D., Beswick T., Bearn J., Rees S. et al. Loss of tolerance and overdose mortality after inpatient opiate detoxification: follow up study. *BMJ.* 2003; **326** (7396): 959–60.

8 Green L., Gossop M. Effects of information on the opiate withdrawal syndrome. *British Journal of Addiction.* 1988; **83**: 305–9.

9 National Treatment Agency for Substance Misuse. Drug Misuse: Opioid Detoxification. NICE, 2007.

10 Nosyk B., Sun H., Evans E., Marsh D. C., Anglin M. D., Hser Y.-I. et al. Defining dosing pattern characteristics of successful tapers following methadone maintenance treatment: results from a population-based retrospective cohort study. *Addiction.* 2012; **107** (9): 1621–9.

11 Connock M., Juarez-Garcia A., Jowett S., Frew E., Liu Z., Fry-Smith A. et al. Methadone and buprenorphine for the management of opioid dependence: a systematic review and economic evaluation. *Health Technology Assessment.* 2006; **11** (9): 1–171.

12 Simpson D., Sells S. B. *Opioid Addiction and Treatment: A 12-Year Follow-Up.* Malabar, FL: Robert E. Krieger Publishing Co., 1990.

13 Krantz M. J., Martin J., Stimmel B., Mehta D., Haigney M. C. P. QTc interval screening in methadone treatment. *Annals of Internal Medicine.* 2009; **150** (6): 387–95.

14 Recovery Orientated Drug Treatment Expert Group. Medications in Recovery: Re-Orientating Drug Dependence Treatment. National Treatment Agency, 2012.

15 Dole V. P., Nyswander M. E. Heroin addiction – a metabolic disease. *Archives of Internal Medicine.* 1967; **120** (1): 19–24.

16 White W., Mojer-Torres L. Recovery-Oriented Methadone Maintenance. Northeast Addiction Technology Transfer Center, 2010.

17 Simpson D. D. A conceptual framework for drug treatment process and outcomes. *Journal of Substance Abuse Treatment.* 2004; **27**: 99–121.

18 Prochaska J. O., DiClemente C. C. Transtheoretical therapy: Toward a more integrative model of change. *Psychotherapy Theory Research and Practice.* 1982; **19** (3): 276–88.

19 Moos R. H. Theory-based active ingredients of effective treatments for substance use disorders. *Drug and Alcohol Dependence.* 2007; **88** (2–3): 109–21.

20 Petry N. M. Contingency management treatments. *British Journal of Psychiatry.* 2006; **189**: 97–8.

21 Meyers R. J., Miller W. R. *A Community Reinforcement Approach to Addiction Treatment.* Cambridge: Cambridge University Press, 2001.

22 Day E. *Routes to Recovery via the Community.* Public Health England, 2013.

23 Substance Abuse and Mental Health Services Administration: Centre for Substance Abuse Treatment. Treatment for stimulant use disorders. In: Treatment Improvement Protocol (TIP) Series. US Department of Health and Human Services, 1999.

24 White W. L. *Pathways from the Culture of Addiction to the Culture of Recovery.* Center City, MN: Hazelden, 1996.

25 US Department of Health and Human Services (HHS): Office of the Surgeon General. Facing Addiction in America: The Surgeon General's Report on Alcohol, Drugs, and Health. HHS, 2016.

26 UK Drug Policy Commission Recovery Consensus Group. A Vision of Recovery. UK Drug Policy Commission, 2008.

27 Ashton M. The new abstentionists. *Druglink.* 2007; Special Insert (Dec/Jan 2008): 1–16.

28 Ashford R. D., Brown A. M., Ryding R., Curtis B. Building recovery ready communities: The recovery ready ecosystem model and community

framework. *Addiction Research and Theory.* 2020; **28** (1): 1–11.

29 Achara-Abrahams I., Evans A. C., King J. K. Recovery-focused behavioral health system transformation: A framework for change and lessons learned from Philadelphia. In: *Addiction Recovery Management: Theory, Research and Practice* (eds. J. F. Kelly, W. L. White): 187–208. New York: Humana Press, 2011.

30 Kirk T. A. Connecticut's journey to a statewide recovery-oriented health-care system: Strategies, successes, and challenges. In: *Addiction Recovery Management: Theory, Research and Practice* (eds. J. F. Kelly, W. L. White): 209–34. New York: Humana Press, 2011.

31 Davidson L., White W. The concept of recovery as an organizing principle for integrating mental health and addiction services. *Journal of Behavorial Health Services and Research.* 2007; **34** (2): 109–20.

32 National Institute on Drug Abuse. Principles of Drug Addiction Treatment: A Research-Based Guide. NIDA, 2018. [Available from: https://bit.ly/39twZYf.]

33 Simoneau H., Kamgang E., Tremblay J., Bertrand K., Brochu S., Fleury M.-J. Efficacy of extensive intervention models for substance use disorders: A systematic review. *Drug and Alcohol Review.* 2018; **37** (S1): S246-S62.

34 Kelly J. F., Bergman B., Hoeppner B. B., Vilsaint C., White W. L. Prevalence and pathways of recovery from drug and alcohol problems in the United States population: Implications for practice, research, and policy. *Drug and Alcohol Dependence.* 2017; **181**: 162–9.

35 White W. L. Recovery/Remission from Substance Use Disorders: An Analysis of Reported Outcomes in 415 Scientific Reports, 1868–2011. Philadelphia Department of Behavioral Health and Intellectual Disability Services and Great Lakes Addiction Technology Transfer Center, 2012.

Addiction to Prescription Medication: Benzodiazepines, Z-Drugs and Gabapentinoids

Emma Rourke and Fergus Law

Introduction

Benzodiazepines, Z-drugs and gabapentinoids are prescription medications that have recognised potential for dependence and misuse. Benzodiazepines (including diazepam, lorazepam, temazepam) and Z-drugs (zopiclone, zolpidem) are sedative-hypnotics, and both benzodiazepines and gabapentinoids (pregabalin, gabapentin) are used as anxiolytics. Prescription drug misuse is a particular concern for professionals who issue prescriptions, as all prescribers have a responsibility to minimise the risk of misuse and dependence. These medications are widely misused and are readily available on the illicit drugs market, as well as through online pharmacies and internet drug sellers.

These drugs, which all have misuse or dependence-forming potential, may be clinically indicated in some situations and may still be the best available treatment option. The majority of problems with benzodiazepines, Z-drugs and gabapentinoids appear with longer-term use or use in combination with other drugs. When considering prescribing these drugs, it is good practice to undertake a full history and examination to identify any risk factors, and to monitor the patient for any signs of evolving misuse and dependence.

Online Pharmacies and Importation of Drugs

The advent of online retail has enabled people to obtain medications more easily than ever before. People may buy medication online because they don't want to bother the doctor, they may be too embarrassed to ask or they may know that the doctor won't want to give it to them. In 2007 approximately 2 million people in the UK were estimated to be already using online pharmacies to obtain legitimate or illicit medication, and this is likely to have increased significantly. There is an increased risk associated with the use of online pharmacies, as there may be fewer controls, less advice and more risk of counterfeit products. The WHO estimates that 10 per cent of medicines sold worldwide are counterfeit: 1 per cent in developed countries, and up to 30 per cent in parts of Africa.

Buying drugs from abroad in large quantities or without a prescription for personal use is not in itself illegal in the UK. However, if the website originates in the UK, then those operating the website are in contravention of the law. Individuals in possession of large quantities of benzodiazepines may be arrested on the assumption of intent to supply, but they are likely to be released if they can prove the drugs were obtained from abroad and are for personal use. In the UK, the Medicines and Healthcare products Regulatory Agency (MHRA) works with internet providers to force closure of UK websites selling drugs illegally, but they have no authority outside the UK. There are also easily accessible commercial dark web markets that facilitate the sale of illicit drugs. These sites are not indexed, and are hosted on an encrypted network. They have proved popular as buyers are able to leave reviews about the potency of products and reliability of the seller. Drugs are typically delivered by post, allowing a degree of anonymity.

Benzodiazepines

Introduction
Originally marketed as safer alternatives to barbiturates in the 1960s, benzodiazepines have become one of the most widely prescribed classes of drugs. Although benzodiazepines have existed for a long time, the understanding of how they work, how and why they are misused and models for predicting their effects have advanced considerably in recent years. Benzodiazepines and Z-drugs are Schedule 4 under the Misuse of Drugs Regulations 2001 and Class C under the Misuse of Drugs Act 1971, with the exception of temazepam and midazolam which are Schedule 3.

Epidemiology
Rates of dependence are uncertain among users of prescribed benzodiazepines. One large survey found that about 40 per cent of people using benzodiazepines for more than 12 months were dependent [1]. Estimates in the UK suggest 0.5 to 1.0 million people may be dependent, although some estimates have been as high as 1.5 million.

Rates of dependence among illicit benzodiazepine users are even more uncertain. The National Treatment Outcome Research Study (NTORS) found that 22 per cent of individuals entering addiction treatment in the UK were dependent on benzodiazepines, and suggested that 44,000 of the 200,000 illicit benzodiazepine users in the UK are likely to be dependent [2]. In this study, more than half (54 per cent) of those entering treatment had used benzodiazepines in the past three months, 34 per cent were using them weekly or more frequently and 4 per cent had injected them.

Clinical Indications
The primary medical uses of benzodiazepines are in the management of treatment-resistant anxiety and insomnia, as anticonvulsants and for muscular spasm. They may be hazardous in some groups, such as the elderly and those with sleep apnoea, and should be used cautiously in several other groups: people with a past history of sedative-hypnotic or alcohol misuse/dependence; where interference with emotional processing may occur such as in grief or depression; and in people with poorly developed coping skills, chronic stress and anxious-type personality disorders (cluster C). They should also be rapidly stopped in those who get only non-specific effects from them (e.g. 'feeling better') if there is no reduction in the core target symptoms of the disorder being treated.

Benzodiazepines may be conceptualised as symptomatic treatments only, as indicated by the high relapse rate in anxiety disorders when they are stopped. Unless the underlying cause of the problem is resolved by another mechanism, the anxiety often returns as the dose is reduced or stopped. In this sense they differ from antidepressants used for the treatment of anxiety disorder where the relapse rate is much lower following termination of treatment, suggesting that the underlying mechanism giving rise to the symptoms has been treated. The principal implication of this is that benzodiazepines should be used for short-term treatment only, such as during an acute or anticipated crisis where the precipitating factors will resolve quickly. This may include psychological crises, flying or exam phobia and activation syndrome when starting a selective serotonin reuptake inhibitor (SSRI). There is also evidence, reflected in the NICE treatment guidelines, that using benzodiazepines in the treatment of anxiety disorders does not result in the best long-term outcome for the patient, compared to antidepressants or psychological treatments [3].

Long-term use of benzodiazepines is rarely justified clinically, but may occur if the balance of risk and benefit favours them when compared with other treatments (including no treatment), and if benzodiazepine treatment remains effective in the longer term against the core symptoms of the disorder. Where tolerance to the benzodiazepine has occurred, it must be incomplete such that the size of the treatment effect continues to be clinically significant. Most problems arising from the use of benzodiazepines are due to longer-term use and polydrug use, and the adverse effects that need to be considered include the risk of tolerance, misuse, dependence and diversion, as well as the more subtle adverse effects on memory, coping and emotional suppression. One problem is the presence of a large non-specific treatment effect, where people feel better on treatment even when the core symptoms of the disorder have not improved. When this is the case, benzodiazepines should not be used long term, and should be stopped as soon as any acute crisis has passed. It is important to be clear and explicit about the boundaries and expectations of treatment at the time of initiation of the benzodiazepines, in order to avoid subsequent problems and short-term use inadvertently developing into longer-term use.

Anxiety

Although benzodiazepines are highly effective in the symptomatic treatment of generalised anxiety disorder, social phobia and panic disorder (with or without agoraphobia), they are not recommended for first line use, except short term (two to four weeks maximum) in the context of an acute crisis [3]. They may be used in treatment-resistant anxiety as the fourth- or fifth-line drug treatment, after two antidepressants (an SSRI and a serotonin noradrenaline reuptake inhibitor [SNRI]), gabapentin and buspirone. When psychological interventions such as cognitive behavioural therapy (CBT) or applied relaxation are included, benzodiazepines become at least a fifth- or sixth-line intervention. Benzodiazepines have a much faster onset of action relative to alternatives such as SSRIs, which may be a key consideration in a crisis situation. Tolerance to the anxiolytic effects of benzodiazepines, when used to treat anxiety alone, is considered unlikely to occur (see under 'Tolerance' later in this chapter). Guidance from the joint report of the working group from the British Association for Psychopharmacology and the Royal College of Psychiatrists states that treatment with benzodiazepines for longer than four weeks should not necessarily be regarded as a deviation from good clinical practice, but patients should be made aware of the risks of dependence [4].

Insomnia

Evidence exists for the efficacy of all licensed hypnotic drugs in the management of short-term insomnia. Hypnotics are not indicated in the treatment of chronic insomnia, other than for resetting a sleep rhythm and as an adjunct in other conditions. Melatonin is the only hypnotic with a licence for up to 13 weeks, but is restricted in the UK to those aged 55 years and above. Short-acting benzodiazepines, including temazepam (10–15 hours), loprazolam (6–12 hours) and lormetazepam (10–12 hours), are recommended for use in the short-term treatment (maximum four weeks) of insomnia if it is severe, disabling or subjecting the individual to extreme distress. While diazepam is not generally recommended, it may be useful in the context of concurrent daytime anxiety. The National Institute for Health and Care Excellence (NICE) recommends using the most cost-effective short half-life benzodiazepine or Z-drug hypnotic [5]. The half-life of zopiclone (five hours, range 3.5–6.5 hours) and zolpidem (two hours, range 1.5–4.5 hours) is considerably shorter than those of temazepam, loprazolam and lormetazepam. However, tolerance to the hypnotic effect of benzodiazepines can occur within a few days or weeks of regular use. This is important, as tolerance to a hypnotic is unlikely to develop if taken less frequently than once every four half-lives. Studies have shown that tolerance does not necessarily develop to hypnotics even after one year of use for zolpidem, eszopiclone and ramelteon (a melatonin receptor agonist), the latter two of which are not currently available in the UK [6]. To avoid tolerance development, the half-lives mean that zopiclone and zolpidem can be given every night, but that temazepam, loprazolam and lormetazepam should only be taken every second or third night to avoid the development of tolerance.

Illicit Use: Desired Effects

The likelihood of a benzodiazepine being misused is related to a combination of factors relating to the drug, the person and the treatment strategy. The *drug risk* relates to the speed of onset of the drug, the dose and duration of usage. The *person risk* includes the rationale or motivation for using the drug, concurrent use of other drugs, drug use history and psychiatric and physical health comorbidity. The *treatment strategy risk* involves considering the risks and benefits of benzodiazepine treatment or another alternative treatment in the individual concerned, taking into account the degree of monitoring (e.g. frequency of visits and drug screens) and control (frequency of pickup of medication, boundaries of therapy) used during treatment. In general, people with more severe dependence have better outcomes when a higher level of monitoring and control is used in the early stages of treatment.

When taken in sufficient doses, benzodiazepines can produce a positive mood change experienced as a pleasurable high/buzz/euphoria or feelings of comfort (to feel 'floaty', warm and comfortable with no worries), which is usually followed by sedation. Users may take benzodiazepines in pursuit of these effects, although some never experience the high/buzz/euphoria, only the comforting or sedative effect (which interestingly most users also describe as a pleasurable experience). As tolerance develops rapidly to all these effects, users engage in behaviours to try to optimise the benefit they experience from taking the drug. In addition to escalating the dose, they may use it intermittently (binging with gaps in between), speed up the onset of action (crunching the tablets up, taking with hot drinks, dissolving and injecting it), using it in combination with other sedatives or using it in novel environments (where the effects of conditioned tolerance from environmental cues are minimised). The subjective effects of benzodiazepines are affected by the pharmacokinetics of the drug, particularly the speed of absorption and redistribution. People may enhance the effects of benzodiazepines by using them alongside other drugs to potentiate their effects, including alcohol and methadone or other opiates. Benzodiazepines also prevent withdrawal symptoms from cross-tolerant substances such as alcohol, and their non-specific effects improve coping with opiate and other withdrawal symptoms. They may also reduce the anxiety or paranoia associated with cannabis intoxication, or the comedown symptoms associated with the use of stimulants such as amphetamines, crack and MDMA.

Additionally, they may help to manage the side effects of other prescribed or illicit medications.

Illicit benzodiazepine use does not necessarily indicate that the person is using the drug for comforting or pleasurable effects. It is important to explore with all illicit users the reason or motivation underlying their use. The person's initial response should not necessarily be taken at face value, but collated with other information such as their rationale or motivation for using, their pattern of use including the situations in which they increase or reduce their use, and how they respond to the different doses. The 10 questions in Box 4.1 may be useful in identifying the underlying motivation(s) for use and the alternative treatments that may be beneficial.

Box 4.1 An assessment schedule to help to identify an individual's motivations for using benzodiazepines

(1) Is the patient seeking a rapid onset benzodiazepine?

Rapid onset drugs are most abused, as they are associated with the best positive mood change (high/buzz/euphoria or comforting effect). Slow onset drugs are least abused. However, slow onset drugs such as clonazepam may still be abused as these can form a 'base' on which lower doses of a rapid onset drug may be used to achieve an equivalent buzz.

(2) Is the dose being used consistent with the symptoms that are being medicated for?

Low benzodiazepine doses are sufficient to manage the anxiety of generalised anxiety disorder, anticipatory anxiety and phobic anxiety such as social phobia and agoraphobia. High or very high benzodiazepine doses may be required to manage intrusive feelings, thoughts or memories, such as panic attacks, anger, post-traumatic stress disorder (PTSD), abuse memories, hallucinations and negative obsessional thoughts. Such high doses are also used for positive mood change, so it is important to assess for the underlying motivation(s) for use of the higher doses.

(3) Is the frequency of use consistent with the known pharmacological effects of the benzodiazepine?

Patients using benzodiazepines for anxiety will try to maximise the reduction in symptoms during their waking hours – for example, they will take diazepam three to four times/day. Patients using for insomnia will typically take a single dose at night. Patients using for positive mood change will typically use in a way that maximises the high, buzz or euphoria that they get – for example, taking the whole amount as a single dose in the day. This group will often claim to be taking the medication in three to four divided doses to put the clinician off the scent, so it is important to look for evidence that either corroborates or contradicts their claim, such as evidence of anxiety, lack of other alcohol or drug use, or low doses continuing to be effective.

(4) Is the dosing interval less than four times the elimination half-life of the drug?

Using hypnotic drugs intermittently reduces the risk of developing tolerance to the sedative effects. Drugs with an elimination half-life of six hours or less can be used every night – for example, zopiclone five hours (range 3.5–6.5 hours), zolpidem two hours (range 1.5–4.5 hours). Where the dosing interval is more frequent than four times the elimination half-life of the drug, tolerance to sedative effects will occur, although this may be incomplete meaning that it could continue to be effective for night sedation.

(5) Is the development of withdrawal symptoms consistent with the known elimination half-life of the drug?

Withdrawal symptoms typically develop one elimination half-life after the last dose that prevented withdrawal symptoms – for example, 6–12 hours for loprazolam, 10–12 hours for lormetazepam, 10–15 hours for temazepam, 30–40 hours for nitrazepam and 50–93 hours for diazepam. For diazepam, withdrawal symptoms do not develop until two to four days after stopping it. If a patient reports benzodiazepine withdrawal symptoms within a few hours of their last dose, or within one elimination half-life, it is very unlikely to be due to withdrawal symptoms. They are instead likely to be experiencing a lack of comfort, high, anxiolytic or sedative effect, or lack of effect on intrusive feelings, thoughts and memories.

(6) Is there evidence of tolerance, such as reduced effectiveness or dose escalation?

Evidence of tolerance typically indicates use for positive mood change (comfort or pleasure). Rapid tolerance develops to the positive mood change (comfort or buzz/rush/high), sedation and cognitive-motor effects of benzodiazepines, although it is not usually complete. Partial tolerance may develop to the antiepileptic effects of benzodiazepines. Little or no tolerance develops to the anxiolytic, anti-panic and anti-phobic effects of benzodiazepines.

(7) Is the minimum dose of benzodiazepine being used to achieve the desired effect?

If the patient is using the minimum dose required to manage their anxiety symptoms, they are unlikely to be using for positive mood change (comfort or pleasure). Typically, these patients are very willing to consider alternative and more appropriate treatments for anxiety, such as antidepressants or psychotherapeutic interventions. A patient may express a motivation to use the minimum dose but then end up using a higher dose than intended. Being unable to carry through intentions in this way may be due to a lack of motivation to change, but can equally be a hallmark of addiction. Neuroadaptation in addiction leads to a loss of control such that individuals experience unwanted cravings and succumb to taking medication even when they do not want to. Many patients claim to be using the minimum dose, but on further exploration it transpires that they continue to take a higher dose even after the desired effect on anxiety, insomnia or withdrawal symptoms has been achieved. This indicates the presence of more than one motivation for using, and may suggest difficulty controlling use due to psychological dependence.

(8) Is a high dose being used to knock the person out, numb the mind, or cause sedation/oblivion?

High doses may be used in combination with alcohol or other sedative drugs to attain a state of oblivion. This type of use is associated with a high risk of respiratory depression that can result in overdose. In this group of patients, the treatment goal is to help them find and consistently use the minimum dose required to achieve the desired effect, without knocking themselves out completely. This will involve a psychosocial approach, rather than pharmacological intervention. High benzodiazepine doses may also be used to manage intrusive feelings, thoughts or memories. Benzodiazepines may give a sensation of numbing, emotional suppression, derealisation or depersonalisation, or a sense that thoughts are slowed down, which may be considered beneficial by those trying to manage difficult emotions, such as after trauma. Consider introducing alternative psychological and pharmacological (e.g. SSRI, low dose quetiapine for anxiety or insomnia) treatments in order to assist in managing these symptoms more appropriately.

(9) Does the patient say that benzodiazepines are being used to medicate for a comorbid psychiatric or physical health disorder?

From a medical perspective, benzodiazepines are rarely the treatment of choice for psychiatric or physical health conditions, other than as short-term interventions. However, patients often use them to self-medicate as they are easily accessible and provide very rapid short-term benefit for psychiatric symptoms associated with anxiety, depression and auditory hallucinations. Assessment of the rationale or motivation for using benzodiazepines is helpful in providing insight into the patient's state of mind and the issues they are trying to manage – for example, low dose for anxiety, high dose for intrusive thoughts, feelings and memories; and high doses for comfort or pleasure. This is critical information that guides the clinician to the issues that need to be targeted in treatment interventions.

(10) Is the benzodiazepine used for positive mood change or comfort (to feel 'floaty', warm and comfortable with no worries), or to manage low mood, low self-confidence or low self-esteem (rather than to remove an anxious state)?

If benzodiazepines are being used in the absence of anxiety to provide comfort or positive mood change, there is a high risk of rapidly developing tolerance and misuse, which may lead to development of the dependence syndrome. High dose users are more likely to be male and under thirty years of age, and to be using alcohol and/or other illicit substances as well. To maximise the buzz, benzodiazepines will often be used in combination with other sedatives such as alcohol and methadone. Where misuse is occurring in the absence of the dependence syndrome, the most appropriate treatment is typically a harm reduction approach. Where the dependence syndrome is present a more in-depth approach is required i.e. treatment for addiction.

Pharmacokinetics

Benzodiazepines are well absorbed when administered orally, with peak plasma concentrations typically occurring at around one to three hours post dose, although there is considerable variation within the class. As benzodiazepines are lipophilic they are rapidly absorbed, and after absorption are quickly redistributed into the fatty tissues of the body. The duration of action of such lipophilic drugs is determined by a combination of the alpha (redistribution) half-life and the beta (elimination) half-life. The duration of clinical action of a drug relates to the length of time above a threshold plasma level, which needs to be higher in order to achieve a sedative effect than it is to achieve an anxiolytic effect. Therefore, although diazepam has an elimination half-life of two to four days, the sedative effect may last for two hours or so, the anxiolytic effect for six to eight hours, and the prevention of withdrawal symptoms for two to four days.

Benzodiazepines with greater lipid solubility, low plasma-binding capacity and low rates of ionisation will typically have a greater volume of distribution. Diazepam and midazolam are more lipophilic benzodiazepines with a greater volume of distribution, while oxazepam and lorazepam are less lipophilic with a smaller volume of distribution. Regular dosing may lead to saturation of the volume of distribution, especially for drugs that have a smaller volume of distribution. This may then extend the duration of clinical action of the drug.

Metabolism of Benzodiazepines

All benzodiazepines are metabolised by the liver. Most undergo both phase I and phase II metabolism. Phase I metabolism involves oxidation, and phase II metabolism involves glucuronide conjugation so that they can be renally excreted. The three benzodiazepines that are predominantly metabolised by phase II metabolism are lorazepam, oxazepam and temazepam. These three drugs, the 3-hydroxy-substituted benzodiazepines, are therefore more suitable for use in patients with impaired liver function as phase II metabolism is less subject to the effects of liver disease, aging and enzyme inducers/inhibitors than phase I metabolism.

Most benzodiazepines that undergo oxidation do so via cytochrome P450 enzymes, primarily CYP3A enzymes. Diazepam and clobazam also undergo oxidation via CYP2C19 enzymes. Some benzodiazepines are oxidised to active metabolites – for example, desmethyldiazepam (also known as nordazepam, nordiazepam and desoxydemoxepam) is an active metabolite of a number of benzodiazepines, including diazepam and chlordiazepoxide.

Drug Interactions, Overdose and Adverse Effects

Drug Interactions

A range of medications interact with benzodiazepines, particularly other CNS depressants such as alcohol, opioids and sedating antidepressants, antihistamines and antipsychotics. Potentially serious consequences of these interactions include excessive sedation (where aspiration becomes a risk), respiratory depression and cognitive and psychomotor impairment (possibly leading to accidents). Among the most dangerous interactions are those with alcohol and barbiturates, as these increase the affinity of benzodiazepines for the benzodiazepines receptor, resulting in potentiation of their effects. Antacids and food may reduce the rate, but not the extent, of benzodiazepine absorption from the GI tract.

Hepatic enzyme inhibitors result in reduced drug clearance, leading to increased plasma levels and an increased risk of side effects. Drugs that inhibit CYP3A4 include macrolide antibiotics (e.g. erythromycin), antifungals (e.g. ketoconazole), fluvoxamine and cimetidine. Inhibitors of CYP2C19, including fluoxetine, isoniazid and proton pump inhibitors, may result in reduced clearance of diazepam. Conversely, hepatic enzyme induction can lead to lower drug levels, and so elimination of benzodiazepines undergoing oxidative metabolism may be increased by carbamazepine, rifampicin and phenobarbital.

Overdose

Benzodiazepines rarely cause life-threatening overdose in the absence of concomitant sedating medications or underlying respiratory disease, and so the most likely presentation of overdose is sedation with normal vital signs. Signs of intoxication with sedative-hypnotic drugs are not specific to the drug class, and may include drowsiness ('nodding'), slurred speech, ataxia, respiratory depression, stupor, coma and death. Flumazenil is a competitive antagonist at the GABA-A receptor, which can be administered parenterally to reverse the benzodiazepine contribution to the overdose. However, reversal using flumazenil is not without risk, as it may cause seizures and cardiac arrhythmias, so in most situations the risks of using flumazenil outweigh the benefits.

Overdose rates associated with benzodiazepines began to decline in England in the 1990s, reaching an all-time low in 2006. However, since then the rate has rapidly increased, with benzodiazepines now found at post mortem in nearly 400 people per year [7]. During the period 2006–19, overdose rates increased by 235 per cent, while benzodiazepine prescriptions reduced by 20 per cent (Figure 4.1). Scotland, which has a population less than 10 per cent of England and Wales, has nearly 900 drug-related deaths per year associated with benzodiazepines, with an increase of more than 450 per cent between 2015 and 2019. Etizolam, an imported benzodiazepine, was associated with nearly 85 per cent of all benzodiazepine deaths in Scotland in 2019. Over the decade 2009 to 2019 the proportion of all drug-related deaths associated with benzodiazepines has remained at around 9 per cent in England and Wales although it did peak at 11.6 per cent in 2013, but in Scotland rose from 22 per cent to 64 per cent between 2009 and 2019. The number of benzodiazepine-associated deaths per million population has risen over the same period from 4.7 to 6.7 in England and Wales, and from 30 to 164 in Scotland, a massive and alarming five times increase [7, 8, 9]. The increase in deaths despite the declining prescribing of benzodiazepines is likely to be related to more frequent, more complex and higher risk polydrug use.

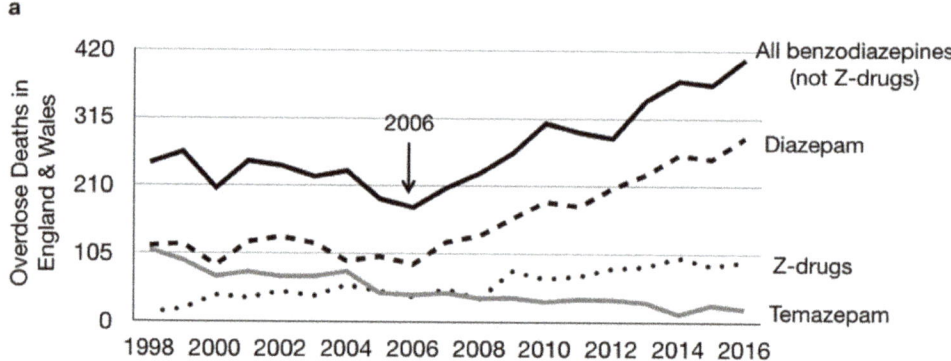

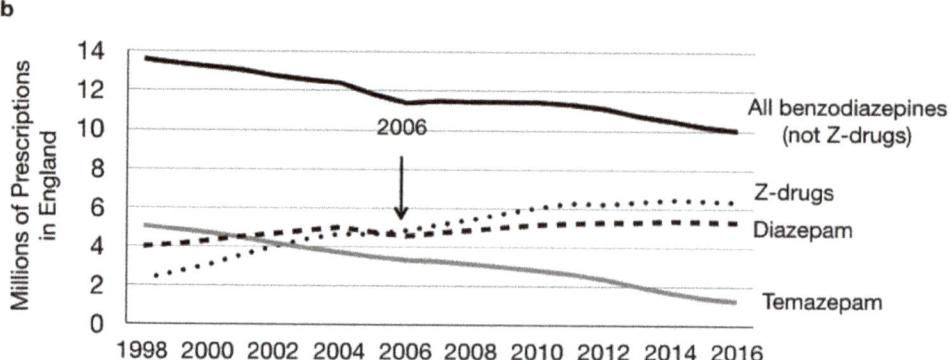

Figure 4.1 Number of benzodiazepine overdoses annually (Fig 1a) in England and the number of prescriptions for the same benzodiazepines (Fig 1b), showing a more than doubling of overdoses associated with diazepam and all benzodiazepines between 2006 and 2019, despite a falling number of benzodiazepine prescriptions and a minimal increase in diazepam prescriptions (Sources: Deaths related to drug poisoning in England and Wales, 2019. ONS, 2020; Prescription cost analysis - England 2019, NHS BSA, 2020, open government licence v3.0)

Side Effects

The commonest side effects of benzodiazepines are drowsiness, sedation, dizziness and unsteadiness. They have been associated with hip fracture in elderly populations, with the first two weeks of treatment having the highest risk [10]. Falls may be associated with lack of tolerance and peak plasma levels of benzodiazepines, in which case more rapid-onset medications and higher doses are likely to pose a greater risk. Accordingly, low doses of slower-onset, shorter-acting medications may be the most appropriate choice in the elderly. Disorientation, confusion and memory impairment are more common side effects in older patients. There are also more subtle effects in benzodiazepine users of all ages that become increasingly important with prolonged benzodiazepine use, including emotional suppression and a reduced ability to cope leading to increased anxiety, agoraphobia, panic attacks and low mood [11]. These are often new symptoms which were not present when the drug was first prescribed. A number of side effects are highlighted below:

- *Disinhibition:* Although laboratory studies have shown disinhibition in association with peak plasma levels of benzodiazepines, clinical studies rarely find this to be a significant effect. Disinhibition is rare at therapeutic dose levels, but may occur on initiation of treatment, with dose increases or high-dose usage, in children, the elderly and people with psychiatric disorders. A 'paradoxical' behavioural activation involving excitement, talkativeness, restlessness, agitation, irritability, increased anxiety and argumentativeness may occur. Where patients are chronically suppressing their own reactions in an effort to control themselves, benzodiazepines can result in other 'paradoxical reaction' due to disinhibition, including loss of impulse control, aggression, violence, reduced mood and suicidal behaviour.

- *Memory issues:* Loss of memory for biographical events (anterograde amnesia) occurs particularly in association with peak plasma levels of the benzodiazepines. This occurs even with patients who have been taking low doses for a considerable time. High benzodiazepine doses may cause loss of all the previous day's events (transient global amnesia), even though the patient behaved normally at the time. This is no doubt why flunitrazepam (Rohypnol) has been used in 'date rape'. A similar effect has been observed with high dose zopiclone (30 mg+), and it is possible that alcohol-related blackouts occur via a similar mechanism. At high doses disinhibition may occur, where the patient feels invincible and invisible, and may commit crimes in front of police, security guards or security cameras (the 'Rambo syndrome'), but not subsequently remember doing so.

- *Emotional suppression:* Benzodiazepines are sedative drugs that suppress emotions. In the long term this leads to a reduced capacity to resolve emotional issues to the same degree, which is thought to be one of the main mechanisms leading to increased anxiety and reduced mood in people taking benzodiazepines long term. When the dose is reduced, not only is there an increase in anxiety, but unresolved emotional issues may come to the surface. These patients will therefore be likely to benefit from an increase in psychosocial support as the dose is reduced.

- *Reduced coping:* Benzodiazepines may be used as a coping strategy to deal with stress. Individuals come to rely on the medication, and as a consequence do not employ other coping skills to the same degree to manage challenging emotional situations. Over time this will lead to a deficit in coping skills, the second of the two main mechanisms leading to increased anxiety and reduced mood with longer-term use of benzodiazepines. When the dose is reduced, this coping deficit becomes more apparent, and is associated with increased anxiety, poorer self-esteem, lower self-confidence and vulnerability. Good psychosocial support is therefore required to support the patient as the dose is reduced.

- *Dementia, cancer and all-cause mortality:* Benzodiazepine use and particularly hypnotic use has been associated with a 25 per cent increased risk of many types of cancer, a 43 per cent increased risk of dementia and a 60 per cent increased risk of all-cause mortality [12, 13]. Although the risk is dose-related, it is unlikely to be a direct causal relationship as benzodiazepines are not known to be carcinogenic in animal models, and even very occasional doses were associated with increased all-cause mortality, suggesting it is a non-pharmacological effect. All hypnotics, independent of chemical class, appear to have a similar effect, including benzodiazepines, Z-drugs, barbiturates and antihistamines. Adjusting for possible confounders often failed to reduce the strength of the association.

- *Pregnancy, foetal and neonatal effects:* Benzodiazepines may be associated with an increased risk of foetal harm such as cleft lip and palate during the first trimester. A benzodiazepine may be used if the benefits are thought to outweigh the risks provided it has a long safety record – for example, diazepam, chlordiazepoxide [14]. Preterm delivery, low birth weight, hypotonia, depression and withdrawal are described in neonates but long-term effects are controversial and poorly understood. Using the lowest effective dose for the shortest period of time reduces the risk to the newborn and tapering the dose reduces the severity of foetal withdrawal. Benzodiazepines pass into breast milk and can cause hypotonia, somnolence and apnea, so neonates should be monitored for increased sedation.

- *Driving:* Benzodiazepines are the second commonest drug found in the blood of impaired drivers (after alcohol). Even therapeutic doses of benzodiazepines impair driving and increase the risk of road traffic accidents by 60–80 per cent. Patients need to be informed about the risk of impairment, and that they may still be impaired the following morning due to the duration of effects from the drug. While it is acceptable to the Driving and Vehicle Licensing Agency (DVLA) for licensing purposes to drive when prescribed benzodiazepines within the BNF limits (even if the dependence syndrome or physical dependence on benzodiazepines exists), the driver is committing an offence if they are impaired (e.g. sedated), if there is any non-prescribed use or if they are using above BNF limits (e.g. above 30 mg diazepam in the UK, even if prescribed). They may also be committing an offence if their blood levels exceed a specified cut-off, although they can use the statutory defence if they are following medical or dental advice.

Tolerance, Misuse and Dependence

Tolerance

Factors that influence the time taken to develop tolerance to benzodiazepines include the indication or rationale for treatment, the dose taken and the frequency of dosing relative to the elimination half-life of the drug. Tolerance develops to the various effects of benzodiazepines at different rates – for example, tolerance develops most rapidly to comforting, euphoric, sedative and cognitive-motor effects, but little tolerance develops to anxiolytic and anti-panic effects. These differential rates for developing tolerance indicate different mechanisms of action for the various effects. In contrast to all other benzodiazepines, which are licensed for short-term use only, clobazam and clonazepam are licensed for long-term use in epilepsy, typically as adjunctive therapy alongside other anti-epileptic medication. This indicates that tolerance is not thought to develop fully to the anti-epileptic effects.

Intermittent use of drugs reduces the risk of developing tolerance, and based on data from ultra-short acting benzodiazepines and Z-drugs, the authors suggest that tolerance to sedative effects is unlikely to develop if a drug is used no more frequently than every four to five half-lives. This means that zaleplon (half-life 1.5–4.5 hours) and zopiclone (3.5–6.5 hours) can be taken every 24 hours, temazepam (10–15 hours) every 2–3 days, nitrazepam (30–40 hours) every 5–7 days and diazepam (54 hours, but with the active metabolite desmethyldiazepam, 93 hours) every 10–16 days. The half-life of a drug does vary between individuals, so longer periods may be needed to avoid development of tolerance in some people.

Tolerance is much less likely to develop to the anxiolytic effects. Benzodiazepines interact with the anxiety pathways in the brain to reduce anxiety, and stimulation of these pathways alone is not particularly psychologically reinforcing. However, when benzodiazepines are used in the absence of anxiety, or when a higher dose is taken than is necessary to treat the anxiety, a positive mood change may occur as the pleasure pathways are stimulated. This is much more highly psychologically reinforcing. Therefore, a dose that enhances mood is reinforcing and potentially addictive, whereas a dose that purely reduces anxiety is not. This model is illustrated in Figure 4.2. Patients seeking comfort or pleasure will typically escalate the dose to manage the developing tolerance, while the group using for anxiety alone will not escalate the dose, as the low dose continues to be effective as an anxiolytic.

Misuse

It is a common misconception that short half-life benzodiazepines are the most abused, while long half-life benzodiazepines are least abused. In fact, it is the rapid-onset benzodiazepines that are most abused (whether they have a short or long half-life – see Figure 4.3). Diazepam has a very long half-life, but is widely misused. Although slow-onset benzodiazepines are least abused (e.g. clonazepam, chlordiazepoxide, oxazepam), they may still be abused when used as a 'base' on which to use a rapid-onset drug (another benzodiazepine, alcohol or other sedative drug). A lower dose of the rapid-onset drug is required to achieve the same buzz.

Typically a 10 mg (blue) diazepam tablet, which costs the NHS around 2.4 pence, will retail on the street for £1, with the 5 mg (yellow) and 2 mg (white) tablets costing proportionally less. Benzodiazepines bought on the Internet and imported from abroad are generally cheaper, as there is less certainty that what is ordered is the same as what is received. Importation of unlicensed benzodiazepines is an increasingly common practice in the UK, especially etizolam (half-life, 3.5 hours, with active metabolite alpha-hydroxyetizolam, 8.2 hours, but may be 7–17 hours depending on the rate of metabolism), delorazepam (60–140 hours), diclazepam (42 hours), phenazepam (6–18 hours, with active metabolite, 60 hours), flubromazolam (10–20 hours), flubromazepam (106 hours) and pyrazolam (16–18 hours).

Dependence

The dependence syndrome is characterised by the presence of three or more features as described in ICD-10. These comprise four psychological features and two biological features

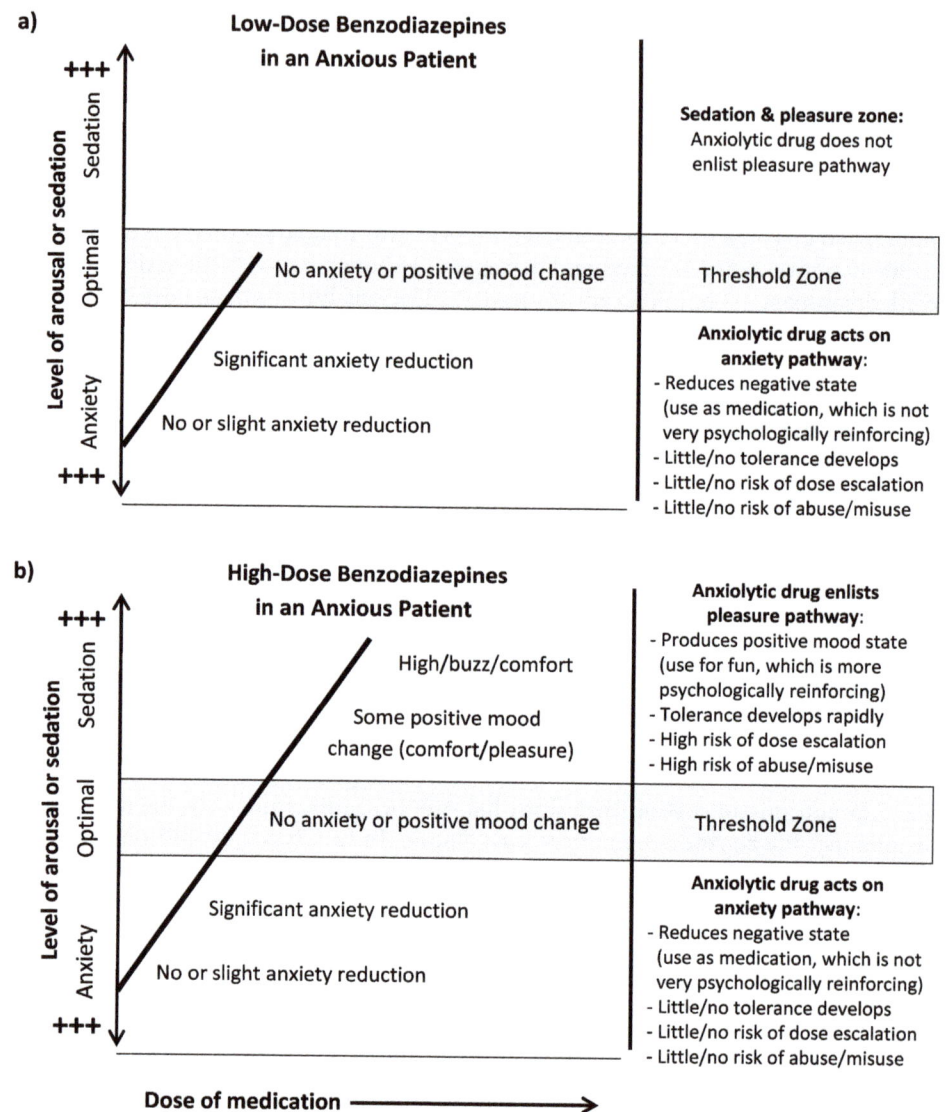

Figure 4.2 Model of tolerance development for anxiolytic drugs including benzodiazepines and antidepressants. Fig 2a: Low dose benzodiazepines in an anxious patient. Fig 2b: High dose benzodiazepines in an anxious patient. Fig 2c: Low or high dose benzodiazepines in a non-anxious patient. Fig 2d: Antidepressants in an anxious patient, e.g. SSRIs, SNRI or TCA.

(tolerance and withdrawal). This means that someone can meet the criteria for the dependence syndrome without physical dependence or evidence of tolerance being present, indicating that dependence is primarily a psychological state. The treatment of dependence is therefore primarily psychological, with medications being used when necessary as an adjunct to psychological treatment. Neither the ICD-10 nor DSM-5 dependence criteria make any mention of the frequency, amount or duration of benzodiazepine use. These factors should therefore not be used to determine whether dependence is present, and

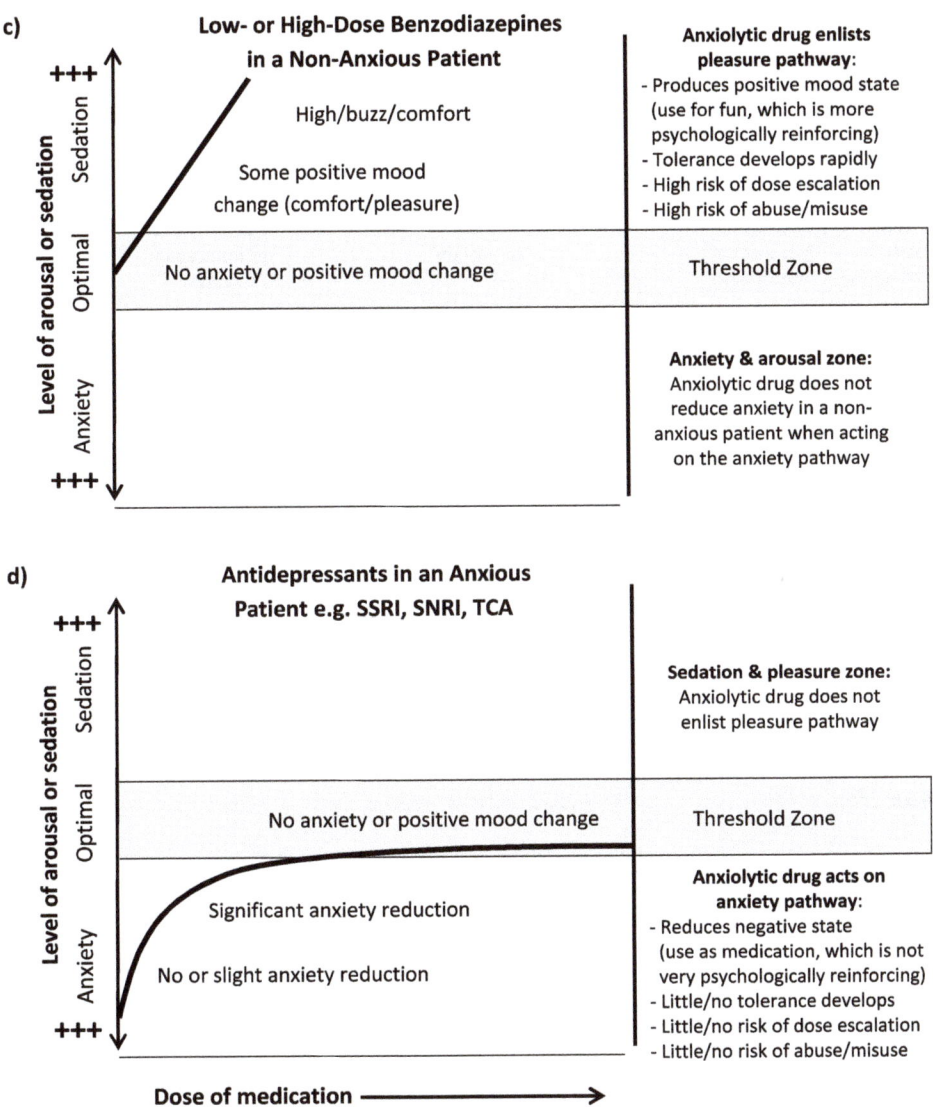

Figure 4.2 (cont.)

instead the criteria specified for the dependence syndrome should be sought. A multidimensional self-report measure of the presence and severity of benzodiazepine dependence (Bendep-SRQ) exists [15].

Dependence on benzodiazepines develops slowly, with one large population study finding that only 15 per cent had developed dependence within six months of regular use, increasing to about 40 per cent after one year, 50 per cent after two years, 60 per cent after three years and 70 per cent after four years of use [1]. People using higher doses for longer

	Rapid Onset	Intermediate Onset	Slow Onset
Ultra short half-life (< 8 hours)	Midazolam Zopiclone[s] Zolpidem[s]		
Short half-life (8-24 hours)	Flunitrazepam[s] Temazepam[s] (oral solution or caplets)	Lormetazepam[s] Lorazepam[a,s] Temazepam[s] (tablets)	Oxazepam[a] Loprazolam[s]
Long half-life (≥ 24 hours)	Diazepam[a,s] Nitrazepam[s] Flurazepam[s]	Alprazolam[a]	Chlordiazepoxide[a] Clonazepam[e] Clobazam[a,e]

Fig 4.3a Classification of benzodiazepines licensed in the UK by speed of onset and elimination half-life (licenced indications: a=anxiolytic, e=antiepileptic, s=hypnotic for sleep)

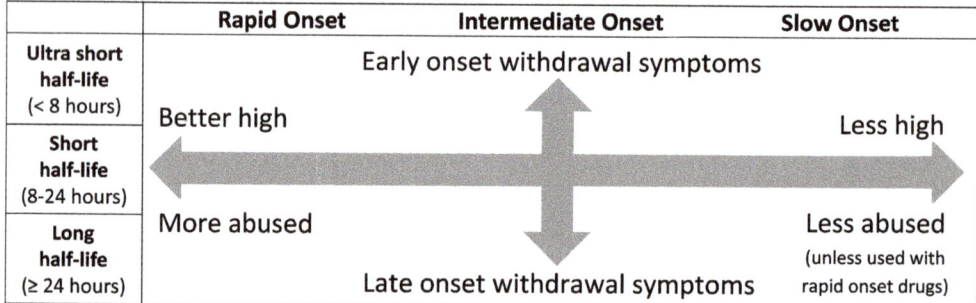

Fig 4.3b Effect of speed of onset and elimination half-life on abuse potential and onset of withdrawal symptoms.

	Note: Limited data exists for most of these drugs. Half-life estimated from published data or reported duration of action. Those in bold have been associated with deaths in the UK
Ultra short half-life (< 8 hours)	Adinazolam, Bentazepam (thiadipone, tiadipone), Brotizolam, Eszopiclone, Fluclotizolam, Flunitrazolam, Flutazolam, Tofisopam, Triazolam, Zaleplon
Short half-life (8-24 hours)	Bromazepam, Bromazolam, Camazepam, Cinazepam, Clonazolam, Cloniprazepam, Clotiazepam, Deschloroetizolam (Etizolam-2), Estazolam, **Etizolam, Flubromazolam,** Fludiazepam, **Flualprazolam,** Flunitrazepam, Halazepam (paxipam), 3-Hydroxyphenazepam, Lormetazepam, Meclonazepam (3-methylclonazepam), Metizolam (desmethyletizolam), Nifoxipam, Nimetazepam, Nitemazepam, Nitrazolam, Pinazepam, **Pyrazolam,** Tetrazepam
Long half-life (≥ 24 hours)	Chlorazepate, Cloxazolam, **Delorazepam, Diclazepam, Flubromazepam,** Gidazepam, Haloxazolam, Ketazolam, Medazepam, Nordiazepam (Desmethyldiazepam, nordazepam, desoxydemoxepam), Norfludiazepam (Norflurazepam, desalkylflurazepam), Oxazolam, **Phenazepam,** Prazepam
Unknown half-life or duration of effects	Alprazolam triazolobenzophenone derivatives, Clobromazolam (Phenazolam), 4'-Chlorodiazepam (Ro 5-4864), Difludiazepam, Fonazepam, Ro 7-4065, Thionordazepam (Thionordiazepam)

Fig 4.3c Classification of imported and designer benzodiazepines by estimated elimination half-life, including the active metabolites (ACMD reports on Novel Benzodiazepines (2000) and Designer Benzodiazepines (2016), BNF, Wikipedia, Tripsit, Erowid) (Limited data exists for most drugs. Half-life estimated from published data or reported duration of action. Those in bold have been associated with deaths in the UK.)

Figure 4.3 Factors affecting misuse and abuse of prescribed and imported benzodiazepines

periods of time are more likely to develop dependence. The observation that nearly 30 per cent of people did not develop dependence even after four years of use, strongly suggests that dependence is not inevitable, and that it may be related to the interaction of the drug with the person's psychology and how the drug is used. One hypothesis is that when the benzodiazepine is used as a coping strategy a stronger psychological conditioning to the drug develops, whereas people who use it just as 'a medicine', independent of their mental state or circumstance may avoid such conditioning, and therefore not develop the dependence syndrome. Benzodiazepine dependence is much more likely to develop in those with a history of alcohol and other sedative-hypnotic dependence. Benzodiazepine liking has been found to be higher in moderate social drinkers (consuming an average of 12 units of alcohol/week), compared to minimal drinkers (4 units or fewer/week) [16]. An alternative hypothesis is therefore that alcohol leads to a change in the subunit structure of the GABA-A receptor, thus leading to increased liking of benzodiazepines and therefore an increased risk of dependence. Both these factors are likely to be operating together.

Clinical Assessment and Treatment

Assessment

Following comprehensive assessment, there are three phases of treatment with clear goals at each stage: stabilisation, withdrawal and aftercare. The assessment process for benzodiazepines is similar to that for Z-drugs and gabapentinoids and is described in Box 4.2.

Box 4.2 A summary of the comprehensive process to follow in assessing benzodiazepine, Z-drug or gabapentinoid use disorder

Assessment

Addiction is a complex problem with biological, psychological and social components. Assessment of a patient who desires treatment or wishes to reduce their drug use should be comprehensive and include the following:

- Primary diagnosis: *many users of benzodiazepines will be using another drug as their primary drug of choice or have another psychiatric disorder.*

- Current use of substances: *including methadone, buprenorphine, heroin, crack, cocaine, benzodiazepines, gabapentinoids, other sedatives and anxiolytics, stimulants, nicotine, cannabis and hallucinogens. For each substance note the rationale and underlying motivation for use, the amount used, whether prescribed or obtained illicitly, the route of administration, frequency of use and when last used. A history of early repeat prescription requests, reporting lost prescriptions, over-utilisation of emergency and out of hours services, or requesting different members of staff suggest potential misuse. This information will allow contextualisation of the drug use and stratification of risk.*

- Alcohol history: *including current and historic use, withdrawal symptoms or seizures.*

- Injecting status: *current or previous intravenous drug use, blood borne virus status if known, any complications such as venous thromboembolism, abscess, etc.*

- Previous experience of withdrawal, treatment and abstinence.

- Support services involved.
- Psychiatric history: *including any formal diagnoses, current symptoms and past psychiatric history, contact with mental health services, screening for any symptoms of anxiety or depression and any history of suicide attempts or deliberate self-harm.*
- Medical history: *including any prescribed medication and allergies.*
- Family history: *including who they live with, any childcare concerns, any social work involvement, family history of substance misuse.*
- Social history: *living arrangements, employment, relationships. In women of childbearing age ask about pregnancy and offer a pregnancy test.*

Examination
Clinical examination may yield useful information about general health, well-being and self-care, as well as identifying any physical effects of drug dependence and injecting drug use.

Investigations
A urine drug test is useful to confirm recent benzodiazepine use and to screen for any other substance use, but cannot in itself indicate dependence. However, a benzodiazepine negative urine sample in the last three months suggests that the patient is unlikely to be dependent. In this situation, consider if there is any possibility it may not be their urine, or if they may be using the more potent benzodiazepines that are not detected on point-of-care (instant) urine tests. There are specific point-of-care tests for the Z-drugs, and for pregabalin (which also tests positive for gabapentin), but they are not widely used.

The urine test remains positive for benzodiazepines for two to four days after short-term use, and up to four to six weeks after long-term use, as it slowly leaches out of the fatty tissues of the body. Standard immunological point-of-care tests will typically identify diazepam, chlordiazepoxide, temazepam, oxazepam and nitrazepam. Zopiclone may also result in a positive urine benzodiazepine test if concentrations in the urine are sufficiently high. The more potent benzodiazepines clonazepam, lorazepam and alprazolam will not test positive on point-of-care tests unless present in high concentrations in the urine. The standard tests do not distinguish subtypes of benzodiazepines, and in the rare instances where substitute benzodiazepine prescribing occurs, point-of-care tests are not helpful in distinguishing prescribed from illicit use. More specific laboratory testing to subtype the benzodiazepines will be beneficial in this context.

Stabilisation and Substitute Prescribing
There is little evidence to support maintenance prescribing of benzodiazepines in illicit drug users, although it may reduce illicit benzodiazepine use in some patients [17]. This is summarised in the UK Orange Guidelines [18]:

> Many drug misusers misuse benzodiazepines, but the majority do not require long-term replacement prescribing or high doses ... To prevent symptoms of benzodiazepine withdrawal, the clinician should continue a current prescription but the dose should be gradually reduced to zero. Only very rarely should doses of more than 30 mg diazepam equivalent per day be prescribed ... While most patients in receipt of structured drug treatment will either not require benzodiazepine replacement, or will be provided with a time-limited detoxification programme, there will be exceptional cases ... Any such longer-term

prescribing of benzodiazepines should adhere to general principles of management of dependence (including identifying clear indications of benzodiazepine dependence, clear intermediate treatment goals and milestones, regular review of the approach and use of methods to prevent diversion).

Services providing psychological interventions may exclude benzodiazepine users from treatment, fearing that patients will fail to engage emotionally to a sufficient degree. Benzodiazepines may reduce emotional engagement in some users, but in others may have a beneficial effect on the outcome of psychological interventions if the medication acts to reduce anxiety to a level where the patient is better able to engage with therapy. Rules excluding all benzodiazepine users from psychological treatment are not justified.

Where the dependence syndrome on opiates and benzodiazepines coexists, the initial focus should be the evidence-based intervention, namely opioid agonist treatment with methadone or buprenorphine. The combination of benzodiazepine and buprenorphine is less likely to cause overdose than the same combination with methadone. Drug and psychosocial treatment for opioid dependence should be optimised before considering a prescription for benzodiazepines. Often the need for a benzodiazepine prescription disappears following adequate treatment of opioid dependence, suggesting that benzodiazepines were being used to manage emotional issues without true psychological dependence. Where the benzodiazepine dependence syndrome persists despite optimised opioid treatment, short-term stabilisation with benzodiazepines followed by gradual withdrawal is the standard treatment.

Benzodiazepines used in combination with opioids may cause QT interval prolongation on the ECG. Diazepam alone does not prolong the QT interval, and buprenorphine also has little effect, but the combination of diazepam and methadone can have a significant effect. Methadone has a combination of effects, prolonging the QT interval by blocking the hERG potassium channel while exerting a simultaneous protective effect by blocking sodium and calcium channels. However, when diazepam and methadone are combined the protective effect of sodium channel blocking may be lost, especially at higher diazepam doses [19]. This means there is an increased risk of cardiac arrhythmia (torsade de pointes), especially if the QT interval is already prolonged. Torsade de pointes may degenerate into sustained ventricular tachycardia and ventricular fibrillation, which is a life terminating arrhythmia.

Detoxification and Withdrawal

A well-characterised benzodiazepine withdrawal syndrome occurs in patients who are physically dependent on benzodiazepines and either stop or reduce the dose. A range of physical and psychological symptoms occur, attributed to increased glutamate excitatory activity in the brain. If a patient has benzodiazepine withdrawal symptoms, it is useful to distinguish three types of benzodiazepine withdrawal symptoms: anxiety symptoms, distorted perceptions and major incidents such as seizures, delirium or psychosis (which can occur in someone physically dependent and stopping high doses abruptly). Anxiety symptoms could be due to a recurrence of the anxiety that was being treated with the benzodiazepine, but distorted perceptions such as hypersensitivity to stimuli and abnormal body sensations are much more characteristic of benzodiazepine withdrawal. Look in particular for objective evidence of benzodiazepine withdrawal, such as anxiety signs, tachycardia, hypersensitivity to light, etc. Each case must be assessed individually, and detailed guidance for patients on how to withdraw is available [20]. Several measures of benzodiazepine withdrawal exist e.g. [33–36], although it is unclear which is best.

The Orange Guidelines

The guidelines [18] state:

> The rate of withdrawal is often determined by an individual's capacity to tolerate symptoms … While full detoxification can proceed without difficulty within weeks or within 2–3 months for some patients, NICE expert review has noted that withdrawal may take 3 months to a year or longer in some cases … Good assessment and care planning – and adherence to local protocols – are prerequisites for considering prescribing benzodiazepines.

When physical withdrawal symptoms from benzodiazepines are problematic, the use of smaller increments or a benzodiazepine with a longer elimination half-life (e.g. diazepam) may be beneficial. When other difficulties in reducing the benzodiazepine occur, switching to a slower-onset benzodiazepine (e.g. oxazepam, chlordiazepoxide) is often beneficial. The rapid-onset reinforcing effects of benzodiazepines lead to psychological conditioning, which can make it difficult to reduce the dose even if the patient is keen to do so. Switching to a slow-onset benzodiazepine can have the benefit of bypassing this issue. Although the slower-onset drugs will be equally effective at preventing benzodiazepine withdrawal symptoms, a period of adaptation to the less reinforcing medication may be useful, before slowly reducing it. Equivalent doses to 5 mg diazepam are 15 mg chlordiazepoxide and 15 mg oxazepam.

Treatment recommendations for those with mild or early dependence include advice, providing information and involving the General Practitioner (GP). For those with established dependence, a gradual dose reduction is suggested. There is little evidence that routinely switching from a short half-life benzodiazepine to a long half-life benzodiazepine is of benefit; however, this should be assessed on an individual basis for those experiencing significant withdrawal symptoms [17]. Some patients describe severe withdrawal symptoms from stopping the last milligram or two of the benzodiazepine, and one hypothesis is that this is due to inadequate endogenous benzodiazepines or related to the protracted withdrawal syndrome.

High dose illicit benzodiazepine users will need more active treatment, including the requirement for urine drug screens to monitor for use of other drugs, and being alert to the risks of polydrug use and overdose (particularly in those dependent on alcohol or opioids). Seizures may occur if high doses of benzodiazepines are stopped abruptly, but only if the patient is physically dependent on the benzodiazepine. Patients stopping or running out of high doses of benzodiazepines obtained illicitly may claim to experience seizures if they run out, and demand equivalent prescribed doses. Where possible, corroborative evidence for seizures should be sought, and other possible explanations explored, including stimulant and tramadol misuse, stopping gabapentinoids or baclofen abruptly, as well as alcohol, benzodiazepine and barbiturate withdrawal. Doses greater than 30 mg diazepam are rarely necessary, as 30 mg is sufficient to prevent most withdrawal effects and seizures even in very high dose users [17]. Doses of up to 60 mg may very rarely be used short term to engage the patient in treatment, with the goal of rapidly reducing the dose down to 30 mg daily over a few weeks. Doing a two-stage detox may be useful for high dose users, by reducing initially to a therapeutic dose level (e.g. 30 mg diazepam daily), and stabilising at this level before reducing further [17].

If the patient is using different amounts each day or bingeing, then the level of supervision of the medication may need to be increased. This can be achieved by increasing the frequency of medication pickup, and an FP10MDA prescription can be used to ensure collection from the pharmacy on a daily basis. Alternatively, relatives or pharmacists may be willing to provide additional support and supervision of the medication consumption.

Success rates for treatment vary with both the severity of dependence and the context of treatment. Among primary care patients, routine care has a 5–10 per cent chance of successful withdrawal, with the addition of a structured brief intervention increasing the rate of success by 15 per cent to 20–25 per cent [17]. For those receiving secondary care input, 15–20 per cent withdraw successfully with routine care only, and an additional 20–35 per cent are able to withdraw with a gradual reduction regimen. The efficacy of gradual reduction can be enhanced with additional psychological therapies, particularly in individuals with panic disorder and insomnia [17]. The use of additional medication to support gradual withdrawal (e.g. antidepressants, melatonin, valproate or flumazenil) does not increase the effectiveness of gradual dose reduction, but can be considered on an individual basis.

Aftercare and the Maintenance of Abstinence

A patient with benzodiazepine dependence will have a high risk of relapse, and so will need aftercare. If the patient has only been physically dependent (i.e. without meeting criteria for the dependence syndrome) the rate of relapse will be low. Where the dependence syndrome has been present, psychosocial interventions should be continued to help the patient adapt to a drug-free life and develop relapse prevention strategies. The patient should also be monitored for the development of psychiatric problems, as there is a significant risk of developing an anxiety or depressive disorder during high stress periods such as the first few months and years of abstinence.

Protracted withdrawal symptoms from benzodiazepines may occur, especially if high doses have been used and if there are comorbid issues. This is thought to be caused by persisting drug-induced receptor changes, psychological factors and possibly structural neuronal damage. Symptoms typically last six months to one year before gradually improving, but may persist for years. Longer-lasting symptoms occur in a minority of patients, and there are typically a multitude of symptoms affecting many organ systems. Common protected symptoms include anxiety, depression, tinnitus, paraesthesia, muscle jerking and irritable bowel. Reduced concentration, memory, energy, insomnia, metallic taste, blurred vision, eye soreness, light/touch/noise sensitivity, derealisation, cramps, pins and needles, severe pains and many other neurological symptoms may also occur. One way of understanding this is that benzodiazepines act on GABA-A, the main inhibitory neurotransmitter system of the brain. When the dose is reduced, this inhibition is reduced, and all the organ systems (including the brain) can become overstimulated. These patients may feel generally unwell but have normal test results. A central issue for patients is that professionals typically do not understand what they are going through, why they have such difficulty describing their bewildering array of symptoms and how they could possibly be having symptoms in so many organ systems simultaneously. Patients often feel unheard, misunderstood and marginalised, rejected or abandoned, when they need understanding, support, encouragement and reassurance. A model to overcome these issues and to facilitate communication between patients and clinicians has been developed (Figure 4.4).

	The Benzodiazepine Dose is Reduced	Overactivity in the Brain and Body Occurs	A Sense of Bewilderment Occurs	Fear Feeds Fear in a Vicious Cycle	Feelings of Depression Occur
The Patient's Experience of Benzodiazepine Withdrawal:	• Benzodiazepines act on the GABA-A system of the brain, which is the main inhibitory brain system. • When the dose is reduced, the brain can get over-activated.	• Psychological effects– over activity of the brain and all organ systems occur. • Psychological effects – over activity of thinking and emotions occur.	• Lack of understanding of what is going on - why you feel so ill. • Feeling lost/alone, that there is no way out. • Bewilderment breeds fear and low confidence.	• It feels like no one understands you, that you will never get better, and you are "going mad". • Becoming obsessed with "how I am today?" & "will I ever recover?"	• Emotional exhaustion. • Poor concentration, can't think clearly, can't listen or absorb advice. • Symptom levels fluctuate from hour to hour and day to day.
Helpful Analogies to Relate to the Patient:	**Taking "Your Foot Off the Brake"** Reducing the benzodiazepine dose is like taking your foot off the brake of a car, where the accelerator is being pushed at the same time. Your brain is like an engine that is constantly being "over-revved".	**Brain Becomes "Over-Revved"** Your brain speeds up, and you feel out of control. All your nerves become "sensitised", so you over-react to anxiety provoking things. You feel ill but are not ill, as you are suffering from benzodiazepine withdrawal.	**Stuck in the Mud or in a Pit** Your wheels are spinning helplessly in the mud which threatens to engulf you, or in a deep pit with no way out. Stay calm and trample down anything bad thrown at you, so it builds up until there is enough for you to climb out of the pit.	**The Taut Rubber Belt or Elastic Band** You have become stretched like an elastic band, and feel ready to snap. You experience "tightness" in your nerves and a feeling of unease. This over-stretching is due to the withdrawal and so can take a long time to return to normal.	**The Dark Tunnel or Fog** Your brain feels so tired, depleted, emotionally wrecked and exhausted. You feel like you're in a dark tunnel and your mind has become like a fog where thinking is like wading through treacle or thick mud.
Useful Advice for Coping with these Issues:	**Reduce the Dose More Slowly** If your engine tends to "over-rev", you need to feather the brakes, taking your foot off the brake more gradually. Reduce the dose slower, to avoid a surge of acceleration. Aim for a more achievable target to help confidence e.g. 50% dose reduction.	**"Go with the Flow, Float, Don't Fight"** You feel bad and ill, but this is due to benzodiazepine withdrawal, and it will pass. Be like a reed in the wind, an oak tree in a storm, or a palm tree in a hurricane – accept that the bad weather is there for a time but will pass. "Relax into the anxiety".	**Share Your Symptoms and Empower Yourself** Find someone who will listen, understand your symptoms, and support you (e.g. PostScript 360). Share your experiences. Accept that they are normal during withdrawal. Seek out information that helps you and your symptoms to empower yourself.	**Aim to Disrupt or Break the Fear Cycle** Expect to feel fearful. Try not to over-react to fears/triggers. Practice relaxation regularly to "desensitise", e.g. breathe out for twice as long as you breathe in. Face the fear when able, to empower yourself - even provoking it to regain a sense of control.	**Accept that Recovery is Erratic but Gradual** Recovery is a marathon, never a sprint, so plan for this. Levels of symptoms fluctuate, so it is normal for progress to be erratic. Function "as though" you don't care about the symptoms. The light at the end of the tunnel will gradually get brighter.

Figure 4.4 A language for clinicians to assist them in relating to the patient's experience of protracted benzodiazepine withdrawal (developed in conjunction with Don Macpherson)

Z-Drugs

Zopiclone and zolpidem are non-benzodiazepine hypnotics, often referred to as 'Z-drugs'. The Z-drugs, like benzodiazepines, are agonists at the GABA-A receptor, although they are thought to be more selective with higher affinity for the alpha-1 binding site. They are licensed for short-term use of up to four weeks in the management of insomnia, when non-drug measures have failed [22]. Z-drugs and indeed all licensed hypnotics reduce time to fall asleep and improve self-reported sleep quality [22]. Benzodiazepines suppress rapid eye movement sleep and reduce deep sleep, but Z drugs have much less impact on sleep architecture especially at lower therapeutic doses.

Z-drugs have shorter half-lives than any oral benzodiazepine, resulting in less hangover, daytime sedation and a reduced propensity to accumulate, making them safer in the elderly and those with renal or hepatic impairment. Crucially, although they can be misused and be addictive, Z-drugs are thought to create less physical and psychological dependence and are less subject to misuse than benzodiazepines. Patients taking the Z-drugs describe a different type of subjective effect to the benzodiazepines, with a rapid sleep-inducing ('knockout') effect, without much buzz, rush or high, and generally without the desirable 'dopey' feelings or sedation on drug onset. There is also little hangover on waking in the morning, with patients often describing awaking fully alert – which is considered to be a rather unpleasant effect by many drug using patients.

There have been case reports of withdrawal symptoms on abrupt termination of high dose usage of zolpidem and with both high and low doses of zopiclone. Withdrawal symptoms typically do not occur or are very mild in clinical studies even after several months of use at a therapeutic dose, and indeed tolerance may not develop to hypnotics such as eszopiclone or zolpidem even after a year of use [22]. Benzodiazepines such as diazepam are commonly abused at one to three times the therapeutic dose, and sometimes at much higher dose levels. Z-drugs rarely give a high, buzz or euphoria at therapeutic dose levels, and the small proportion of patients who abused them did so on average at 40 times the therapeutic dose level for zolpidem and at several times the therapeutic dose level for zopiclone.

Gabapentinoids

Introduction

The gabapentinoids, pregabalin and gabapentin, are used in a number of specialties for a variety of clinical indications. Initially marketed as antiepileptic drugs, they are now licensed for use in neuropathic pain and generalised anxiety disorder. As these drugs have become prescribed more frequently, their potential for misuse has become increasingly apparent. Gabapentinoids are Class C drugs, which were reclassified under Schedule 3 in April 2019, because of concern about their misuse.

Epidemiology

Despite growing concerns about misuse potential, pregabalin prescribing has risen by 150 per cent and gabapentin prescribing by 130 per cent during the five-year period from 2015–19, to 7.4 million and 7.3 million prescriptions respectively in 2019 in England [8, 9]. Recent reports suggest that the number of people administering high doses of gabapentinoids in pursuit of euphoric effects continues to increase, with a corresponding increase observed in the number of documented adverse effects including death [16]. In 2011, there were already more than 5 million prescriptions for gabapentin and pregabalin issued annually even before many overdoses involving gabapentinoids occurred (Figure 4.5). In April 2019, following advice from the Advisory Council for the Misuse of Drugs, the UK Government reclassified both pregabalin and gabapentin as Class C drugs under the Misuse of Drugs Act 1971. Pregabalin has been classified in the USA as a Schedule-V controlled substance since its release in 2005, but gabapentin remains a non-schedule medication in most states.

Risk factors found to predispose to dependent use of gabapentinoids include male sex, young age and current or previous substance misuse disorders [24]. Gabapentinoids are often used to potentiate the effects of opiates, alcohol and other sedative-hypnotics. Opiate users are at a particularly high risk of developing gabapentinoid misuse, with prevalence ranging from 3 per cent to 68 per cent in this group, compared with 1.6 per cent in the general population [23]. Gabapentinoids are widely misused in prison populations, which can present prescribing dilemmas, particularly in individuals reporting chronic neuropathic pain.

Clinical Indications

Epilepsy

The gabapentinoids were initially developed for the treatment of epilepsy. In this context, their main use is as adjunctive therapy for focal seizures, with or without secondary generalisation.

Neuropathic Pain

In the UK, NICE recommends gabapentin and pregabalin as first-line agents for the treatment of neuropathic pain, including painful diabetic neuropathy [25]. Amitriptyline (off-label) and duloxetine are also considered first-line treatment options. All four drugs were found to be consistently superior to placebo in reducing neuropathic pain, and considered safe and cost-effective. There is evidence that a small number of patients benefit very significantly from treatment with gabapentinoids, and a larger number will experience a moderate improvement in symptoms, although up to 60 per cent will experience some adverse effects as a result of their treatment. There is no evidence to support the use of gabapentinoids in the management of acute pain, or pain that isn't neuropathic [25].

Generalised Anxiety Disorder (GAD)

Pregabalin has been licensed in the EU for use in the treatment of GAD since 2006. Onset of anxiolytic action is faster than with other classes of drugs, such as SSRIs, with most patients achieving significant reduction in symptoms by day seven of treatment. Those who do not show any response at two weeks are likely to require either an increase in dose or an alternative medication [26].

Other Uses

There are a number of off-label indications for which pregabalin and gabapentin may be prescribed, such as migraine prophylaxis and the treatment of menopausal symptoms in women with breast cancer. In the USA and Canada, gabapentinoids are licensed for the management of fibromyalgia.

Illicit Use: Desired Effects

Euphoria, increased sociability and dissociative effects are commonly reported with both gabapentinoids, with sedative/opiate-type and psychedelic or MDMA-like effects less common [27]. Traditionally, drugs of misuse and their subjective effects have been classified into four types (depressants, stimulants, analgesics, hallucinogens), and this works well for most drugs. However, the gabapentinoids have several types of subjective effects, and The Drug Wheel by Mark Adley has expanded on the traditional classification to include seven types of drugs of misuse and their subjective drug effects (www .thedrugswheel.com). While the benzodiazepines are classified as pure depressants, the gabapentinoids fall into at least four of the seven categories as depressants, empathogens, dissociatives and analgesics.

Euphoria has been reported as a side effect of pregabalin even at therapeutic doses, although tolerance develops quickly to this effect. Those who misuse gabapentinoids often do so with other substances, including alcohol, cannabis, GHB and opiates [27, 28]. They are also used to self-medicate opiate withdrawal, and to manage insomnia associated with problematic alcohol and benzodiazepine use. When taken recreationally, doses may be up to 20 times in excess of the recommended daily maximum. The commonest route of administration is by mouth; however, reports also exist of intranasal, intramuscular, rectal and intravenous administration [27].

Pregabalin has a greater abuse potential than gabapentin, as it has a greater affinity for the $\alpha2$-δ subunit of voltage-activated calcium channels and is much more rapidly absorbed with higher bioavailability. This may explain why pregabalin ('pregabs') is more commonly associated with euphoria, why is it anecdotally perceived as more powerful among drug users and why it is associated with a higher level of overdose deaths despite a similar level of prescribing [27].

Mechanism of Action

Despite being structural analogues of the endogenous neurotransmitter GABA, neither pregabalin nor gabapentin bind to GABA receptors. In contrast to benzodiazepines, which increase the effect of the inhibitory neurotransmitter GABA, the gabapentinoids act to decrease central neuronal excitability. They exert this effect by binding to $\alpha2$-δ protein subunits of voltage-activated calcium channels on the neuronal membrane. The action of binding to the calcium channels of hyperexcited neurons leads to a reduction in the release of excitatory neurotransmitters, including glutamate, noradrenaline and substance P. It has been suggested that these drugs may have GABA-mimetic properties. In common with a number of other substances of misuse, the gabapentinoids may also have effects on the dopaminergic reward system.

Pharmacokinetics

Although gabapentin and pregabalin have similar mechanisms of action, important differences exist between their pharmacokinetic profiles. Gabapentin is typically absorbed slowly following oral administration, with peak plasma concentrations occurring at three to four hours post dose [29]. When taken orally, gabapentin has non-linear zero-order kinetics, whereby the rate of elimination is constant and independent of the total plasma concentration of the drug. Crucially, this elimination mechanism is saturable and results in the pharmacokinetics of gabapentin being somewhat less predictable. Furthermore, the plasma concentration of gabapentin does not increase proportionately with increased doses.

Pregabalin is much more rapidly absorbed following oral administration, with peak plasma concentrations occurring around one hour post dose, with steady state concentrations being achieved within 24–48 hours of regular dosing. For gabapentin the absolute bioavailability reduces from 60 per cent to 33 per cent with increased dosage (from 900 mg to 3,600 mg per day), but for pregabalin the absolute bioavailability remains consistently at 90 per cent and above, at any given dosage [29].

Gabapentinoids have a relatively short elimination half-life of around six hours, and both gabapentin and pregabalin are renally excreted, with 90–98 per cent of pregabalin eliminated unchanged in the urine. Renal clearance is directly related to creatinine clearance in patients not on dialysis. Neither gabapentin nor pregabalin undergo hepatic metabolism. Importantly, they do not induce or inhibit hepatic enzymes involved in the metabolism of other drugs and as a result have relatively few drug interactions.

Drug Interactions, Overdose and Adverse Effects

Drug Interactions

The gabapentinoids undergo minimal metabolism and are excreted largely unchanged in the urine. As a result, they are unlikely to have many true pharmacokinetic drug interactions. The key interaction to be aware of is the potential synergistic effect when taken with other CNS depressant medications. This includes alcohol, antidepressants, antihistamines, hypnotics, opiates and skeletal muscle relaxants such as baclofen. The risk is of additive CNS depression, leading to sedation and potentially respiratory depression and death.

Misuse of non-prescribed gabapentinoids is a particularly important consideration in the prison setting and in the context of detoxification or maintenance prescribing. Reports exist of people using gabapentinoids to potentiate the effects of heroin, methadone and buprenorphine [29].

Overdose

Symptoms experienced in an isolated gabapentinoid overdose may include drowsiness, dizziness, nausea, confusion, agitation, restlessness, tachycardia and hypotension, although a significant proportion of patients are likely to remain asymptomatic. There is one reported fatality as a consequence of intentional gabapentin overdose as a sole substance, associated with post-mortem blood gabapentin concentration of 88 μg/mL. There have been no reports of death as a result of isolated pregabalin overdose. By contrast, gabapentinoid overdose in combination with other CNS depressants is highly dangerous and may result in drowsiness, respiratory depression, coma and death. Treatment for overdose consists of general supportive measures, and may include haemodialysis if necessary. There is evidence that most people who die from gabapentinoid overdose have used them in combination with opiates, and there is convincing animal evidence that gabapentinoids reverse any tolerance that has developed to opiates [30].

Adverse Effects

Gabapentinoids are generally well tolerated. The commonest adverse effects are somnolence and ataxia, which typically resolve within the first few weeks of treatment. Pregabalin may be

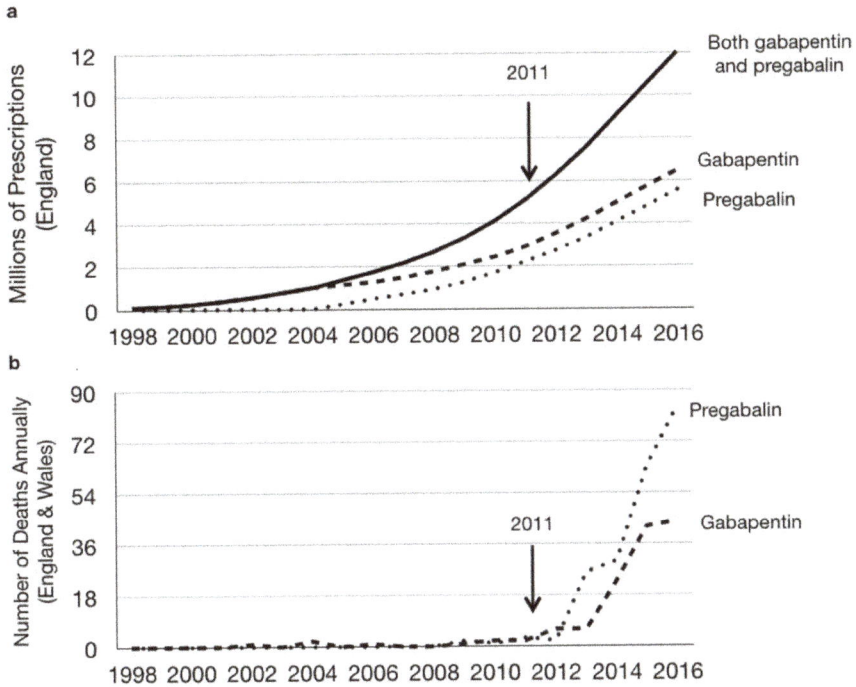

Figure 4.5 Overdoses on gabapentin and pregabalin (Fig 5a) and prescriptions (Fig 5b) in England 1998–2019, showing minimal overdoses until 2011 when there were already more than 5 million prescriptions for gabapentinoids annually, and that pregabalin overdoses occur twice as often as gabapentin overdoses, despite a similar number of prescriptions (Sources: Deaths related to drug poisoning in England and Wales, 2019. ONS, 2020; Prescription cost analysis – England 2019, NHS BSA, 2020, open government licence v3.0)

associated with peripheral oedema, dry mouth, weight gain, blurred vision and altered cognition and concentration. Although a rare side effect, both pregabalin and gabapentin are associated with an increased risk of suicidal thoughts and suicidal behaviour, irrespective of indication. The longer-term effects of gabapentinoid use are yet to be fully elucidated, as the drugs are still relatively new, but may include effects on spermatogenesis and fertility in males.

Tolerance, Misuse and Dependence

The potential to develop tolerance and dependence with the gabapentinoids, particularly in the context of recreational use, is increasingly recognised. Tolerance to gabapentinoids develops quickly with regular use and as a result, users may need to escalate their dose to achieve ongoing effects. This behaviour is more commonly observed in those with a history of recreational substance misuse. Risk of euphoric and dissociative effects, as well as misuse or dependence, are typically much more common with higher doses [27].

While the gabapentinoids are most certainly misused, whether a true dependence syndrome develops is less clear. Other sedative medications are misused even when they are clearly not addictive – for example, sedative antipsychotics. The presence of physical withdrawal symptoms in some patients does not necessarily indicate the dependence syndrome, as is the case with the SSRI discontinuation syndrome which is related to the receptors having to adapt so rapidly. Psychological dependence may also develop in patients with difficulty coping when the medication that assists their coping is reduced or withdrawn. However, if the standard criteria for dependence syndrome are applied, a small proportion of patients will meet these criteria. Most will have comorbid psychiatric conditions and/or a previous history of alcohol, cocaine or opioid misuse [16, 23].

Detoxification and Withdrawal

Physical withdrawal symptoms occur in a small proportion of patients, and it is generally not advisable to abruptly discontinue gabapentinoid medication, with most guidelines advising a minimum taper period of seven days. Withdrawal symptoms may still occur, even with slow tapering of the drug. It is good clinical practice when initiating treatment to advise the patient of the possibility of withdrawal symptoms when it is reduced or stopped. It is now recognised that a level of physical dependence may develop, and occasionally a psychological dependence with continued use of these substances.

There is a low incidence of withdrawal symptoms even when long-term therapy is stopped [26, 29]. The onset of withdrawal symptoms correlates with the elimination half-life of the medication. The commonest withdrawal symptoms include insomnia, nausea, anxiety, diarrhoea, dizziness and nervousness. Occasionally, akathisia, catatonia and seizures occur.

Treatment of gabapentinoid misuse and dependence typically focuses on gradual dose reduction and psychological therapies. Some have suggested short courses of benzodiazepines to manage withdrawal. However, interestingly, in many cases benzodiazepines fail to resolve gabapentinoid withdrawal symptoms, with the only option being to wait for the symptoms to resolve on their own, or if the withdrawal is severe, to recommence the drug and to reduce more slowly with additional support.

Use of Gabapentinoids in the Treatment of Addiction

Studies have considered the potential utility of gabapentinoids in the treatment of other substance misuse disorders, including mitigation of the symptoms of alcohol withdrawal and supporting alcohol relapse prevention, with comparable efficacy to naltrexone [31]. Gabapentinoids may reduce withdrawal symptoms from cocaine, opiates, benzodiazepines, nicotine and cannabis, although it is unclear whether this is a specific or non-specific effect. There may be some utility in the management of behavioural addictions [32]. Research is still ongoing in this evolving area.

References

1 de las Cuevas C., Sanz E., de la Fuente J. Benzodiazepines: more 'behavioural' addiction than dependence. *Psychopharmacology*. 2003; **167** (3): 297–303.

2 Gossop M., Marsden J., Stewart D., Kidd T. The National Treatment Outcome Research Study (NTORS): 4–5 year follow-up results. *Addiction*. 2003; **98**: 291–303.

3 National Institute for Health and Care Excellence. Generalised anxiety disorder and panic disorder in adults: management (CG113). In: Clinical Guideline. NICE, 2011.

4 Baldwin D. S., Aitchison K., Bateson A., Curran H. V., Davies S., Leonard B. et al. Benzodiazepines: Risks and benefits – A reconsideration. *Journal of Psychopharmacology*. 2013; **27** (11): 967–71.

5   National Institute for Health and Care Excellence. Guidance on the use of zaleplon, zolpidem and zopiclone for the short-term management of insomnia: Technology appraisal guidance (TA77). In: Technology Appraisal. NICE, 2004.

6   Wilson S., Anderson K., Baldwin D., Dijk D.-J., Espie A., Espie C. et al. British Association for Psychopharmacology consensus statement on evidence-based treatment of insomnia, parasomnias and circadian rhythm disorders: An update. *Journal of Psychopharmacology*. 2019; **33** (8): 923–47.

7   Office for National Statistics. Deaths Related to Drug Poisoning in England and Wales, 2019. ONS, 2020.

8   National Records of Scotland. Drug-Related Deaths in Scotland in 2019. National Statistics for Scotland, 2020.

9   NHS Business Services Authority. Prescription Cost Analysis – England 2019. NHSBSA, 16 April 2020.

10 Cumming R. G., Le Couteur D. G. Benzodiazepines and risk of hip fractures in older people: A review of the evidence. *CNS Drugs*. 2003; **17** (11): 825–37.

11 Ford C., Law F. Guidance for the Use and Reduction of Misuse of Benzodiazepines and Other Hypnotics and Anxiolytics in General Practice. SMMGP, 2014.

12 Parsaik A. K., Mascarenhas S. S., Khosh-Chashm D., Hashmi A., John V., Okusaga O. et al. Mortality associated with anxiolytic and hypnotic drugs: A systematic review and meta-analysis. *Australian and New Zealand Journal of Psychiatry*. 2016; **50** (6): 520–33.

13 Zhang T., Yang X., Zhou J., Liu P., Wang H., Li A. et al. Benzodiazepine drug use and cancer risk: A dose–response meta-analysis of prospective cohort studies. *Oncotarget*. 2017; **8** (60): 381–91.

14 Iqbal M. M., Sobhan T., Ryals T. Effects of commonly used benzodiazepines on the fetus, the neonate, and the nursing infant. *Psychiatric Services*. 2002; **53** (1),39–49.

15 Kan C. C., Breteler M. H., van der Ven A. H., Timmermans M. A., Zitman F. G. Assessment of benzodiazepine dependence in alcohol and drug dependent outpatients: a research report. *Substance Use and Misuse*. 2001; **36** (8): 1085–109.

16 de Wit H., Doty P. Preference for ethanol and diazepam in light and moderate social drinkers: A within-subjects study. *Psychopharmacology* (Berl). 1994; **115**: 529–38.

17 Lingford-Hughes A. R., Welch S., Peters L., Nutt D. J., Ball D., Buntwal N. et al. BAP updated guidelines – Evidence-based guidelines for the pharmacological management of substance abuse, harmful use, addiction and comorbidity: recommendations from BAP. *Journal of Psychopharmacology*. 2012; **26** (7): 899–952.

18 Independent Expert Working Group. Clinical Guidelines on Drug Misuse and Dependence Update, 2017. Drug Misuse and Dependence: UK Guidelines on Clinical Management. Department of Health, 2017.

19 Kuryshev Y. A., Bruening-Wright A., Brown A. M., Kirsch G. E. Increased cardiac risk in concomitant methadone and diazepam treatment: Pharmacodynamic interactions in cardiac ion channels. *Journal of Cardiovascular Pharmacology*. 2010; **56** (4): 420–30.

20 Ashton C. H. *Benzodiazepines: How They Work and How to Withdraw*. Newcastle University Institute of Neuroscience, 2002.

21 Busto U. E., Sykora K., Sellers E. M. A clinical scale to assess benzodiazepine withdrawal. *Journal of Clinical Psychopharmacology*. 1989 **9** (6): 412–16.

22 Wilson S., Anderson K., Baldwin D., Dijk D.-J., Espie A., Espie C. et al. British Association for Psychopharmacology consensus statement on evidence-based treatment of insomnia, parasomnias and circadian rhythm disorders: An update. *Journal of Psychopharmacology*. 2019; **33** (8): 923–47.

23 Evoy K. E., Morrison M. D., Saklad S. R. Abuse and misuse of pregabalin and gabapentin. *Drugs*. 2017; **77** (4): 403–26.

24 Gahr M., Freudenmann R., Kölle M., Schönfeldt-Lecuona C. Pregabalin and addiction: Lessons from published cases. *Journal of Substance Use*. 2013; **19** (6): 448–9.

25 National Institute for Health and Care Excellence. Neuropathic Pain – Drug Treatment. 2020. [Available from: https://cks.nice.org.uk/topics/neuropathic-pain-drug-treatment/#!scenario.]

26 Baldwin D. S., den Boer J. A., Lyndon G., Emir B., Schweizer E., Haswell H. Efficacy and safety of pregabalin in generalised anxiety disorder: A critical review of the literature. *Journal of Psychopharmacology*. 2015; **29** (10): 1047–60.

27 Schifano F., D'Offizi S., Piccione M., Corazza O., Deluca P., Davey Z. et al. Is there a recreational misuse potential for pregabalin? Analysis of anecdotal online reports in comparison with related gabapentin and clonazepam data. *Psychotherapy and Psychosomatics*. 2011; **80** (2): 118–22.

28 Smith R. V., Havens J. R., Walsh S. L. Gabapentin misuse, abuse and diversion: A systematic review. *Addiction*. 2016; **111** (7): 1160–74.

29 Bockbrader H. N., Wesche D., Miller R., Chapel S., Janiczek N., Burger P. A comparison of the pharmacokinetics and pharmacodynamics of pregabalin and gabapentin. *Clinical Pharmacokinetics*. 2010; **49** (10): 661–9.

30 Lyndon A., Audrey S., Wells C., Burnell E. S., Ingle S., Hill R., Hickman M., Henderson G. Risk to heroin users of polydrug use of pregabalin or gabapentin. *Addiction*. 2017; **112** (9): 1580–9.

31 Freynhagen R., Backonja M., Schug S., Lyndon G., Parsons B., Watt S. et al. Pregabalin for the treatment of drug and alcohol withdrawal symptoms: A comprehensive review. *CNS Drugs*. 2016; **30** (12): 1191–200.

32 Olive M. F., Cleva R. M., Kalivas P. W., Malcolm R. J. Glutamatergic medications for the treatment of drug and behavioral addictions. *Pharmacology Biochemistry and Behavior*. 2012; **100** (4): 801–10.

33 Tyrer P, Murphy S, Riley P. The Benzodiazepine Withdrawal Symptom Questionnaire. *Journal of Affective Disorders* 1990; **19** (1): 53–61.

34 de las Cuevas C, Sanz E. J., de la Fuente J.A., Padilla J., Berenguer J.C. The Severity of Dependence Scale (SDS) as screening test for benzodiazepine dependence: SDS validation study. *Addiction*. 2000; **95** (2): 245–50.

35 Kobayashi, M., Okajima, I., Narisawa, H., Kikuchi T., Matsui K., Inada K., et al. Development of a new benzodiazepine hypnotics withdrawal symptom scale. *Sleep and Biological Rhythms* 2018; **16**: 263–71.

36 Narisawa H., Inoue Y., Kobayashi M., Okajima I., Kikuchi T., Kagimura T., et al. Development and validation of the Benzodiazepine Hypnotics Withdrawal Symptom Scale (BHWSS) based on item response theory. *Psychiatry Research* 2021; **300**: 113900.

Alcohol Use Disorders: Epidemiology and Prevention

Paul Bogowicz, Eilish Gilvarry, Andrea Hearn and Eileen Kaner

Overview

Alcohol misuse is a major public health problem in the United Kingdom (UK). It is associated with many biopsychosocial harms. There is some evidence that these harms are borne disproportionately by those in more deprived areas [1]. The costs associated with alcohol-related harm were thought to be approximately £21 billion in England in 2012 [2], which equates to 1.3 per cent of gross domestic product (GDP) [3]. This is consistent with earlier estimates of 1.3 to 3.3 per cent for six middle- and high-income countries [4]. Alcohol is the third most important risk factor in terms of overall global burden of disease [5].

Epidemiology

The WHO has defined alcohol misuse as drinking excessively, beyond the recommended limits specified by medical guidelines [6]. In the UK, the limits are 14 units per week for both men and women, consumed evenly over three or more days (Box 5.1) [7]. It is worth noting that prior to 2016, the limits were 21 units per week for men and 14 units for women. The lower limit of 14 units for men is used throughout this chapter, for consistency. The guidelines do not specify absolute limits for single occasion drinking. The UK government defines heavy single occasion (binge) drinking as consuming eight or more units for men and six or more units for women [2]. Individuals who are at risk of alcohol-related harm are deemed to be hazardous users, whereas those whose drinking is causing harm to their health are said to be harmful users [6]. The concept of alcohol dependence is covered in Chapter 1 of this book.

Data on alcohol use and misuse in the general population may be obtained from a number of different sources, including government and academic surveys. Advantages of using government survey data over data from academic surveys include more rigorous study design, relatively unbiased sampling, larger sample sizes and the ability to track trends over time. In this chapter, data from government surveys is presented in lieu of academic survey data, where available. Disadvantages to both government and academic survey data include coverage bias (excluding individuals that are homeless or not in school), non-response bias (respondents differ from non-respondents in terms of alcohol use) and social desirability bias (respondents under-report their alcohol use).

General Population – Adults

Great Britain

Alcohol use trends in England, Scotland and Wales are captured by the Opinions and Lifestyle Survey [8]. Past week alcohol use was reported by 57 per cent of adults (aged 16 and over) in

---

Box 5.1 A comparison of the relative strengths of various alcoholic drinks

14 units of alcohol =
140 ml or 112 g of pure ethanol
6 pints of 4% ABV beer or cider
4 pints of 6% ABV beer or cider
3 pints of 8% ABV beer or cider
8 glasses of 10% ABV wine
6 glasses of 13% ABV wine
14 measures of 40% ABV spirits

Alcohol units; 1 glass = 175 ml, 1 measure = 25 ml, 1 pint = 568 ml, ABV = alcohol by volume.

2017. More men (62 per cent) reported drinking than women (52 per cent). The prevalence of past week use was lowest among those aged 16 to 24 (48 per cent) and highest among those aged 45 to 64 (65 per cent). The prevalence of past week use was 64 per cent in 2005 and has been decreasing since 2008. Past week use was least prevalent in Wales (50 per cent) and Scotland (53 per cent) and ranged from 55 per cent to 61 per cent in England.

The prevalence of teetotalism was 20 per cent in 2017 (i.e. consuming no alcohol at all). More women (23 per cent) reported being teetotal, compared to men (18 per cent). The prevalence of teetotalism was highest among those aged 16 to 24 (23 per cent) and 65 and over (24 per cent). Although the overall prevalence of teetotalism has been static over time, there is an increasing prevalence among those aged 16 to 44 with a decreasing prevalence among those aged 65 and over. Teetotalism was most prevalent in London (27 per cent) and least prevalent in the South-West of England (15 per cent). The prevalence of teetotalism ranged from 17 per cent to 24 per cent in other regions.

Past week heavy single occasion drinking was reported by 16 per cent of those surveyed in 2017. More men (18 per cent) reported this form of misuse than women (13 per cent). The prevalence of past week heavy single occasion drinking was highest among those aged 16 to 24 (20 per cent) and lowest among those aged 65 and over (6 per cent). The prevalence is decreasing among those aged 16 to 44. The fall is most marked among males aged 16 to 24, from 32 per cent in 2005 to 20 per cent in 2017. There was marked variation in the prevalence of past week heavy single occasion use, with some evidence of a north–south divide (Figure 5.1).

The Opinions and Lifestyle Survey does not consider weekly alcohol consumption. Data on this variable is captured at national level by the Health Survey for England [9], the Scottish Health Survey [10] and the National Survey for Wales [11]. Alcohol use trends in Northern Ireland are discussed separately.

In England, drinking in excess of 14 units per week was reported by 23 per cent of adults (aged 16 and over) in 2016 (Table 5.1) [9]. More men (31 per cent) reported this form of misuse than women (16 per cent). Drinking in excess of 14 units per week was least common among those aged 16 to 24 (18 per cent) and 75 and over (18 per cent) and highest among those aged 55 to 64 (30 per cent). The prevalence of drinking in excess of 14 units per week was slightly lower than it was in 2011 (26 per cent). The survey report did not consider regional variation for this variable.

In Scotland, drinking in excess of 14 units per week was reported by 26 per cent of adults (aged 16 and over) in 2016 (Table 5.1) [10]. The difference between men and women was

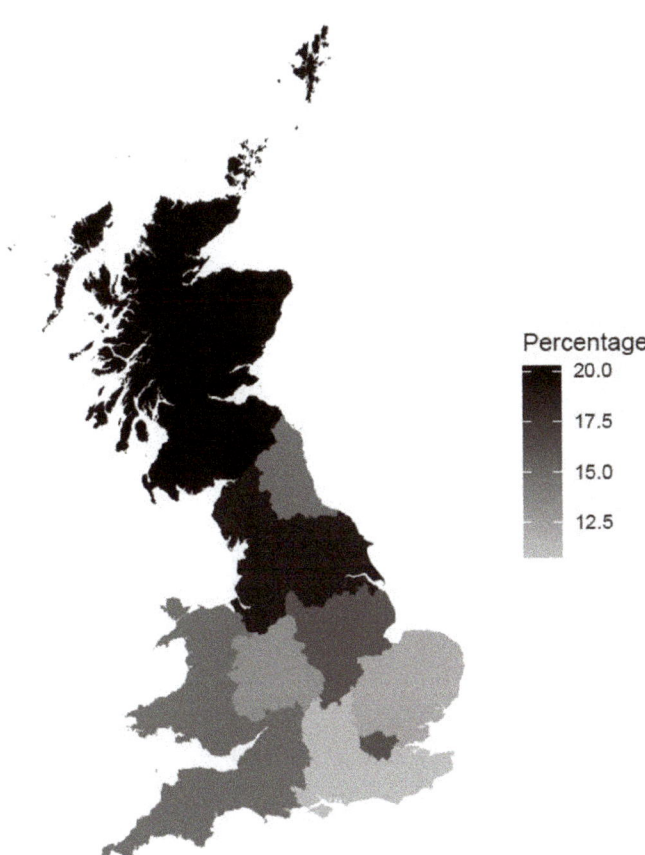

Figure 5.1 The prevalence of heavy single occasion (binge) drinking among adults (aged 16 and over) in 2017 in Great Britain, by country/English region. This figure contains National Statistics and OS data. (Both © Crown copyright and database right.)

Percentage
20.0
17.5
15.0
12.5

similar to that in England. In contrast, drinking in excess of 14 units per week was much more common among those aged 16 to 24 (29 per cent) in Scotland. The prevalence of drinking in excess of 14 units was 34 per cent in 2003 and has decreased steadily since then. The prevalence was lowest in the most deprived quintile (19 per cent) and ranged from 26 per cent to 30 per cent in other areas.

In Wales, drinking in excess of 14 units per week was reported by 18 per cent of adults (aged 16 and over) in 2017–18 (Table 5.1) [11]. More men (25 per cent) reported this form of misuse than women (12 per cent). Drinking in excess of 14 units was least prevalent among those aged 16 to 24 (14 per cent), 25 to 34 (12 per cent) and 75 and over (12 per cent). The prevalence ranged from 20 per cent to 23 per cent in the other age groups. The prevalence followed an increasing trend from the most deprived quintile (15 per cent) to the least deprived (21 per cent).

Northern Ireland

Alcohol use trends in Northern Ireland are captured by the Health Survey Northern Ireland [12]. The prevalence of teetotalism was 20 per cent among adults (aged 18 and

Table 5.1 The prevalence of drinking in excess of 14 units of alcohol per week among adults in the United Kingdom; by country, gender and age

Age	England		Scotland		Wales		Northern Ireland	
	Men (%)	Women (%)	Men (%)	Women (%)	Men (%)	Women (%)	Men (%)	Women (%)
16–24*	21	14	32	25	17	12	43	17
25–34	28	13	33	13	16	8	32	9
35–44	31	14	37	19	26	15	33	13
45–54	31	19	38	18	29	13	35	15
55–64	39	23	40	23	32	14	33	11
65–74	36	15	38	14	31	13	25	6
≥75	27	11	20	5	18	7	13	3

* 18–24 in Northern Ireland

over) in 2016/17. More women (22 per cent) reported being teetotal, compared to men (16 per cent). The prevalence of being teetotal was similar among all age groups apart from those aged 65 to 74 (33 per cent) and 75 and over (48 per cent). There is no clear trend in terms of the prevalence of teetotalism over the period from 2010 to 2017. The prevalence of teetotalism was lowest in the least deprived quintile (15 per cent) and ranged from 19 per cent to 22 per cent elsewhere.

The prevalence of drinking in excess of 14 units per week was 20 per cent in 2015–16; this data was not captured by the 2016–17 survey (Table 5.1). More men (32 per cent) reported this form of misuse than women (11 per cent). Drinking in excess of 14 units per week was more common among those aged 18 to 24 (29 per cent), less common among those aged 25 to 64 (range 19 to 24 per cent), and least common among those aged 75 and over (6 per cent). The prevalence of drinking in excess of 14 units was 24 per cent in 2010–11 and has been decreasing since then. The prevalence was highest in the least deprived quintile (22 per cent) and ranged from 18 per cent to 21 per cent elsewhere, with no clear trend.

International

Measurements of alcohol consumption vary from country to country. Proxy measures, such as alcohol sales per capita, are often used instead of direct measures of consumption. Per capita alcohol consumption among UK adults (aged 15 and over) was 9.5 l/capita in 2016 (see https://data.oecd.org/healthrisk/alcohol-consumption.htm). Changes in per capita consumption are given in Figure 5.2, for the UK and the other Group of Seven countries.

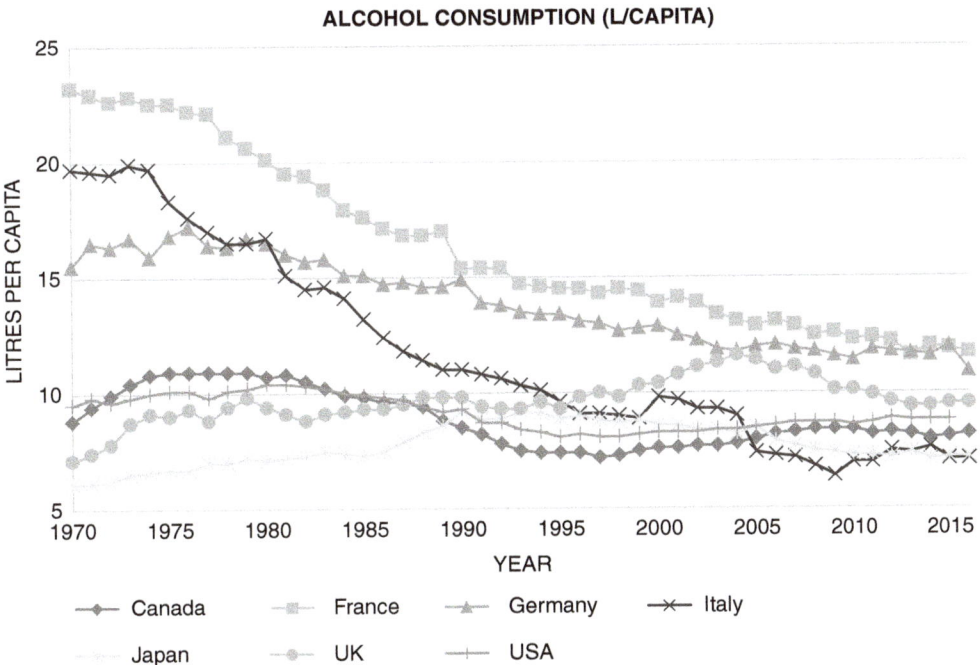

Figure 5.2 Alcohol consumption in litres per capita among adults (aged 15 and over) in the Group of Seven countries, by year from 1970 to 2016 (where available)

Per capita consumption is lower in the UK than in France and Germany. The UK has not experienced as much change in per capita consumption over time, compared to France, Germany and Italy.

General Population – Children

England

The Smoking, Drinking and Drug Use among Young People in England survey examines trends in alcohol use among students in years 7 to 11 (typically aged 11 to 15) [13]. The prevalence of past week drinking was 10 per cent in 2016, and slightly more girls (11 per cent) reported this behaviour than boys (9 per cent). The prevalence of past week drinking ranged from 1 per cent among 11-year-olds to 24 per cent among 15-year-olds. The trend in prevalence of past week drinking had been decreasing from 2004 (23 per cent) to 2014 (8 per cent). The prevalence was lowest among Londoners (6 per cent) and similar elsewhere (10 per cent to 12 per cent).

The prevalence of having been drunk in the past four weeks was 9 per cent in 2016. More girls (11 per cent) reported this behaviour than boys (7 per cent). The prevalence of this behaviour ranged from 0 per cent among 11-year-olds to 23 per cent among 15-year-olds. Girls aged 15 years had the highest prevalence (27 per cent), with 7 per cent reporting that they had been drunk three or more times in the past four weeks. The prevalence of this behaviour has decreased since 2006, when it was 19 per cent. The survey report did not consider regional variation for this variable.

Scotland

The Scottish Schools Adolescent Lifestyle and Substance Use Survey captures trends in alcohol use among S2 and S4 students (typically aged 13 and 15, respectively) [14]. The prevalence of past week drinking was 4 per cent among those aged 13 and 17 per cent among those aged 15 in 2015. Slightly more 15-year-old girls (19 per cent) reported this behaviour compared to boys (16 per cent) The prevalence rose through the 1990s and has been decreasing since around 2002. Among 13-year-old students, drinking in the past week was more prevalent among those living in the most deprived quintile. There was no relationship between this variable and deprivation among 15-year-old students.

The prevalence of having been drunk in the past week was 2 per cent among those aged 13 and 10 per cent among those aged 15. Slightly more 15-year-old girls (11 per cent) reported this behaviour, compared to boys (9 per cent). There was no difference between 13-year-old boys and girls in this regard. There is no clear trend to the prevalence of having been drunk in the past week, though levels in 2015 were generally decreased relative to 2006. The survey report did not consider regional variation for this variable.

Wales

The best available data for trends in alcohol use among young people in Wales is from the Health Behaviour in School-Aged Children 2013/14 survey study [15]. The prevalence of drinking at least once per week was 3 per cent/1 per cent for boys/girls aged 11 years old, 7 per cent/5 per cent for 13-year-olds and 14 per cent/12 per cent for 15-year-olds. The prevalence of having been drunk at least twice for boys/girls was 1 per cent/1 per cent for 11-

year-olds, 8 per cent/9 per cent for 13-year-olds and 28 per cent/34 per cent for 15-year-olds. The survey report did not consider trends or regional variation for these variables.

Northern Ireland

The Young Persons' Behaviour and Attitudes Survey examines alcohol use trends among students aged 11 to 16 in Northern Ireland [16]. The prevalence of past week drinking was 6 per cent among girls and 7 per cent among boys in 2016. Few student (2 per cent) in Year 8 (typically aged 11 to 12) reported this behaviour, compared to 20 per cent of those in Year 12 (typically aged 15 to 16). The prevalence of having been drunk at least twice was 11 per cent. The survey report did not consider demographic breakdowns for this variable or trends for either variable.

Select Clinical Groups

Individuals are said to have a comorbid diagnosis if they have a severe mental illness and misuse alcohol and/or other substances. The epidemiology of comorbidity was explored in a systematic review conducted by the National Collaborating Centre for Mental Health [17]. The prevalence of alcohol misuse or alcohol dependence varied from 7 to 16 per cent among people with severe mental illness living in the UK. It is unclear whether there is a statistically significant difference in prevalence between those with severe mental illness and those without.

The epidemiology of alcohol misuse among people with personality disorder was examined in a systematic review and meta-analysis published in 2018 [18]. The prevalence of lifetime alcohol use disorder, which encompasses the spectrum of harmful alcohol misuse through to dependence, was 59 per cent overall. The prevalence was higher (77 per cent) for those with antisocial subtype. The prevalence of lifetime alcohol dependence among people with personality disorder in the general and treatment-seeking populations ranged from 21 per cent to 47 per cent (no pooled estimate available).

Harms

Alcohol-related harm should be considered in the context of the amount and duration of alcohol use and other factors. These include individual-level factors such as age, gender, ethnicity and genetic predisposition (familial nature of alcohol misuse); and the environment in which alcohol is consumed. In some circumstances it may be not safe to consume any alcohol at all. For example, if it is important that judgement is not impaired such as when driving a car or train or flying a plane. Another important concept is that of the 'alcohol harm paradox': deprived populations consuming similar average levels of alcohol experience greater alcohol-related harm compared to less deprived populations [19].

Health Harms

Physical harm as a result of consuming alcohol may be broadly considered in terms of the harmful effects caused directly through acute intoxication with alcohol, and effects caused through regular heavy alcohol consumption.

Acute intoxication is defined in the 10th edition of the International Classification of Diseases (ICD-10) as a 'transient condition following the administration of alcohol or other psychoactive substance, resulting in disturbances in level of consciousness, cognition, perception, affect or behaviour, or other psychophysiological functions and responses.' Alcohol acts primarily as a central nervous system depressant but the harmful effects of acute intoxication are many and varied including alcohol poisoning, trauma, self-harm and suicide, aspiration, cardiac arrhythmias and amnesic episodes including alcoholic blackouts.

The long-term effects of regular heavy alcohol consumption include death and illness from heart disease, stroke, hypertensive disease and liver disease. It has been known since the 1980s that alcohol is carcinogenic. In addition to the direct cancer-causing effects of alcohol, heavy drinkers are less likely to access preventive services such as cancer screening programmes. Each year in England there are approximately 19,000 new alcohol-attributable cancer cases [20].

Liver disease is the only major cause of death that is increasing in England [21]. Deaths from liver disease are decreasing in the rest of Europe. More than a third of the liver disease deaths in England are alcohol-attributable. Up to 15 per cent of dependent drinkers develop cirrhosis of the liver, and an even larger proportion of harmful alcohol users (not necessarily dependent) develop fatty liver.

Alcohol-related brain damage (ARBD) is now a recognised significant health, social and economic problem. Heavy social drinkers who have no apparent neurological or hepatic problems may have localised brain damage and demonstrable cognitive impairment [22]. The mechanisms underlying the damage are not yet well understood. Changes are more severe in individuals with thiamine (vitamin B1) deficiency, the so-called Wernicke–Korsakoff syndrome. It is likely that ARBD is underdiagnosed relative to other forms of cognitive impairment.

Alcohol impacts upon mental as well as physical health. One study found that 85 per cent of individuals accessing UK-based alcohol treatment services had a diagnosable mental health problem [23]. Another systematic review and meta-analysis found that having an alcohol use disorder was associated with increased risks of suicidal ideation and completed suicide [24]. The National Confidential Inquiry into Suicide and Homicide by People with Mental Illness found that 45 per cent of mental health patients who died by suicide between 2005 and 2015 had a history of alcohol misuse.

Alongside the wealth of evidence for alcohol-related harm is the evidence that moderate drinking may reduce the risk of death from ischaemic vascular disease. The first evidence for this appeared in the 1970s. The concept of a J-shaped curve emerged, where mortality from cardiovascular disease, and indeed total mortality, initially falls as alcohol consumption increases, and then rises with increasing consumption. More recent evidence suggests that the relationship between alcohol consumption and cardiovascular disease is more complicated [25].

In 2017–18, there were 338,000 hospital admissions in England where the main reason for admission was attributed to alcohol (the narrow measure) [26]. This was similar to the previous year, although 15 per cent higher than in 2007–8. On the other hand, there were 1.2 million admissions in 2017–18 where the primary or any secondary reason for admission was linked to alcohol (the broad measure). The drivers behind the large numbers of alcohol-related admissions appear to be cancer and injuries (narrow measure) and cardiovascular disease and mental/behavioural disorders due to alcohol (broad measure).

Alcohol has also been shown to affect life expectancy. In 2016, there were 7,327 alcohol-specific deaths in the UK [27]. Alcohol-specific death rates are higher than they were 15 years ago, but have been relatively static since 2013. The rates of alcohol-specific deaths are

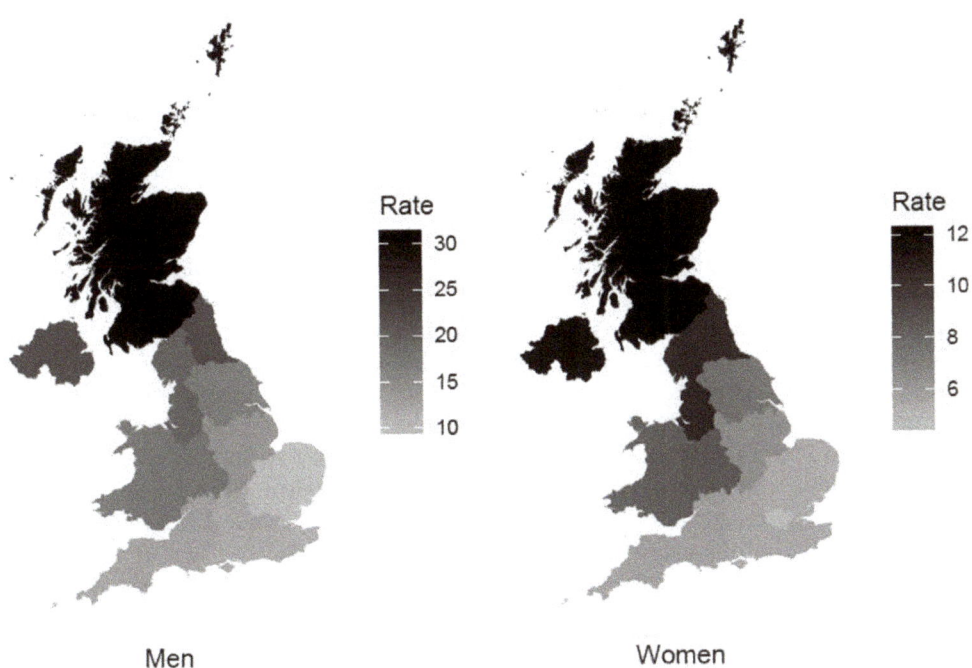

Men Women

Figure 5.3 Age standardised alcohol-specific death rates (per 100,000) in 2016, by country/English region and gender. Note that the scale used for women differs from that of men. This figure contains National Statistics and OS data. (Both © Crown copyright and database right.)

approximately 55 per cent higher among males, compared to females. There is significant regional variation, in terms of alcohol-specific deaths, with clear evidence of a north–south gradient divide (Figure 5.3).

Maternal alcohol consumption is known to have a profound effect on the unborn child and foetal alcohol syndrome (FAS) is well described [28]. FAS was historically thought to encompass a combination of physical health problems, such as craniofacial anomalies and growth retardation, along with developmental delay. It is now known that the damage caused by alcohol can be subtler; the developing brain is particularly vulnerable. This has led to the concept of foetal alcohol spectrum disorders (FASD), of which FAS is one extreme. In addition, maternal drinking has been linked to sudden infant death syndrome (SIDS) [29].

Social Harms

Parental alcohol misuse can affect the health and well-being of children and families in a number of different ways. For example, the frequency and quality of parent–child interaction may decrease, resulting in poor parenting. The parent may be unable to work, and this may have an impact on family finances. There is an association between childhood exposure to parental alcohol misuse and externalising problems, including conduct disorders and substance misuse. Children may take on caring responsibilities, either for their alcohol misusing parent(s) or for siblings. This may have ramifications for school attendance and social development in general. With more alcohol now being consumed in the home (65 per cent/73 per cent of alcohol in England/Scotland is sold in off-trade settings), more children are likely to be exposed to parental drinking and to the potential harms associated with this.

There is a complicated relationship between alcohol consumption and criminality. Alcohol is implicated in public disorder offences, violence (including domestic) and acquisitive crime. In the 2013–14 Crime Survey for England and Wales, more than half of violent incidents involved perpetrators thought to be under the influence of alcohol [30]. This proportion has been static for some time, though the overall number of incidents has been decreasing. The proportion of violent incidents thought to be alcohol-related is higher in the evenings and at night (70 per cent) and at the weekend (70 per cent). There was an association between alcohol-related incidents and more serious injury in the survey data. In 2015, approximately 220 people were killed in drink-driving-related accidents in Great Britain. Some 1,380 people were either killed or seriously injured, among a total of 8,480 drink-drive casualties. The absolute number of alcohol-related fatal road traffic accidents decreased from 2005 to 2010 and has been relatively static since 2010.

The economic consequences of alcohol include absenteeism. Those who die from alcohol-related causes are also clearly unable to participate in the labour market. In England in 2015, approximately 167,000 working years of life (17 per cent of total) were lost due to alcohol misuse [31]. These losses were driven by deaths caused by self-harm, liver disease and accidental poisoning. It is worth noting that the 10 leading causes of cancer accounted for fewer (151,000) working years of life lost.

Preventive Interventions

It is clear that harmful alcohol use is common and is associated with significant morbidity and mortality. Policies aiming to prevent or reduce alcohol-related harm can be targeted at individuals, communities, regions or entire countries. These typically involve legal or public health interventions that aim to limit accessibility, availability and affordability of alcohol. There are seven broad areas of alcohol policies with good evidence of effectiveness in reducing harm. These include: altering the economic context; altering the availability of alcohol through licensing restrictions and opening hours; altering the environmental context; drink-driving control measures; advertising and marketing measures; information, education and awareness campaigns; and early interventions to reduce risk and change alcohol consumption behaviour [32]. The concept of the preventive paradox applies to alcohol use, whereby interventions to reduce alcohol-related harm may be most impactful among the large group of low-level misusers rather than the smaller group of those at highest risk.

The main approach to altering the economic context around alcohol consumption is through the regulation of taxes. Taxation has been an important revenue stream for many countries, particularly developing countries over the past 30 years [32]. Taxes are a broad policy instrument, which tend to be applied to many if not most or all alcohol products. This may impact the heaviest and riskiest drinkers, but also those who drink within recommended limits. Evidence suggests that alcohol prices do have an effect on alcohol consumption and related harm; for example, by reducing violent behaviour, homicides, drink driving and fatal accidents. The price of alcohol is also influenced by cultural and environmental factors. Notably, price increases have been slower in supermarkets, off-licenses and other off-trade environments. Moreover, alcohol has become increasingly more affordable; there has been a rise in affordability of 64 per cent from 1980 to 2017 [26].

More recently, much attention has been centred on alcohol minimum unit pricing (MUP), a mandated price line below which retailers are not legally allowed to sell. This policy instrument targets the cheapest alcohol. The aim is to reduce harm among the heaviest drinkers, particularly those with lower socioeconomic status. In 2012, the Scottish Government introduced legislation to bring in MUP. However, there were appeals to the Scottish Courts and ultimately to the European Court of Justice in 2015. MUP was eventually introduced at a price of 50p per unit in May 2018. England, Wales and Northern Ireland have not adopted MUP at this time. The evidence for MUP comes from observational studies and through academic modelling. An observational study on MUP in the Canadian province of British Columbia (not exactly the same as MUP in Scotland) found that for a 10 per cent increase in minimum price there was a 3 per cent reduction in total alcohol consumption [33]. One modelling study found that a 50p MUP would reduce total alcohol consumption by nearly 5 per cent among male harmful drinkers and lead to a reduction in alcohol-related workplace absenteeism and deaths [34].

Licensing systems are the main control on the availability of alcohol. These include restricting hours of trading, age restrictions, regulation of physical outlets and other geographical conditions placed on the sales of alcohol. Almost all countries limit access of alcohol to young people, though there is variation in terms of age restriction (16 to 21 years of age). There is strong evidence that a higher minimum age is associated with decreased road traffic accident casualties [32]. While reducing availability of alcohol is seen as a key control on levels of alcohol consumption, this is balanced and sometimes conflicted by market forces and influences such as employment and the night-time economy.

Other preventive harm reduction approaches include server training and alcohol service practice and policy (focusing on the management of intoxicated and aggressive people in high-risk environments), use of voluntary codes of practice and community mobilisation approaches. Community approaches can be effective, albeit resource intensive, and need long-term interagency commitment and consistency. Some countries have mandatory warning labels on alcoholic beverages – for example, 'Excessive drinking is harmful to health' in China. Others have suggestions for voluntary use. Suggestions in England include 'UK Chief Medical Officers recommend adults do not regularly drink more than 14 units per week' and 'It is safest not to drink alcohol when pregnant.'

Drink-driving control measures include drink-driving limits and drink-driving campaigns. In England and Wales, the blood alcohol concentration (BAC) limit is 80 mg of ethanol (alcohol) per 100 ml of blood, as set by the Road Safety Act 1967. This level is higher than those of all other European Union countries, apart from Malta. Many countries have a BAC limit of 50 mg per 100 ml and some have an even lower level for novice drivers. Scotland reduced their BAC limit to 50 mg per 100 ml in 2014, with an immediate reduction in offending behaviour noted in the first year following the change. Although drink-driving casualties remain prevalent in England, the proportion of drink-driving casualties as a proportion of all casualties has been falling. In 2015, drink-driving casualties accounted for 13 per cent of all road deaths in the UK. A review published in 2010 found that drivers with BAC level of 20–50 mg per 100 ml are at least three times more likely to die in a road traffic accident, rising to more than six times for those with a BAC level of 50–80 mg per 100 ml [35].

There is much global advertising of alcohol currently on television and in posters, films, at sporting events and at concerts. In addition, there is exposure and the potential for exposure to advertising through social media and the Internet more generally, particularly for younger people. There is evidence of a cumulative influence of alcohol advertising on alcohol behaviour and perceptions. One review found that there is an association between prior alcohol advertising and exposure and subsequent alcohol use in young people [36]. A more recent longitudinal study found a positive association between alcohol advertising exposure and use among this age group [37]. There is little evidence that alcohol industry voluntary regulations are effective in terms of reducing exposure to alcohol in particular populations.

There is much popular consideration of the need for education and awareness-raising approaches to reduce alcohol-related harm, at differing levels and in different contexts. There is a lack of good quality evaluations of this type of approach. The existing evidence suggests that there is a modest effect at best on alcohol behaviour and with little persistence of any effects. Similarly, the impact of mass media campaigns such as those promoting responsible drinking is thought to be limited [32].

Brief Interventions

Much preventive research and implementation work has focused on screening for alcohol misuse paired with the delivery of a brief intervention. The aim of the latter is to reduce consumption and prevent further harmful use and related problems.

Screening is the process used to identify those that are misusing alcohol and who may benefit from a brief intervention. There are a broad range of instruments, including questionnaires, blood tests and structured interviews. Standardised questionnaires are the most sensitive and specific method of detection. The alcohol use disorders identification test (AUDIT) is a 10-item questionnaire that incudes questions addressing frequency, quantity and intensity of alcohol consumption, as well as experience of alcohol-related problems [38]. The shorter version of AUDIT, AUDIT-C, and other short screening tools are generally less accurate, albeit faster to complete. Screening for alcohol misuse can either be universal, aimed at all patients attending a specific service or targeted at specific groups – for example, new attenders or those at higher risk. The cost-effectiveness and acceptability of both approaches continues to be researched.

There are generally two approaches to brief intervention: structured advice with personalised feedback and a more extended intervention, typically employing motivational interviewing techniques. Both use a common strategy with the acronym FRAMES; personalised *feedback*, promoting *responsibility*, *advice*, offering a *menu* of options, *empathy* and promotion of *self-efficacy* [39]. Brief interventions are typically delivered face-to-face. Some interventions include booster sessions. The evidence base for brief interventions is substantial, particularly in primary care settings, including emergency departments. There is also evidence from across a range of population groups and in different contexts – for example, in criminal justice settings and in colleges. Studies have consistently shown that brief interventions are effective in terms of reducing frequency and quantity of alcohol consumption and related harm. In recent years there has been a movement towards mobile and web-based brief interventions. These digital interventions do not appear to have any lasting effect on alcohol consumption, and few trials have directly compared digital interventions to face-to-face interventions.

References

1 Johnston M. C., Ludbrook A., Jaffray M. A. Inequalities in the distribution of the costs of alcohol misuse in Scotland: A cost of illness study. *Alcohol and Alcoholism*. 2012; **47** (6): 725–31.

2 HM Government. *The Government's Alcohol Strategy*. London: Home Office; 2012.

3 Public Health England. *The Public Health Burden of Alcohol and the Effectiveness and Cost-Effectiveness of Alcohol Control Policies: An Evidence Review*. London: PHE; 2016.

4 Rehm J., Mathers C., Popova S., Thavorncharoensap M., Teerawattananon Y., Patra J. Global burden of disease and injury and economic cost attributable to alcohol use and alcohol-use disorders. *The Lancet*. 2009; **373** (9682): 2223–33.

5 World Health Organization. *Global Health Risks: Mortality and Burden of Disease Attributable to Selected Major Risks*. Geneva, Switzerland: WHO; 2009.

6 World Health Organization. Lexicon of alcohol and drug terms published by the World Health Organization. WHO; 1994 [Available from: www.who.int/substance_abuse/terminology/who_lexicon/en.]

7 Department of Health. *UK Chief Medical Officers' Alcohol Guidelines Review: Summary of the Proposed New Guidelines*. London: DH; 2016.

8 Office for National Statistics. Adult drinking habits in Great Britain, 2017. ONS; 2018 [Available from: www.ons.gov.uk/releases/adultdrinkinghabitsingreatbritain2017.]

9 National Statistics. Health Survey for England, 2016: Adult Health-Related Behaviours. NHS Digital; 2017 [Available from: https://digital.nhs.uk/data-and-information/publications/statistical/health-survey-for-england/2018.]

10 Scottish Government. Scottish Health Survey, 2016: Summary. National Statistics for Scotland; 2017 [Available from: www.gov.scot/publications/scottish-health-survey-2016-volume-1-main-report.]

11 Welsh Government. National Survey for Wales, 2017–18 National Statistics; 2018 [Available from: https://gov.wales/sites/default/files/statistics-and-research/2019-01/national-survey-wales-headline-results-2017-18.pdf.]

12 Department of Health NI. Health Survey Northern Ireland: First Results, 2016/17. Information Analysis Directorate; 2017.

13 NHS Digital. Smoking, Drinking and Drug Use Among Young People in England, 2016. National Statistics; 2017 [Available from: https://files.digital.nhs.uk/47/829A59/sdd-2016-rep-cor-new.pdf.]

14 National Statistics for Scotland. *Scottish Schools Adolescent Lifestyle and Substance Use Survey (SALSUS): Alcohol Report 2015*. Edinburgh: The Scottish Government; 2016.

15 Inchley J., Currie D., Young T., Samdal O., Torsheim T., Augustson L., et al. Growing Up Unequal: Gender and Socioeconomic Differences in Young People's Health and Well-Being. Health Behaviour in School-Aged Children (HBSC) Study: International Report from the 2013/14 Survey. Copenhagen, Denmark: World Health Organization, Regional Office for Europe; 2016.

16 Foster C., Scarlett M., Stewart B. Young Persons' Behaviour and Attitude Survey, 2016. Belfast: Department of Health NI; 2017.

17 Megnin-Viggars O., Brown M., Marcus E., Stockton S., Pilling S.. *The Epidemiology, and Current Configuration of Health and Social Care Community Services, for People in the UK with a Severe Mental Illness Who Also Misuse Substances: A Systematic Review*. London: National Collaborating Centre for Mental Health; 2016.

18 Guy N., Newton-Howes G., Ford H., Williman J., Foulds J. The prevalence of comorbid alcohol use disorder in the presence of personality disorder: Systematic review and explanatory modelling. *Personality and Mental Health*. 2018; **12** (3): 216–28.

19 Bellis M. A., Hughes K., Nicholls J., Sheron N., Gilmore I., Jones L. The alcohol harm paradox: Using a national survey to explore how alcohol may disproportionately impact health in deprived individuals. *BMC Public Health.* 2016; **16** (1): 111.

20 Public Health England. Local Alcohol Profiles for England: May 2017. London: PHE; 2017 [Available from: https://bit.ly /2PlWYKe.]

21 Leon D. A., McCambridge J. Liver cirrhosis mortality rates in Britain from 1950 to 2002: An analysis of routine data. *Lancet.* 2006; **367**: 52–6.

22 Harper C. The neuropathology of alcohol-related brain damage. *Alcohol and Alcoholism.* 2009; **44** (2): 136–40.

23 Weaver T., Madden P., Charles V., Timso G. S., Renton A., Tyrer P. et al. Comorbidity of substance misuse and mental illness in community mental health and substance misuse services. *British Journal of Psychiatry.* 2003; **183**: 304–13.

24 Darvishi N., Farhadi M., Haghtalab T., Poorolajal J. Alcohol-related risk of suicidal ideation, suicide attempt, and completed suicide: A meta-analysis. *PLOS ONE.* 2015; **10** (5): e0126870.

25 Day E., Rudd J. H. F. Alcohol use disorders and the heart. *Addiction.* 2019; **114** (9): 1670–8.

26 Health and Social Care Information Centre. Statistics on Alcohol, England, 2019 [PAS]. NHS Digital; 2019 [Available from: https:// bit.ly/3dgQBzO.]

27 Office for National Statistics. Alcohol-Specific Deaths in the UK: Registered in 2016 2017 [Available from: https://bit.ly /31BM59u.]

28 Riley E. P., Infante M. A., Warren K. R. Fetal Alcohol spectrum disorders: An overview. *Neuropsychology Review.* 2011; **21** (2): 73.

29 Phillips D. P., Brewer K. M., Wadensweiler P. Alcohol as a risk factor for sudden infant death syndrome (SIDS). *Addiction.* 2011; **106** (3): 516–25.

30 Office for National Statistics. Violent Crime and Sexual Offences: Alcohol-Related Violence, 2015 [Available from: https://bit .ly/3cEbnKM.]

31 Public Health England. Working Years of Life Lost Due to Alcohol: Ad Hoc Statistical Release, 2016 [Available from: https://bit.ly /3u8pnSB.]

32 Babor T., Caetano R., Casswell S., Edwards G., Giesbrecht N., Graham K. et al. *Alcohol: No Ordinary Commodity.* 2nd ed. Oxford: Oxford University Press; 2010.

33 Stockwell T., Auld M. C., Zhao J., Martin G. Does minimum pricing reduce alcohol consumption? The experience of a Canadian province. *Addiction.* 2012; **107** (5): 912–20.

34 Meier P. S., Holmes J., Angus C., Ally A. K., Meng Y., Brennan A. Estimated effects of different alcohol taxation and price policies on health inequalities: A mathematical modelling study. *PLOS Medicine.* 2016; **13** (2): e1001963.

35 Killoran A., Canning U., Doyle N., Sheppard L. *Review of Effectiveness of Laws Limiting Blood Alcohol Concentration Levels to Reduce Alcohol-Related Road Injuries and Deaths.* Centre for Public Health Excellence: National Institute for Health and Care Excellence; 2010.

36 Smith L. A., Foxcroft D. R. The effect of alcohol advertising, marketing and portrayal on drinking behaviour in young people: Systematic review of prospective cohort studies. *BMC Public Health.* 2009; **9** (1): 51.

37 de Bruijn A., Tanghe J., de Leeuw R., Engels R., Anderson P., Beccaria F. et al. European longitudinal study on the relationship between adolescents' alcohol marketing exposure and alcohol use. *Addiction.* 2016; **111** (10): 1774–83.

38 Saunders J. B., Aasland O. G., Babor T. F., De La Fuente J. R., Grant M. Development of the alcohol use disorders identification test (AUDIT): WHO collaborative project on early detection of persons with harmful alcohol consumption-II. *Addiction.* 1993; **88** (6): 791–804.

39 National Institute for Health and Clinical Excellence. *Alcohol-Use Disorders: Preventing the Development of Hazardous and Harmful Drinking.* NICE; 2010.

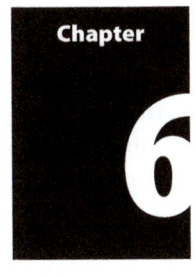

Alcohol Use Disorders: Aetiology and Pathophysiology

Nicola J. Kalk and Mary Thornton

Introduction

More than 80 per cent of the population in England drink alcohol. Yet the prevalence of alcohol dependence is estimated as around 1.4 per cent [1]. Even if we include those who are not dependent but drink at levels exceeding government recommendations, it is only 31 per cent and 16 per cent of the population respectively [2]. This leads us to question what factors increase the vulnerability to developing alcohol dependence. It may also lead us to question why as psychiatrists we encounter harmful use of alcohol and alcohol dependence or in DSM-5 parlance, Alcohol Use Disorders (AUD), so often in our patient population, particularly in those attending emergency services following self-harm and suicidal acts [3] and those who go on to die by suicide [4]. Understanding the aetiology and pathophysiology of alcohol dependence is helpful clinically, because it accounts for why we use certain medications to treat alcohol withdrawal and for relapse prevention, reminds us of the importance of trauma-informed care for this patient group and alerts us that psychiatric comorbidity may not be secondary to the alcohol itself.

The aetiology of alcohol dependence is multi-factorial and incorporates biological, psychological and social elements. In establishing a causal relationship, three criteria need to be established:

- The proposed risk factor must be correlated with outcome.
- There must be a temporal relationship – that is, the risk factor must predate the outcome.
- The relationship should not be better explained by a third factor.

Much of the research regarding risk factors for alcohol dependence falls short of meeting these three criteria.

Family History

AUD in either parent roughly doubles the risk of AUD in children irrespective of other mental health comorbidity [5]. Twin studies have established that the heritability of alcohol dependence is between 40 and 60 per cent [6, 7]. Both genetics and family environmental factors play a role.

Genetic linkage studies (reviewed in [7]) have identified chromosomal regions including 4q, which encodes the alcohol dehydrogenase gene involved in alcohol metabolism, and parts which include the areas encoding for GABA-A receptors and CHRM2, a cholinergic receptor gene; however, multiple peaks have been found in each region suggesting that vulnerability is complex and polygenic. Candidate gene approaches have also found a protective effect of genes encoding isoforms of the enzymes involved in the metabolism of alcohol. Alcohol is metabolised in two steps: first, alcohol dehydrogenase metabolises alcohol to acetaldehyde, and then acetaldehyde is metabolised to acetate by acetaldehyde dehydrogenase. Acetaldehyde is toxic, causing nausea, vomiting, flushing, dizziness, throbbing headache, chest and abdominal discomfort and general hangover-like symptoms. In fact, the relapse prevention medication disulfiram works by inhibiting acetaldehyde dehydrogenase causing the build-up of acetaldehyde when someone drinks, as a deterrent. So it makes sense that isoforms of alcohol dehydrogenase that speed up the conversion of alcohol to acetaldehyde, and isoforms of acetaldehyde dehydrogenase that slow down conversation of acetaldehyde to acetate, have been reported to be protective against alcohol dependence in candidate gene studies [10]. Although an association with genes relating to various neurotransmitter systems (GABA, glutamate, serotonin, opioid) have been reported, effect sizes have been small, dependent on gene–environment interaction and there has been a lack of replication. Genome-wide association studies, a hypothesis-free method, have in the main confirmed the association of genes encoding enzymes involved in alcohol metabolism and other associations found via GWAS await replication.

Family culture around drinking also contributes to the development of drinking patterns: children learn social behavioural patterns from observing their parents' behaviour – so the type of behaviour modelled by parents, particularly mothers, is important. Frequent or increasing maternal drinking during childhood – even early childhood – has been consistently associated with an increased risk of AUD in young adults and this has been quantified as a twofold increase in odds – although sons appear to be more susceptible than daughters [8]. The belief that normalising drinking – by serving young teenagers wine at family dinner, for example – prevents alcohol problems is also flawed. Several studies have reported an association between parental supply of alcohol and increased drinking, binge drinking and alcohol-related harm later in adolescence (summarised in [9]), with no consistent evidence of a protective effect. More recently this association has been quantified: the odds of binge drinking, alcohol related harm and symptoms of AUD more than doubled [10] in those late adolescents whose parents had provided alcohol earlier in adolescence. This is perhaps unsurprising because earlier age of onset of regular drinking (one to two times a week) is associated with an increased risk of developing AUD (reviewed in [8]).

Indirect consequences of parental drinking such as family conflict have also been reported to account for the association between a family history of alcohol dependence and risk of it developing in young adult offspring (see [8]). Other aspects of parenting have been described as protective. Stricter parenting in early childhood and teenage years and parental reward for good behaviour are associated with a reduced frequency of AUDs in young adults [8].

Childhood Circumstances

Large epidemiological studies have established that the odds of alcohol and other drug dependence in those whose childhood was characterised by socioeconomic disadvantage was more than twofold [11]. Beyond socioeconomic disadvantage, up to 22–74 per cent of patients with alcohol dependence report some form of childhood neglect or abuse [12]. There appears to be a dose-dependent relationship between the number of adverse childhood experiences (so-called ACEs) and the risk of alcohol dependence: while having experienced one ACE is associated with twofold odds of 'considering oneself an alcoholic', having experienced two is associated with fourfold odds, three with 4.9-fold odds and four with 7.4-fold odds [13]. Those alcohol-dependent patients with a history of childhood abuse are also reported to transition to alcohol dependence at an earlier age [12], suffer from more severe dependence and shorter periods of abstinence [14].

One possible explanation for this association has been derived from Attachment Theory. According to this theory, the relationship with our primary caregiver determines our attachment style. Attachment styles have been categorised as secure and insecure [15]. It is thought that our pattern of attachment persists into adulthood, giving us a framework upon which future relationships are built, and contributes to our ability to respond to emotional distress. Those who are securely attached are better adjusted [16], and insecure attachments are more common in those who have suffered childhood maltreatment [15]. This attachment style has been associated with a small but significant increase in substance use.

Peer influences during adolescence are also important in determining drinking patterns because of peer pressure. Involvement with peers who use alcohol and engage in deviant behaviour (such as vandalism, truanting, minor theft) is a predictor of AUD in adolescence. Deprivation in childhood, which as just discussed is associated with AUD, is also associated with increased likelihood of entering deviant peer groups. Conversely, feeling involved with school, having high educational expectations and high school achievement appeared to be protective [8].

Childhood Externalising Behaviour

Externalising behaviour is a broad term for problem behaviour related to the external environment – physical aggression, destruction of property, breaking rules, cheating, lying and hyperactivity. Apart from the inclusion of hyperactivity, the features of externalising behaviour are similar to antisocial behaviour in adults. Externalising behaviour in childhood or early adolescence, whether captured via a questionnaire, or via a diagnosis of conduct disorder or oppositional defiant disorder, is predictive of later AUD (reviewed in [8] and [17]). Evidence for the relationship present in some studies only if externalising behaviour was present at two time points, suggesting that early intervention could change this trajectory.

Social and Political Architecture

'In societies which have an extremely high degree of acceptance of large daily alcohol consumption, the presence of any small vulnerability, whether psychological or physical, will suffice for exposure to the risk of addiction.' So wrote E. M. Jellinek in 1960 [18].

Beyond the immediate social network, the broader political and social architecture can determine levels of alcohol use and thereby the potential for AUD. Globally, although the percentage of current drinkers has decreased by 5 per cent between the years 2000 and 2016, the overall total alcohol consumption per capita (APC) has increased. APC is a measure of how many litres of pure ethanol is consumed on average per person in a year. It has increased from 5.7 l to 6.4 l. As this is spread across the total population (current drinkers and current abstainers), this translates to an increase of 4 l (from 11.1 l to 15.1 l) over this period in those who actually consume alcohol [19]. There are distinct regional variations. For example, consumption in the World Health Organization (WHO) Europe region is declining and in the WHO South-east Asia and WHO Western Pacific regions increasing. These trends have been forecasted to continue. While there are many factors that play a role, wealth, religion and alcohol policy have been identified as three key determinants [20].

Worldwide the most striking difference in abstinence rates is seen between the WHO Organisation Eastern Mediterranean Region (EMR) and WHO Region of the Americas, where the rates are 94.9 per cent and 16.9 per cent respectively. Many of the countries residing in the EMR are Muslim-majority, whose laws are based on the rules of the Quran, where alcohol is forbidden [19]. More than half the countries present have a total ban on alcohol [19]. It therefore is comprehendible that the rates of consumption have remained low and resistant to change.

Alcohol is a luxury commodity and for many in lower-income countries is unaffordable. For example, in Jakarta to buy a bottle of whisky costs almost six times the average daily income, compared to Zurich where it costs less than a sixth [21]. Therefore consumption is lower-income countries is lower. Even when the informal or 'unrecorded' market is taken into consideration, this holds true. The informal market consists of any alcohol product that is outside government regulation, such as home brews or black market sales [19]. The increased consumption globally has been strongly linked to economic growth, making alcohol more affordable. Entwined within this is the role the alcohol industry plays in making the product more available, shifting social norms through marketing and influencing policy through self-regulation and assisting in the development of policy [20]. We know that effective alcohol policy can reduce both harmful drinking and dependence, evidence for which is discussed later in this chapter. Low-income countries have less well developed polices, indeed only 15 per cent have a national alcohol policy [19].

WHO's 'best buys' of decreasing availability, increasing taxes and banning advertisement are the most cost-effective interventions [19]. A prime example of these policies being used effectively was seen in Russia. In the early 2000s, one in two working-aged men in Russia died from alcohol-related causes. The Russian government instituted a range of measures, including marketing restrictions, monitoring alcohol production, a ban on internet alcohol sales, a 50 per cent tax increase on ethyl alcohol in 2004, followed by increase in excise tax, minimum unit pricing and reducing the availability of retail outlets in 2011. These changes were associated with a drop of 38 per cent in the prevalence of alcohol-dependent patients in statutory treatment services and a reduction in the prevalence of harmful use of 54 per cent [22]. This demonstrates how the prevalence of both harmful drinking and alcohol dependence is linked to alcohol policy. Other studies have demonstrated the power of policy. A price elasticity study from the United States study using the DSM-IV condition of alcohol abuse (roughly equivalent to ICD-10 harmful use) as an outcome, found that a 10 per cent increase in alcohol prices was associated with a decrease in prevalence of alcohol abuse by around 2 per cent and dependence by around 1 per cent [23].

Psychological Theories of Addiction

The evolution of psychological theories of addiction are summarised by Khantzian [24]. In psychodynamic theory, addiction was initially conceptualised as pleasure-driven and often linked to libidinal drives. For example, Freud theorised that substance addictions replaced the primary addiction of masturbation. Since then many different theories have arisen.

Addiction as a way of 'adapting' to inner psychological life has been prominent, whereby substances are used to manage emotions often from adolescence. It further hypothesises that through this individuals do not develop the ability to cope, thereby increasing the necessity of drugs and chances of dependence.

It has been argued that certain drugs can compensate for precarious ego defences. It is this idea that can explain why certain drugs appeal to certain individuals – for example, the opiates are calming and can reduce internal rage or disgust, which perhaps explains use of heroin in association with sex work. Object relations theory explains how a troubled sense of self, derived from our childhood experiences, affects how we attach to others. It reduces our ability to depend on individuals and increases our chance of turning to substances to maintain our emotional well-being.

The self-medication hypothesis suggests that rather than take substances for the high, they are used to maintain equilibrium. The substance counteracts their psychological pain. Yet, it does not remove it; rather, it creates an existence of continual relief and suffering that feels more controllable. This idea has been developed in the allostasis model of addiction proposed by George Koob (see later in this chapter, Pulling It Together), which has elaborated a neurobiological mechanism for this.

Classical and operant conditions lie at the heart of learning theory models of addiction. Classical conditioning explains how addictions can be maintained, particularly focusing on cravings. An environmental stimulus such as drug paraphernalia is paired with the effect of taking the drug, after a while the drug paraphernalia elicits a cue or craving by itself. In operant conditioning the substance is a reinforcer of behaviour, either positive by creating an enhanced state or negative by reducing an unpleasant state, such as withdrawal. This gave rise to Hull's drive-reduction theory where individuals seek to maintain homeostasis through satisfying their drives, which in this situation would be their cravings. Social learning theory places emphasis on learning behaviours through the observation of others, explaining why if our parents consume high levels of alcohol, we are more likely to. More recent transtheoretical models have sought to bring these principals together. One example is the PRIME model, which explains our motivations as a way of understanding addictive behaviour (see Chapter 2).

Neuropharmacology of Alcohol Dependence

How does the transition to alcohol dependence actually work, on a neurobiological level? We know from animal studies that it is actually quite hard to get an animal dependent on alcohol, because the taste is aversive. Usually alcohol is given in a sweetened mixture to increase the palatability (like a rodent alcopop) but even then only certain strains of rats will drink enough to develop dependence and it is a distinctive enough trait to influence their name – for example, the Sardinian alcohol-preferring rat. One of the compelling pieces of evidence for the neurobiological contribution to dependence is that once it has been established, alcohol-dependent rats will relapse much like any human, starting to consume large volumes of alcohol after a period of abstinence almost immediately.

A consistent association with development of dependence across substances and species is that the greater the dose and frequency of intake, the quicker the development of dependence – the government's advice about two alcohol-free days a week could be considered to guard against this by limiting intake. There is evidence that this association may be in part responsible for the moderate (~50 per cent) genetic association with alcohol dependence and the observed clustering of alcohol dependence in families, although this has multiple mechanisms (see the previous section). About 40 per cent of people with a family history of alcohol dependence have a reduced sensitivity to the effects of alcohol such as sedation and incoordination (versus 8 per cent of controls) (reviewed in [25]). This may lead to a less aversive experience of alcohol and an ability to drink more, with a concomitant increased risk of transition to dependence. Indeed, it has been associated with a fourfold risk of developing alcohol dependence over the next ten years [24] and is in part genetically determined (heritability of 0.4–0.6) (reviewed in [25]). Interestingly, it has been found that people with a family history of alcoholism have a reduced sedative response to thiopental, a barbiturate which acts via GABA-A receptors, suggesting that sensitivity to alcohol transmission is mediated by this pathway (see below) [26]. NMDA-related differences may also pre-date alcohol dependence: ketamine, which inhibits NMDA transmission, produces a greater stimulant effect relative to sedative effect in people with a family history of alcohol dependence.

An acute dose of alcohol has many pharmacological effects. It leads to the release of endorphins, associated with pleasure. It is associated with release of dopamine in the mesolimbic tract, which tells your brain that something important has happened – and a neurobiological event associated with all drugs of abuse. Alcohol also potentiates the action of GABA at GABA-A receptors, the chloride ion channels that mediate inhibition of neurotransmission [27]. At the same time, alcohol reduces NMDA-mediated glutamate transmission [28] – in fact, experimental participants report that moderate intoxication with the NMDA antagonist ketamine (at a dose lower than the range associated with psychotic phenomena) feels a lot like having around 12 units of alcohol.

The brain adapts to chronic drinking, and the adaptations appear to persist in abstinence. You may have noticed that alcohol-dependent patients may relapse to very high alcohol intake immediately and are able to tolerate it. Similarly, rodents exposed to high doses of alcohol exhibit reduced incoordination when re-exposed after weeks of abstinence and in the absence of changes in alcohol metabolism or clearance [29]. Understanding the adaptations that occur in GABA and glutamate transmission is particularly important in understanding alcohol withdrawal – one of the diagnostic criteria, and perhaps more important features of alcohol dependence – and its treatment. Historically, the rewarding experience of acute drug use has been emphasised as being most important for driving relapse – the clinical hallmark of addiction – and withdrawal has been dismissed as unimportant because relapse risk outlasts it. However, this is being re-evaluated with increasing recognition that the affective disturbances and dysregulation of hormonal and neurochemical stress systems that occur during withdrawal outlast the physical signs by several weeks [30].

GABA-A Receptors

GABA is the main inhibitory neurotransmitter in the central nervous system and is widely distributed, binding to both ionotropic and metabotropic receptors. The GABA-A receptor is a large and beautiful ionotropic receptor which looks like a child's drawing of a daisy under the electron microscope. It has five transmembrane proteins – two alpha, two beta and a gamma, arranged around a central pore. There are six different forms of alpha protein and the distribution and function of GABA-A receptors differs according to which kind of alpha protein forms part of the receptor. GABA-A alpha-1 subtype receptors are widely distributed, for example, but alpha-5 receptors, which seem to be important in alcohol-related amnesia, are concentrated in the hippocampus and nucleus accumbens. If you give humans a drug that selectively blocks GABA-A alpha-5 transmission, they get as drunk but remember better [31] – to their potential mortification. The GABA gene subtype most commonly associated with alcohol dependence in genetic studies encodes GABA-A alpha-2 subtype receptor subunit. GABA-A alpha-2 subtype receptors mediate anxiolytic effects of alcohol.

Chronic alcohol intake is associated with a reduction in GABA-A receptor density in brain both preclinically (i.e. in animal models of alcohol dependence – reviewed in [35]) and in alcohol-dependent patients. The sensitivity to GABA is also reduced in animals exposed to chronic alcohol, possibly because less GABA-sensitive subunits are substituted for more GABA sensitive ones, or more sensitive types are internalised [27]. In effect, the 'break on the brain' is removed which accounts for tolerance to sedative effects when large doses of alcohol are being ingested, but has catastrophic results when alcohol is suddenly removed – for example, when someone who is alcohol-dependent runs out of money (see Figure 6.1).

GABA-B Receptors

There has been increasing interest in GABA-B receptors in alcohol dependence in the last decade. GABA-B receptors are metabotropic and modulate release of numerous neuro-transmitters including dopamine. GABA-B agonism reduces release of dopamine in response to drugs of abuse. Chronic alcohol administration is associated with decreased GABA-B receptor expression (reviewed in [33]). Baclofen, a GABA-B agonist, reduces both alcohol drinking in preclinical paradigms exploring escalation of alcohol use, and alcohol seeking in abstinent alcohol-dependent rats (reviewed in [33]), although its clinical efficacy as relapse prevention treatment in patient populations is contested. A recent human challenge study using baclofen as a probe of GABA-B function in alcohol dependence found a reduction in both subjective experience of, and growth hormone response to, baclofen, suggesting that reduced GABA-B function occurs in alcohol dependence as well as rodent models [34].

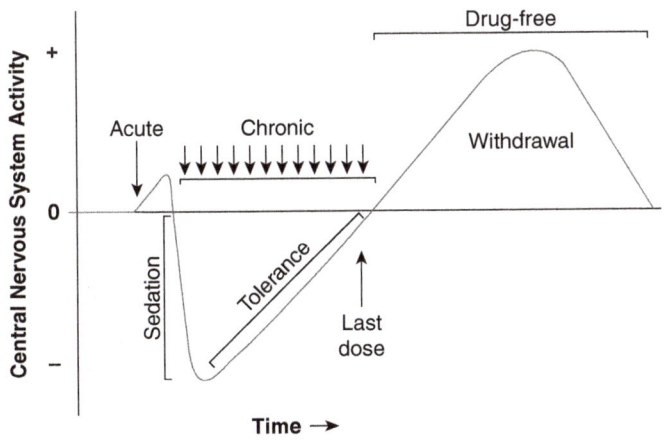

Figure 6.1 Neurobiological mechanism of alcohol withdrawal (reproduced from Finn and Crabbe 1997 (32))

Glutamate Transmission and NMDA Receptors

Glutamate plasticity in the mesolimbic-cortical loop is considered fundamental to the transition to addiction to many substances [35]. This is certainly the case in alcohol dependence and alcohol has direct pharmacological effects on glutamate release and glutamate receptor function across NMDA, kainite, AMPA and, to a lesser extent, metabotropic glutamate receptors (reviewed in [36]).

One of the highest affinity targets for alcohol in the brain is the NMDA receptor, an ionotropic glutamate receptor which is widely distributed [28]. NMDA receptor function is highly regulated – in addition to glutamate binding, opening is determined by a degree of depolarisation of the neuron, phosphorylation and clustering of receptors. Alcohol is an NMDA receptor antagonist – this is why ketamine is considered 'alcohol-like' in terms of its subjective effects. Ketamine's psychotomimetic effects are not seen with alcohol. This is because of alcohol's relatively selective affinity for NR2B and NR2A subtypes of the NMDA receptor, as well as alcohol's effects on other cation channels and neurotransmitter systems. In response to chronic alcohol consumption, NMDA receptors, particularly NR2A and NR2B subunits, are upregulated, as well as kainite and AMPA receptors. NMDA receptors also become less sensitive to the effect of alcohol and other antagonists, such as ketamine. Alcohol-dependent patients in early abstinence show reduced cognitive, perceptual and dysphoric responses to ketamine.

With withdrawal of alcohol, the inhibition of the NMDA system is suddenly released, and with all the adaptations aimed at increasing transmission in the presence of alcohol, the system goes into overdrive. Increased NMDA-mediated calcium influx results in seizures, delirium and neurotoxicity. The seizure threshold is lowered with repeated episodes of withdrawal in animals and humans [37] via a mechanism akin to kindling in epilepsy. Lamotrigine, which reduces glutamate release, memantine, an NMDA antagonist, and topiramate, a kainate and AMPA antagonist, have been tested as alternatives to benzodiazepines for alcohol withdrawal. All have been reported to show equivalent efficacy to diazepam in controlling alcohol withdrawal symptoms.

Opioid System

There are three classical opioid receptors: mu, kappa and delta (MORs, KORs and DORs). All are inhibitory G-protein coupled receptors. Endorphins have a greater affinity for MORs, while enkephalins have a greater affinity for DORs and dynorphins for KORs. Opioid receptor function is synergistic in some areas (e.g. analgesia), but opposing in affective regulation – MOR stimulation is associated with euphoria and KOR dysphoria. Little is known about DOR function in humans.

MORs and KORs appear to have different roles in the pathophysiology of alcohol dependence: MOR transmission appears to be involved in reward driving initial escalation in use in operant conditioning paradigms, while KOR is involved in the dysphoria which occurs during withdrawal and abstinence. MORs are widely expressed in brain areas involved in addiction, such as the VTA, nucleus accumbens, amygdala and prefrontal cortex. In the VTA, release of endorphins inhibits GABA interneurons, which in turn stop inhibits dopamine neurons, facilitating dopamine release. Alcohol is associated with endorphin release, thus stimulating MORs. It is via its action on endorphins that it causes dopamine release, as it can be blocked by naltrexone, an opioid receptor antagonist. Activation of the mesolimbic tract in response to monetary reward is also attenuated by nalmefene, a MOR antagonist, in heavy drinkers receiving alcohol during the challenge [38]. It is therefore unsurprising that there is preclinical evidence that reduced MOR/endorphin function is associated with a lower propensity to addiction. MOR or endorphin knockout mice are resistant to the rewarding effects of alcohol. Operant conditioning related to alcohol can also be blocked by naltrexone. In alcohol-dependent patients, there is a general increase in opioid receptors throughout the brain [39], and an increase in expression of mu-opioid receptors in the nucleus accumbens, which is correlated with craving [40], although this may normalise with protracted abstinence.

KORs are also widely distributed as presynaptic receptors on dopamine efferents to the nucleus accumbens, and the extended amygdala. Dynorphin, the endogenous ligand of KORs, is associated with preclinical depressive phenotypes and can be stimulated by corticotrophin-releasing factor (CRF) (i.e. stress – see the next section) [41]. Dynorphin is released following acute alcohol administration and inhibits dopamine release – suggesting that the opioid system is finely balanced in regulating reward. With chronic drinking, dynorphin expression is increased and is implicated in the dysphoria associated with withdrawal. Dynorphin antagonists and KOR knockout mice do not show alcohol seeking in response to stress [42]. In contrast to MOR antagonists, KOR antagonists block alcohol administration in alcohol-dependent rather than alcohol naïve rats only [43]. Understanding the separate roles of MOR and KOR in the aetiology of alcohol dependence is of clinical importance when considering anti-craving medications. Nalmefene, a novel opioid antagonist, may be expected to perform better with respect to stress-induced craving than naltrexone, because it is a partial agonist at the KOR and binds to it with greater affinity than naltrexone. A recent indirect meta-analysis suggested that nalmefene may perform better than naltrexone with respect to quantity and frequency of alcohol intake, which may relate to its action at the KOR [44].

Stress, HPA Axis, CRF and Alcohol Dependence

As well as childhood stress already described, stressful events in young adulthood are associated with an increase in alcohol use and alcohol is used as a means of coping with occupational stress and following catastrophic events (cited in [45]). In addition, alcohol has a direct influence on HPA axis function, as well as extra-hypothalamic corticotrophin releasing factor and glucocorticoid expression [46]. While acute alcohol only causes an increase in cortisol at high dose, chronic heavy drinking is associated with changes in HPA axis function. Intoxicated alcohol-dependent patients and patients in alcohol withdrawal have raised morning cortisol, but cortisol is higher in withdrawal than during drinking, suggesting that withdrawal represents an acute-on-chronic stressor. ACTH and cortisol levels have been found to decrease after two to six weeks of abstinence [47].

Dexamethasone suppression tests are also abnormal in a proportion of alcohol-dependent patients, most commonly in early abstinence (reviewed in [48]). CRF stimulation tests show an impaired cortisol response in alcohol dependent men, but not women. HPA axis hyporesponsiveness has also been found in alcohol-dependent patients using psychological and physiological stimulation paradigms (e.g. [47, 49]).

Chronic elevation in corticosterone – the rodent equivalent of cortisol – has been associated with persistent changes in glucocorticoid receptor and corticotrophic-releasing-factor expression both within and outside the hypothalamus, with implications for stress responsiveness. The extended amygdala is an organ (based on shared neuronal composition and connections) composed of the amygdala, the bed nucleus of the stria terminalis and the transition zone in the posteromedial shell of the nucleus accumbens. It is important in the emotional response to stress and to stress-related learning. CRF mRNA expression is increased in the extended amygdala while it is decreased in the hypothalamus. This accounts for the apparently counter-intuitive observation that alcohol-dependent patients exhibit an attenuated HPA axis response to stress while simultaneously showing an exaggerated emotional response to stress, and stress-induced craving and relapse [50]. CRF1 receptor antagonists blocked alcohol-withdrawal-related anxiety and stress-induced reinstatement of alcohol seeking in preclinical models of alcohol dependence [51]. These insights have driven much clinical interest in developing CRF1 antagonists for the treatment of alcohol dependence, but early proofs of concept experimental pharmacology studies have not demonstrated any effect on cue-related or stress-related craving or anxiety in alcohol-dependent patients. This may relate to pharmacokinetic problems or differences in experimental paradigms between preclinical and clinical research: CRF antagonists inhibited stress-related but not cue-related reinstatement. Alternatively, plasticity that may occur between the phase of addiction that animal models of alcohol dependence represent (animal research is necessarily relatively short term) and the phase at which patients present following many years of drinking may account for this failure of translation.

Putting It Together: Allostasis as a Model of Addiction

The theory of **allostasis** developed by George Koob proposes that stress is as important for the development of addiction as reward (see Figure 6.2). Allostasis is derived from

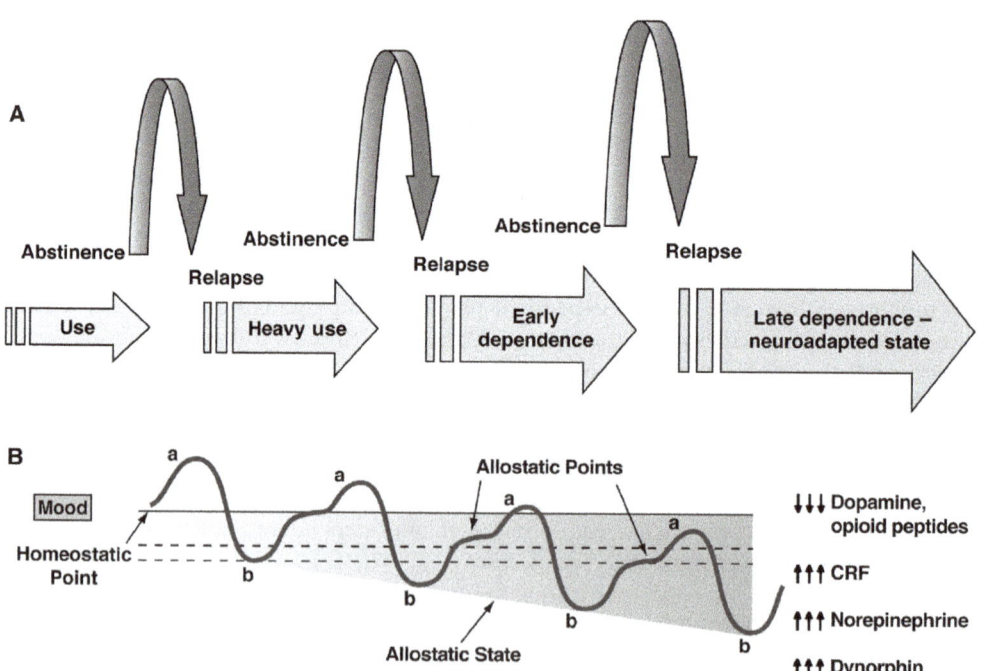

Figure 6.2 Schematic of allostasis model of addiction (from Koob, 2019 [46])

homeostasis – the tendency for the body to self-correct in order to maintain conditions within a physiological range. The term 'allostasis' itself means a chronic deviation from homeostasis. With respect to alcohol dependence, the reduced reward responsiveness coupled with increased stress responsiveness results over time in a chronic dysphoric state, where alcohol use is an attempt to return to baseline, thereby driving increased consumption/dependence. This theory addresses the clinical observation that affective changes, sleep disturbance and stress responsiveness associated with withdrawal outlast physical withdrawal symptoms by weeks to months and that relapse often relates to stress, poor sleep or low mood, rather than euphoric recall [30].

Mental Disorders and Risk of Alcohol Dependence

There is an increased prevalence of alcohol dependence in patients suffering from a variety of psychiatric conditions (see Chapter 9). Any trainee psychiatrist will recognise that patients with alcohol dependence often present because of psychiatric symptoms or in psychiatric crisis. For example, 55 per cent of those detained under Section 136 of the Mental Health Act are intoxicated with alcohol. Globally, alcohol dependence carries a ninefold increase in risk of suicide [52]. The relationship between alcohol dependence and other mental disorders is complex. Broadly speaking, there are three hypotheses relating to the relationship:

- **Self-medication:** people drink to excess in order to medicate their symptoms, and this then develops its own momentum.
- **Shared vulnerability:** psychiatric disorder and alcohol dependence involve a shared genetic, psychological or environmental risk factor.
- **Reverse causality:** alcohol dependence precipitates the psychiatric disturbance.

As this chapter considers the aetiology of alcohol dependence, we will only consider evidence for the first two.

Anxiety Disorders

Family studies have demonstrated that relatives of patients with anxiety disorders have higher odds of alcohol dependence and that those of patients with alcohol dependence have higher odds of having an anxiety disorder. Among the anxiety disorders, the relationship between social anxiety and PTSD and alcohol dependence are most clearly demonstrated.

Forty-eight per cent of patients with a lifetime diagnosis of social anxiety in the United States have a lifetime diagnosis of alcohol dependence [53]. In longitudinal studies, social anxiety predates alcohol dependence or hazardous alcohol use, although in some studies this only applies to women [54]. Social anxiety increases the risk of alcohol dependence relative to other anxiety disorders [55] and the relationship remains where there are other comorbid psychiatric disorders [56]. The relationship is accentuated in women – they show higher rates of alcohol use disorder than men with social phobia.

The mechanism whereby social anxiety increases the risk of developing harmful use of alcohol or alcohol dependence may relate to the increased sensitivity of socially anxious people to peer pressure, as socially anxious people are more likely to drink in response to peer pressure. The direct effect of alcohol in reducing social anxiety seems accentuated in women.

Post-Traumatic Stress Disorder (PTSD)

PTSD and alcohol dependence are highly comorbid. Genetic model fitting studies of large twin samples suggest that a shared genetic vulnerability accounts for at least some of this (reviewed in [57]). There is also some support for the self-medication hypothesis: data primarily from the United States provides consistent evidence that there are stronger associations between trauma experienced as an adult and AUD in men who develop PTSD following in trauma than in those who do not. The increased risk of AUD in the absence of PTSD appears to be present for women only.

Depression

Depression in the context of alcohol dependence is often attributed to its physiological effects and the associated consequences for relationships, work and finances. However, there is also a small body of longitudinal research examining depression as an antecedent of frequent alcohol use and AUD in adolescence and young adulthood. A Finnish twin study found that having depression aged 14 increased the odds of frequent alcohol use and recurrent intoxication twofold, providing support for the self-medication model [58]. However, in two studies, the relationship was moderated by personality factors – that is, more consistent with a shared vulnerability model. In one, depression increased the risk of alcohol abuse and alcohol dependence around twofold, but only in those adolescents with Conduct Disorder [17]. In another, the relationship between depression and increase in drinking was accounted for by the personality traits associated with neuroticism [59]. A large US twin study also supports a shared vulnerability – both genetic and environmental factors which predisposed to depression overlapped with alcohol dependence although these shared factors appeared to be sex-specific [60].

Bipolar Disorder

A recent international systematic review and meta-analysis of AUD in Bipolar Disorder found a point prevalence of 25–30 per cent in patient samples [61]. A meta-analysis of lifetime prevalence of AUD in people with Bipolar Disorder estimated a mean prevalence of 35 per cent in men and 16.9 per cent in women – that is, an odds of AUD of 2.8 relative to the general population [61]. The risk is present across the spectrum of Bipolar Disorder, including Bipolar II Disorder. Forty-one per cent of people with Bipolar Disorder report self-medication – the use of alcohol to control mood symptoms – when asked [62], more commonly for mania than for depression. They also report drinking for different reasons when manic, depressed or euthymic.

There is also evidence of a common neuropharmacological mechanism. Young men at high risk of developing bipolar disorder show the same attenuated behavioural response to alcohol as those with a family history of alcohol dependence [63]. The novel antidepressant, ketamine, also seems to be more effective in those patients with depression in bipolar disorder and those with a positive family history of alcoholism.

Personality and Personality Disorder

Is there an addictive personality? Longitudinal data suggest that several personality profiles are at risk of alcohol dependence: those who have low conscientiousness and high extraversion, who drink in association with positive affective states; those with low emotional stability, who drink to manage negative affective states; and those with low conscientiousness and low agreeableness – that is, aligned with antisocial personality traits [64]. Another birth cohort (n = 1,100) found that the single personality trait of novelty seeking predicted development of alcohol dependence with the risk in the highest quartile double that in the lowest quartile [65]. Another study demonstrated that personality traits, particularly impulsivity, moderated the association between depression and increase in alcohol use [59].

These associations are accentuated when they relate to personality disorder, rather than traits. Epidemiological studies show high rates of comorbidity between personality disorder, particularly Emotionally Unstable and Antisocial Personality Disorders, and alcohol dependence. This has long been recognised in alcohol research, to the extent that Cloninger's typology of alcohol dependence based on adoption studies characterised Type II alcohol dependence as being highly heritable, having high novelty seeking tendencies and displaying criminal behaviour, with onset before the age of 25 [66]. Investigation into whether particular aspects of EUPD and ASPD is associated with risk, a large prospective study examining each diagnostic criterion, found that childhood history of conduct disorder was associated with a threefold increase in the odds of developing an alcohol use disorder, while impulsive self-harm was associated with a fivefold increase in odds [67]. Taken together, it seems that the most consistent finding is an association with impulsivity – in the general population and in those with personality disorders and an increased odds of developing alcohol use disorders.

References

1 Public Health England. Estimates of alcohol dependent adults in England. 2017.

2 NHS Digital. Statistics on Alcohol, England, 2018. Office for National Statistics.

3 Ness J., Hawton K., Bergen H., Cooper J., Steeg S., Kapur N. et al. Alcohol use and misuse, self-harm and subsequent mortality: An epidemiological and longitudinal study from the multicentre study of self-harm in England. *Emergency Medicine Journal.* 2015; 32: 793–9

4 Windfuhr K., Kapur N. Suicide and mental illness: A clinical review of 15 years' findings from the UK National Confidential Inquiry into Suicide. *British Medical Bulletin.* 2011; **100** (1): 101–21.

5 Holst C., Tolstrup J. S., Sørensen H. J., Pisinger V. S. C., Becker U. Parental alcohol use disorder with and without other mental disorders and offspring alcohol use disorder. *Acta Psychiatrica Scandinavica.* 2019; 1–10.

6 Reilly M. T., Noronha A., Goldman D., Koob G. F. Genetic studies of alcohol dependence in the context of the addiction cycle. *Neuropharmacology.* 2017; **122**: 3–21.

7 Tawa E. A., Hall S. D., Lohoff F. W. Overview of the genetics of alcohol use disorder. *Alcohol and Alcoholism.* 2016; **51** (5): 507–14.

8 Meque I., Salom C., Betts K. S., Alati R. Predictors of alcohol use disorders among young adults: A systematic review of longitudinal studies. *Alcohol and Alcoholism.* 2019; **54** (3): 310–24.

9 Kaynak Ö., Winters K. C., Cacciola J., Kirby K. C., Arria A. M. Providing alcohol for underage youth: What messages should we be sending parents? *Journal of Studies on Alcohol and Drugs.* 2014; **75** (4): 590–605.

10 Mattick R. P., Clare P. J., Aiken A., Wadolowski M., Hutchinson D., Najman J. et al. Association of parental supply of alcohol with adolescent drinking, alcohol-related harms, and alcohol use disorder symptoms: A prospective cohort study. *Lancet Public Health.* 2018; **3** (2): e64–71.

11 Melchior M., Moffitt T. E., Milne B. J., Poulton R., Caspi A. Why do children from

socioeconomically disadvantaged families suffer from poor health when they reach adulthood? A life-course study. *American Journal of Epidemiology.* 2007; **166** (8): 966–74.

12   Dom G., De Wilde B., Hulstijn W., Sabbe B. Traumatic experiences and posttraumatic stress disorders: Differences between treatment-seeking early- and late-onset alcoholic patients. *Comprehensive Psychiatry.* 2007; **48** (2): 178–85.

13   Felitti J., Ana R.F., Nordenberg D., Williamson D. F., Spitz A. M., Edwards V., Koss M. P., Marks J. S. Relationship of childhood abuse and household dysfunction to many of the leading causes of death in adults: The Adverse Childhood Experiences Study. *American Journal of Preventive Medicine.* 1998; **14** (4): 245–58.

14   Schwandt M. L., Heilig M. D., Hommer D. W., George M. D., Ramchandani V. A. Childhood trauma exposure and alcohol dependence severity in adulthood: Mediation by emotional abuse severity and neuroticism. *Alcoholism: Clinical and Experimental Research.* 2013; **37** (6): 984–92.

15   Baer J., Daly Martinez C. Child maltreatment and insecure attachment: a meta-analysis. *Journal of Reproductive and Infant Psychology.* 2006; **24** (3): 187–97

16   Fairbairn C. E., Briley D. A., Kang D., Fraley R. C., Hankin B. L., Ariss T. A meta-analysis of longitudinal associations between substance use and interpersonal attachment security. *Psychological Bulletin.* 2018; **144** (5): 532–55.

17   Pardini D., White H. R., Stouthamer-Loeber M. Early adolescent psychopathology as a predictor of alcohol use disorders by young adulthood. *Drug and Alcohol Dependence.* 2007; **88** (S1): S38–S49.

18   Jellinek E. M. *The Disease Concept of Alcoholism.* New Haven, CT: Hillhouse Press; 1960.

19   World Health Organization. *Global Status Report on Alcohol and Health, 2018.* Geneva: WHO; 2018.

20   Manthey J., Shield K. D., Rylett M., Probst C., Rehm J. Global alcohol exposure between 1990 and 2017 and forecasts until 2030: A modelling study. *Lancet.* 2019; **393** (10190): 2893–502.

21   Kan M., Lau M. Comparing alcohol affordability in 65 countries worldwide. *Drug and Alcohol Review.* 2014; **32**: 19–26.

22   Lancet. Russia's alcohol policy: a continuing success story. *Lancet* [Internet]. 2019; **394** (10205): 1205.

23   Farrell S., Manning W. G., Finch M. D. Alcohol dependence and the price of alcoholic beverages. *Journal of Health Economics.* 2003; **22** (1): 117–47.

24   Khantzian E. Understanding addictive vulnerability: an evolving psychodynamic perspective. *Neuropsychoanalysis.* 2013; **5** (1): 5–21.

25   Schuckit M. A., Smith T. L., Kalmijn J., Danko G. P. A cross-generational comparison of alcohol challenges at about age 20 in 40 father-offspring pairs. *Alcoholism: Clinical and Experimental Research.* 2005; **29** (11): 1921–7.

26   Petrakis I. L., Kerfoot K., Pittman B., Perrino A., Koretski J., Newcomb J. et al. Subjective effects of thiopental in young adults with and without a family history of alcoholism. *Journal of Addiction Research and Therapy.* 2012; **S7** (2): 6336–49.

27   Krystal J. H., Staley J., Mason G., Petrakis I. L., Kaufman J., Harris R. A. et al. γ-aminobutyric acid type A receptors and alcoholism: Intoxication, dependence, vulnerability, and treatment. *Archives of General Psychiatry.* 2006; **63** (9): 957–68.

28   Krystal J. H., Petrakis I. L., Mason G., Trevisan L., D'Souza D. C. N-methyl-D-aspartate glutamate receptors and alcoholism: Reward, dependence, treatment, and vulnerability. *Pharmacology and Therapeutics.* 2003; **99** (1): 79–94.

29   Rimondini R., Sommer W. H., Dall'Olio R., Heilig M. Long-lasting tolerance to alcohol following a history of dependence. *Addiction Biology.* 2008; **13** (1): 26–30.

30.   Heilig M., Egli M., Crabbe J.C., Becker H. C. Acute withdrawal, protracted

abstinence and negative affect in alcoholism: Are they linked? *Addiction Biology* . 2010; **15** (2): 169–84.

31 Nutt D. J., Besson M., Wilson S. J., Dawson G. R., Lingford-Hughes A. R. Blockade of alcohol's amnestic activity in humans by an α5 subtype benzodiazepine receptor inverse agonist. *Neuropharmacology.* 2007; **53**(7): 810–20.

32 Finn D. A., Crabbe J. C. Exploring Alcohol Withdrawal Syndrome. *Alcohol Health and Research World* . 1997; **21**(1): 149–56.

33 Maccioni P., Colombo G. Role of the GABAB receptor in alcohol-seeking and drinking behavior. *Alcohol.* 2009; **43** (7): 555–8.

34 Durant C. F., Paterson L. M., Turton S., Wilson S. J., Myers J.F. M., Muthukumaraswamy S. et al. Using Baclofen to explore GABA-B receptor function in alcohol dependence: Insights from pharmacokinetic and pharmacodynamic measures. *Frontiers in Psychiatry.* 2018; **9** (December): 1–17.

35 Kalivas P. W., LaLumiere R., Knackstedt L., Shen H. Glutamate transmission in addiction. *Neuropharmacology.* 2009; **56** (Suppl. 1): 169–73.

36 Alasmari F., Goodwani S., McCullumsmith R. E., Sari Y. Role of glutamatergic system and mesocorticolimbic circuits in alcohol dependence. *Progress in Neurobiology.* 2018; **171** (May): 32–49.

37 Becker H. C. Kindling in alcohol withdrawal. *Alcohol Health and Research World.* 1998; **22** (1): 25–33.

38 Quelch D., Mick I., McGonigle J., Ramos A. C., Flechais R. C., Bolstridge M., Rabiner E., Wal M. B., Newbould R. B., Steiniger-Brach B., van den Berg F., Boyce M., Østergaard Nilausen D., Lingford-Hughes A. A. Nalmefene reduces reward anticipation in alcohol dependence: An experimental functional magnetic resonance imaging study. *Biological Psychiatry.* 2017; **81** (11): 941–8.

39 Williams T. M., Davies S. J. C., Taylor L. G., Daglish M. R. C., Hammers A., Brooks D. J., Nutt D. J., Lingford-Hughes A. R. Brain

opioid receptor binding in early abstinence from alcohol dependence and relationship to craving: An [11C]diprenorphine PET study. *European Neuropsychopharmacology.* 2009; **19** (10): 740–8.

40 Heinz M. D., Reimold M. D., Wrase J., Croissant B., Mundle G., Dohmen B. M., Braus D. H., Schumann G., Machulla H. J., Bares R., Mann K. Correlation of stable elevations in striatal mu-opioid receptor availability in detoxified alcoholic patients with alcohol craving. *Archives of General Psychiatry.* 2005; **62**(1): 57–64.

41 Lam M. P., Gianoulakis C. Effects of corticotropin-releasing hormone receptor antagonists on the ethanol-induced increase of dynorphin A1-8 release in the rat central amygdala. *Alcohol.* 2011; **45** (7): 621–30.

42 Funk D., Coen K., Le A. D. The role of kappa opioid receptors in stress-induced reinstatement of alcohol seeking in rats. *Brain and Behavior.* 2014; **4** (3): 356–67.

43 Walker B. M., Koob G. F. Pharmacological evidence for a motivational role of kappa-opioid systems in ethanol dependence. *Neuropsychopharmacology.* 2008; **33**: 643–52.

44 Soyka M., Friede M., Schnitker J. Comparing nalmefene and naltrexone in alcohol dependence: Are there any differences? Results from an indirect meta-analysis. *Pharmacopsychiatry.* 2016; **49** (2): 66–75.

45 Ramchandani V. A., Stangl B. L., Blaine S. K., Plawecki M. H., Schwandt M. L., Kwako L. E. et al. Stress vulnerability and alcohol use and consequences: From human laboratory studies to clinical outcomes. *Alcohol.* 2018; **72**: 75–88.

46 Koob G. F., Schulkin J. Addiction and stress: An allostatic view. *Neuroscience and Biobehavorial Reviews.* 2019; **106**: 245–62.

47 Errico A. L., King A. C., Lovallo W. R., Parsons O. A. Cortisol dysregulation and cognitive impairment in abstinent male alcoholics. *Alcoholism: Clinical and Experimental Research.* 2002; **26** (8): 1198–204.

48 Besemer F., Pereira A. M., Smit J. W. Alcohol-induced Cushing syndrome: Hypercortisolism caused by alcohol abuse. *Netherlands Journal of Medicine*. 2011; **69** (7): 318–23.

49 Junghanns K., Horbach R., Ehrenthal D., Blank S., Backhaus J. Cortisol awakening response in abstinent alcohol-dependent patients as a marker of HPA-axis dysfunction. *Psychoneuroendocrinology*. 2007; **32** (8–10): 1133–7.

50 Ramchandani V. A., Umhau J., Pavon F. J., Ruiz-Velasco V., Margas W., Sun H. et al. A genetic determinant of the striatal dopamine response to alcohol in men. *Molecular Psychiatry*. 2011; **16** (8): 809–17.

51 Koob G. F. Brain stress systems in the amygdala and addiction. *Brain Research*. 2009; **13** (1293): 61–75.

52 Ferrari A. J., Norman R. E., Freedman G., Baxter A. J., Pirkis J. E., Harris M. G., Page A., Carnahan E., Degenhardt L., Vos T., Whiteford H. A. The burden attributable to mental and substance use disorders as risk factors for suicide: Findings from the Global Burden of Disease Study 2010. *PLOS ONE*. 2014; **9** (4): e9136.

53 Grant B. F., Hasin D. S., Blanco C., Stinson F. S., Chou S. P., Goldstein R. B. The epidemiology of social anxiety disorder in the United States: Results from the National Epidemiologic Survey on Alcohol and Related Conditions. *Journal of Clinical Psychiatry*. 2005; **66** (1351–61).

54 Buckner J. D., Turner R. J. Social anxiety disorder as a risk factor for alcohol use disorders: A prospective examination of parental and peer influences. *Drug and Alcohol Dependency*. 2009; **100** (1–2): 128–37.

55 Kessler R.C., Crum R. M., Warner L. A., Nelson C. B., Schulenberg J., Anthony J. C. Lifetime co-occurrence of DSM-III-R Alcohol Abuse and Dependence with other psychiatric disorders in the National Comorbidity Survey. *Archives of General Psychiatry*. 1997; **54** (313–21).

56 Buckner J. D., Schmidt N. B., Lang A. R., Small J., Schlauch R. C., Lewinsohn P. M. Specificity of social anxiety disorder as a risk factor for alcohol and cannabis dependence. *Journal of Psychiatric Research*. 2008; **42**: 230–9.

57 Breslau N. The epidemiology of trauma, PTSD, and other posttrauma disorders. *Trauma, Violence, and Abuse*. 2009; **10** (3): 198–210.

58 Sihvola E., Rose R. J., Dick D. M., Pulkkinen L., Marttunen M., Kaprio J. Addictive substances in adolescence: A prospective study of adolescent Finnish twins. *Addiction*. 2008; **103** (12): 2045–53.

59 Mackie C. J., Castellanos-Ryan N., Conrod P. J. Personality moderates the longitudinal relationship between psychological symptoms and alcohol use in adolescents. *Alcoholism: Clinical and Experimental Research*. 2011; **35** (4): 703–16.

60 Prescott C. A., Aggen S. H., Kendler K. S. Sex-specific genetic influences on the comorbidity of alcoholism and major depression in a population-based sample of U.S. Twins. *The Primary Care Companion to The Journal of Clinical Psychiatry*. 2000; **2** (5): 186.

61 Hunt G. E., Malhi G. S., Cleary M., Lai H. M. X., Sitharthan T. Prevalence of comorbid bipolar and substance use disorders in clinical settings, 1990–2015: Systematic review and meta-analysis. *Journal of Affective Disorders* . 2016; **206**: 331–49.

62 Bolton J. M., Robinson J., Sareen J. Self-medication of mood disorders with alcohol and drugs in the National Epidemiologic Survey on Alcohol and Related Conditions. *Journal of Affective Disorders*. 2009; **115** (3): 367–75.

63 Yip S. W., Doherty J., Wakeley J., Saunders K., Tzagarakis C., de Wit H., Goodwin G. M., Rogers R. D. Ethanol Administration among young men with a broad bipolar phenotype. *Neuropsychopharmacology*. 2012; **37**: 1808–15.

64 Mezquita L., Bravo A. J., Ortet G., Pilatti A., Pearson M. R., Ibanez M. I. Cross-cultural examination of different personality pathways to alcohol use and misuse in

emerging adulthood. *Drug and Alcohol Dependence*. 2018; **192**: 193–200.

65 Foulds J. A., Boden J. M., Newton-Howes G. M., Mulder R. T., Horwood L. J. The role of novelty seeking as a predictor of substance use disorder outcomes in early adulthood. *Addiction*. 2017; **112** (9): 1629–37.

66 Cloninger C. R., Sigvardsson S., Bohman M. Type I and type II alcoholism: An update.

Alcohol Health and Research World. 1996; **20** (1): 18–23.

67 Rosenström T., Torvik F. A., Ystrom E., Czajkowski N. O., Gillespie N. A., Aggen S. H. et al. Prediction of alcohol use disorder using personality disorder traits: A twin study. *Addiction*. 2018; **113** (1): 15–24.

Alcohol Use Disorders: Clinical Features and Treatment

Duncan Raistrick and Gillian Tober

The Scope of Alcohol Misuse

Alcohol misuse is a common cause and complicating factor for both physical and mental health disorders. In the course of their careers, psychiatrists will see many patients and probably a colleague, family member or friend with a drinking problem. Psychiatrists will be more effective and empathic in their chosen specialty if the management of alcohol use disorders is embedded in their practice during training. It has been estimated that, of patients attending community psychiatric services, 25 per cent have a past year history of harmful drinking and 25 per cent are abstinent [1]. The high incidence of abstinence is indicative of a sizeable group of ex-drinkers. It is, however, striking that psychiatrists are often parsimonious with diagnoses describing alcohol use disorders and related problems. Notwithstanding the availability of empirical classifications, it is deemed sufficient simply to say that there is an alcohol problem, and yet psychiatrists are competent diagnosticians. Psychiatrists are also guardians of clinical governance, have a key role in treatment planning and have the repertoire of skills needed to deliver sophisticated interventions, including for alcohol use disorders with comorbidity. They have a responsibility to collect accurate health data and, to this end, have a role within their teams to encourage usage of correct terminology and to ensure that a scientific approach to understanding the clinical features and treatment of alcohol use disorders prevails. Elaborating on the basics of someone's alcohol use problem is clinically rewarding and need not be onerous.

A useful starting point for delivering on the roles and responsibilities of the psychiatrist is to have a familiarity with the World Health Organization International Classification of Diseases (ICD-11), which is used in the UK to codify health disorders and produce national statistics. An advantage of ICD-11 compared to the other major classification system, the Diagnostic Statistical Manual (DSM), is that it is clinician friendly – each disorder has a description which is meaningful to practitioners and open to clinical interpretation whereas DSM, perhaps because of its roots in research, is prescriptive of criteria that must be applied to determine the presence of a disorder. Moreover, DSM has a tendency to over-medicalise conditions which many consider to be normal behaviours. ICD-11 lists 13 alcohol use disorders, which nicely describe the scope of drinking problems from a mental health practitioner perspective. What follows are the definitions and ICD codes.

1 Disorders Directly Related to Consumption

Acute Intoxication (6C40.3) is the consequence of the pharmacological effects of alcohol and it includes impaired consciousness and cognition, disturbances of perception, lability of mood often accompanied by aggressive behaviour, impaired judgement and poor coordination. The most common complications are accidents, inhalation of vomit, gastritis and socially inappropriate behaviour of varying degrees. Intoxication, even if repeated often, does not necessarily lead to enduring harms. ICD-11 recognises a *Single Episode of Harmful Use (6C40.0)* and a *Harmful Pattern of Use (6C40.1)* as separate problems with consequences for the physical or mental health of an individual. Symptoms of neuro-adaptation develop after protracted or intense periods of drinking. Typically *Alcohol Withdrawal (6C40.4)* builds to a peak after some 8–12 hours of abstinence or significantly reduced consumption and is characterised by tremulousness, sweating, insomnia, anxiety, agitation and dysphoria. Withdrawal symptoms are generally not specific and so their recognition as withdrawal can be difficult – the most specific symptoms are whole body shakes and facial tremors. Withdrawal may be complicated by *Seizures (6C40.42)*, which peak around 24–36 hours, and *Delirium (6C40.4Z)*, which peaks around 48–72 hours and is thought to be distinct from the more common withdrawal syndrome in that some add-itional organic triggers such as concurrent infection or autonomic hyper-arousal are probably required. Some see the manifestation of withdrawal symptoms as a watershed, tantamount to a disorder called 'physical dependence', but this is confusing terminology and it is clearer to use the term 'neuro-adaptation' to refer to tolerance and withdrawal.

2 Alcohol Dependence Syndrome

The *Dependence Syndrome (6C40.2)* arises from repeated or continuous alcohol consump-tion and includes: a strong desire for alcohol sometimes referred to as craving, difficulty controlling its use and continued drinking in the face of adverse consequences. Neuro-adaptive changes of tolerance and withdrawal are commonly present but not an essential part of the syndrome. Dependence is best considered a psychological state, experienced as a need, which is the result of repeated reinforcement of drinking in varied circumstances, including the relief of withdrawal symptoms, if these are present. It is not uncommon for individuals who are heavy drinkers to have low levels of dependence. Dependence is a stressful condition, which is easily mistaken for anxiety or depression – dependence rather than consumption per se is likely to lead people to seek help. It is important because it is a predictor of difficulty in making changes to drinking. ICD-11 recognises that dependence may be in full or partial remission: in other words, recovery is a proper and achievable treatment goal.

3 Alcohol Induced Mental Health Disorders

In addition to *Delirium*, ICD-11 describes alcohol-induced disorders that cannot be explained by intoxication or withdrawal alone and are of sufficient severity to warrant independent clinical attention: *Psychotic Disorder (6C40.6)*, which includes pathological jealousy; *Mood Disorder (6C40.70)*; and *Anxiety Disorder (6C40.71)*. A further diagnostic criterion is that these disorders are not better explained by an alternative aetiology. The important treatment implication is that there is a good probability that alcohol-induced, sometimes referred to as secondary, disorders will resolve after a period of abstinence. What this means is that there should be no hurry to treat – for example, by prescribing anti-depressants – but there should also be a readiness to treat should the severity of the problem require it, or if resolution does not follow from a reasonable period of abstinence. The psychiatrist may well find it challenging to reconcile the expectations of patients who want immediate symptom relief with the need to avoid unnecessary treatment.

Amnestic Disorder due to high blood alcohol levels *(6D72.10)* may be fragmented or continuous and is usually short lived, but occasionally complex and protracted behaviours occur while in an amnesic state. The *Wernicke-Korsakoff Syndrome (5B5A.1)* is caused by thiamine deficiency. *Wernicke's Encephalopathy (5B5A.10)*, which is often subclinical, is characterised by a low-grade confusional state, severe amnesia, diplopia and ataxia. *Korsakoff's Psychosis (5B5A.11)* typically follows on from Wernicke's Encephalopathy and is characterised by severe short-term memory problems, the transposition in time of older memories and confabulation, the invention of memories to fill gaps. Korsakoff's is a form of permanent brain damage commonly requiring 24-hour supervision, and so prevention and urgent treatment of thiamine deficiency is a highly cost-effective intervention which saves the individual from a catastrophic event. *Dementia* due to alcohol use *(6D84.0)* refers to persistent impairment of cognitive function such as memory problems, coarsening of the personality and a mix of other deficits.

ICD-11 codes can easily be applied in routine psychiatric practice and they mirror succinctly the scope of disorders that arise from alcohol misuse; they serve as anchor points, or the skeleton upon which to build the whole picture of what is happening in the person's life. Categorical data, such as diagnoses, are useful but have limitations – in particular, most things biological exist along continua: quantity and frequency of alcohol consumption, dependence, severity of withdrawal symptoms and severity of mental illness are all examples. This is fine – the assessment tools and investigations used to flesh out the diagnoses will identify their ramifications.

Alcohol is noteworthy for the catalogue of health and social problems that it can cause. For people with an alcohol misuse problem there is often a sense of insurmountable obstacles to lifestyle change and life running out of control; for others there is no recognition of a problem at all. It follows that the expectations of patients are quite variable: some want to be told that there is no problem, others want to know the root cause of their problem, others come with a ready-made treatment plan and a few want to know their diagnosis. The task of the psychiatrist is to make sense of all this in a way that will engage and energise the patient.

Assessing Alcohol Misuse

The main purpose of the assessment is to gather baseline data: (i) to inform treatment planning; (ii) to enable progress and outcomes to be measured. An assessment package should be responsive both to these needs and to the circumstances in which it will be used. The setting – for example, a hospital ward, a clinic or patient's home – and the mental state of the patient will be delimiting. A full assessment may need to be conducted over a number of occasions; equally, there are situations where a short form of assessment is all that is required.

Assessment of Addiction

Screening

It is policy in the UK for primary care and acute hospital teams to screen for alcohol misuse problems and there are times when screening will be useful for psychiatrists. The Alcohol Use Disorder Identification Test (AUDIT) is a widely used, brief screening tool that is sensitive to change at the lower end of alcohol consumption, and it rates dependence and alcohol-related problems. The characteristics that make it a good screening tool mean it lacks detail and is less responsive to change at high levels of alcohol use. The implication is that AUDIT data will be insufficient for a specialist service and cannot simply be incremented to make up part of a full assessment. A single screening question has been suggested for use in non-specialist settings [2]. However, the advantage of the AUDIT is that it generates scores that suggest what action should be taken in response to the screening.

Full Assessment

It is usual to assess alcohol use within the broader context of addiction. The extent and priorities for data collection will be a function of the clinical team and the circumstances in which data are collected. The essential elements of addiction are:

- substance use
- dependence
- psychological well-being
- social well-being

Substance Use

The problem substance, in this case alcohol, is the most important part of the overall picture because it is the indicator of successful treatment which is expected by problem drinkers, their family and friends, and commissioners of services; moreover, the other elements of alcohol use disorders are related to levels of drinking. This is not to say that an obsession with the detail of drinking is productive. There is no very satisfactory way of summarising and presenting drinking data. Frequency of drinking is a more accurate measure than quantity. The simplest method is an ordinal ranking of the frequency of drinking: the category chosen – 'daily', 'weekly', or 'monthly', for example – will limit the precision of this method. A more accurate and equally simple approach is to ask the individual how many times they drank alcohol in a given time period – the 'past month' achieves a balance between a period long enough to be representative and short enough to be recalled. Accurate quantity data, usually estimated in standard 'units' equivalent to 8 gm of alcohol in the UK, are difficult to collect.

Biological markers have the advantage of being objective but are neither very specific nor sensitive to alcohol use. Currently there are a number of markers that merit consideration [3]: (i) blood or breath alcohol concentration; (ii) mean corpuscular volume (MCV); (iii) serum gamma-glutamyltransferase (GGT); (iv) aspartate aminotransferase (AST); (v) alanine aminotransferase (ALT); (vi) carbohydrate deficient transferrin (CDT); (vii) HDL-cholesterol; and (viii) uric acid. Given the changes in neuro-transmitter activity and physiology caused by alcohol, it is probable that better markers will be found in the future.

An assessment of alcohol use should include enquiry about prescribed and illicit drug use. It is unusual, particularly in younger drinkers, for alcohol to be the only substance taken. The effects of stimulant drugs such as amphetamine or cocaine, and of hallucinogens and cannabis can all mimic mental illnesses. Prescribed drug effects are unlikely to mimic mental illness but will affect the mental state of people with alcohol use disorders and interact with other medications – poly-pharmacy is a common complication for people with addiction problems [4].

Dependence

Dependence is at the heart of addiction. It is a condition in its own right and it separates what is normal, even heavy, drinking from a disorder that people recognise as problematic and behaviour that is out of control. It indicates the need for a comprehensive, structured treatment and is a predictor of less good outcomes. The stress associated with dependence means that scales designed to screen for anxiety and depression will produce false positives.

Psychological Well-Being

Psychological distress is associated with dependence and also with the multifarious conse-quences of drinking alcohol. The greater the involvement with alcohol the greater the distress, which itself is a trigger to further drinking, thereby creating a vicious circle. It is important to separate expected alcohol-related distress from comorbidities.

Social Well-Being

Social well-being is more loosely associated with drinking alcohol than dependence and psychological well-being because there are more protective factors in play – for example, socioeconomic status, support networks and educational achievement. The life-style change, upon which sustained recovery from an alcohol problem depends, is a crucial part of treatment planning.

Choosing an Assessment Package

For patients, their first contact is not only an assessment, it is also an intervention and they expect to leave with something helpful. Data collection, whether in the form of history taking, self-completion questionnaires or blood tests, should have a clear purpose, and, from an ethical perspective, should be undertaken to benefit the patient.

The principle of collecting Patient Reported Outcome Measures (PROMs) forms a solid basis to assessment. In clinical practice PROMs are typically questionnaires; these must meet validation standards [5] and should be able to measure clinically significant change [6], the gold standard of outcome evaluation. PROMs are themselves informative but, more than this, they signal that the patient's views are important to the psychiatrist. Practitioners need to understand the significance of each PROM question and use the patient's responses as the pegs on which to hang the structure of the assessment, which ideally should take the form of a conversation expanding on the points of interest. Self-report has been shown to be reliable [7] but there are situations where questionnaires or history alone cannot be used: for example, if a patient is unable to read or understand the content of a questionnaire, or if the patient's responses might be coloured by child protection or criminal justice proceedings.

The mix of PROMs needs to be carefully considered – there are many scales for both addictive behaviours and related problems to choose from [8]. Many scales are poorly validated and do not have published values for reporting clinically significant change. A shortcut to putting together a bespoke package is to use a composite assessment tool. The *Addiction Severity Index* is widely used in the USA and Australia while in the UK the *Treatment Outcomes Profile* (TOP) has been used. A weakness of composite measurement tools is that components are predetermined and may lack the sensitivity or detail desired for the target population. They are often designed with a particular function in mind – research or performance management, for example – which may not be what is required. An alternative is a service user derived scale, such as the *Addiction Recovery Questionnaire* [9], as a brief assessment tool designed to inform treatment planning and measure outcomes.

In a demonstration study of 1,470 participants, a full addiction outcome evaluation package, capable of assessing clinically significant change, combined the Leeds Dependence Questionnaire (LDQ), a measure of alcohol dependence; the Clinical Outcomes in Routine Evaluation 10 item scale (CORE-10), an indicator of psychological well-being; and the Social Satisfaction Questionnaire (SSQ), an indicator of social well-being. The outcomes for LDQ, CORE-10 and SSQ showed that there was 'reliable deterioration' in 4.7 per cent, 7.0 per cent and 14.2 per cent of patients respectively; 'reliable improvement' in 60.9 per cent, 47.2 per cent and 30.7 per cent; and 'reliable improvement with clinically significant change' in 42.5 per cent, 22.7 per cent and 23.3 per cent. Positive change was most likely in people with problems of alcohol misuse compared to other substance misuse [10]. When added to measures of drinking, drug use and prescribed medications, there is a comprehensive picture of treatment outcomes, proven to be achievable in routine clinical practice, accessible to all stakeholders and yet using sophisticated statistical methodology.

Mental health teams will collect a core data set which can then be supplemented by some form of addiction severity rating. Conversely, specialist addiction teams will have occasion to supplement the addiction assessment with ratings for specific conditions. For example, teams might want to screen for personality disorder, or have a special interest in PTSD, or undertake brief physical health checks, or assess brain damage with a graphical test such as the *Montreal Cognitive Assessment*. The art is to select assessment tools that patients will find interesting and relevant, and which help the clinician plan treatment.

The Assessment Interview

The effective psychiatrist is empathic, knowledgeable, supportive, goal-directed, helping, understanding and encouraging of patient autonomy; less effective practitioners are psychologically distant, overwhelmed, belittling and blaming, intrusive and controlling, avoid difficult issues and are self-interested [11]. Practitioners with the positive characteristics listed will deliver better outcomes and the more so when combined with those therapeutic techniques that are effective at bringing about change and maintaining it into the future. In a landmark study of people with alcohol misuse problems attending an Emergency Room in the United States, it was found that 1.1 per cent of those seen by the regular staff were referred to and attended five or more sessions at a local alcohol treatment centre compared to 42 per cent of those seen by staff from the alcohol treatment centre who were motivated to see these people again and had a positive therapeutic attitude [12]. The findings of this classic study have been replicated over the past five decades. Talking therapies delivered by poorly skilled practitioners with negative attitudes are damaging to patients and their treatment prospects.

An efficient and convenient way of undertaking an assessment is for patients to complete questionnaires and factual information, preferably with family or friends, prior to their assessment so that form filling does not get in the way of achieving the assessment goals which are: first, to build a therapeutic alliance [13]; second, to synthesise the questionnaire responses into a formulation that becomes a hypothesis as to what the alcohol use is all about; third, to find the one thing that the patient is unhappy with and use this as the motivational hook with which to engage them. Helping someone who may be ambivalent about whether they want to come into treatment at all calls for a collaborative approach – drawing a social network map together, for example – and using a motivational style of conversation [14]. If the assessment has been well done then significant risks, ICD-11 codes, and the material for writing a formulation will readily flow. The formulation can usefully be written or updated under the headings: (i) predisposing factors, (ii) precipitating factors, (iii) perpetuating factors and (iv) protective factors. A good way to close the session is for the psychiatrist to play back their initial conclusions in order to check that they accurately empathise with the patient and to help the patient make sense of any seemingly contradictory thoughts and feelings. It is crucial that the patient leaves their first appointment feeling hopeful and confident in their psychiatrist.

Reducing Harms

People with high dependence scores or comorbidity will benefit most from abstinence, while those with lower scores and fewer problems will be able to aim for a goal of drinking in moderation. Not everyone is ready to engage in making the lifestyle changes required to achieve the ideal goal for them, in which case setting interim, or harm-reduction, goals is the best way forward. Harm-reduction goals can be associated with attenuating drinking or targeting the harmful consequences of drinking. When people are resistant to changing drinking behaviour it is tempting to suggest a host of different things that they might do and refer on to a variety of support services. It is better to concentrate on spotting the one thing that the patient minds most about their drinking and focus on changing motivation while helping to reduce specific harms.

As a general principle, it is important to stay in contact with patients; otherwise, the opportunity to keep concerns about their drinking uppermost in their thoughts is lost. Patients will usually vote with their feet if a clinic does not fulfil their expectations. However, for some there are perverse benefits from attending a clinic even though everything possible to help has been tried without success – it is a judgement when to say that, for now, no more can be done. Giving information on population level drinking patterns, risks and harms, repeating questionnaire ratings, repeating liver function tests are all ways of expressing concern. Follow-up with feedback on any investigations is justification for offering further appointments and will have an impact on the patient's motivation to reduce drinking. Another strategy is to agree and ensure that there are times and activities that the patient sees to be incompatible with drinking – driving, cooking, looking after the children, going to work, for example. Another strategy is to look at the type of alcohol consumed, work out the units of alcohol and calories taken in a typical week and see if the patient might want to change the beverage or reduce the frequency of drinking. For some people drinking only on alternate days is an acceptable first goal.

A strategy to deal with the consequences of problem drinking is to involve people close to the problem drinker, and this has many benefits. Family and friends increase their own sense of well-being if they are helped to develop coping skills – for example, discussion of ways to keep themselves and the problem drinker safe in spite of continued drinking. The general principle here is to support the problem drinker as an individual while rejecting their drinking. Engaging the family or concerned others in supportive activities, mutual aid groups and coping skills training, which can also be offered to children, gives the harm-reduction initiatives a broader basis. Each of these interventions might seem insignificant in isolation but cumulatively they will increase the likelihood that the problem drinker will start to think differently about their drinking and reduce their alcohol consumption independently or through formal help seeking.

Drunkenness De-escalation Techniques

It is useful to distinguish between intoxication, which is the result of a particular blood alcohol level, and drunkenness, which refers to a range of behaviours that are somewhat independent of blood alcohol levels. Alcohol is a drug with a moderate degree of plasticity meaning that its effects can be shaped to some extent by drinkers' beliefs and perceptions of their internal and external environment – witness national stereotypes of drinking and how these cultures lead to people behaving differently, even though they are consuming equivalent amounts of alcohol.

It follows that for any incident of drunkenness, the impact of culture and the environment on behaviour can be modified. For example, where the environment and the people in it are perceived as hostile, then aggressive or defensive behaviour is likely to ensue. Calm and unthreatening behaviour by staff will minimise the risk to all present and facilitate de-escalation. There are some key points to follow: (i) make sure that both staff and patient can see an easy escape route; (ii) introduce yourself and call the patient by their name; (iii) get the patient to sit down and sit down yourself to avoid towering over them; (iv) describe what you need the patient to do in order to de-escalate the situation; (v) make facilitating rather than rejecting statements – for example, instead of saying, 'You cannot be seen now,' say, 'Wait over here and I will see you in twenty minutes.' The psychiatrist may be the senior practitioner present and should be competent to take a lead in managing patients exhibiting drunken and possibly aggressive behaviour. Training and a consistent team response are important for dealing effectively with these situations.

Harm Reduction Medications

Vitamin deficiencies are common among regular heavy drinkers. Deficiencies include: pyridoxine (B6), which can cause confusion, depression, seizures, neuropathy; folate, which can cause depression, dementia, neuropathy; riboflavin, which can cause depression, lethargy; and nicotinic acid, which can cause depression, psychosis, seizures, ataxia, tremor, deafness, neuritis, neuropathy. Most important, however, is thiamine (B1) deficiency, which causes the Wernicke-Korsakoff Syndrome, necrotising encephalomyopathy, neurasthenia, depression and neuropathy.

Heavy drinkers are vulnerable to thiamine deficiency because they have a poor intake of vitamins, poor absorption due to gastritis and high demand because the metabolism of alcohol depends upon thiamine as a co-enzyme. Only 25–30 mg of thiamine is stored in liver, heart, brain and kidneys to meet a normal daily requirement of approximately 1 mg. In healthy individuals the absorption from 10 mg of thiamine or more is 4–5 mg, but in heavy drinkers this falls to 0.75–1.5 mg.

Evidence is mixed on the benefits of prophylactic multivitamin supplements. Where there is either a high risk or diagnosis of Wernicke's, then parenteral vitamins that include high-dose thiamine should be given urgently [15]. The risk of anaphylaxis is very low (one per 5 million doses) and has to be balanced against the risk of Wernicke's Encephalopathy. Practice-based evidence puts regular heavy drinkers with a history of weight loss, vomiting and diarrhoea, general ill health or unexplained hypotension or hypothermia to be at risk of Wernicke's. A presumptive diagnosis can be made with a history of the classic triad of ophthalmoplegia, ataxia and acute confusion.

Management of Medically Assisted Withdrawal (MAW)

Medically assisted withdrawal (or detoxification) is the process of rapidly achieving an alcohol-free state. In 80–90 per cent of cases MAW is a straightforward and uncomplicated procedure and so there is always the danger of complacency and missing complications, which, at the extreme, can be life-threatening. There are a number of scales, of which CIWA is commonly used [16], for rating the severity of alcohol withdrawal in order to determine medication requirements and have early warning of complications. The purpose of medication is to minimise the severity of withdrawal symptoms and to prevent progression to seizures or delirium. Withdrawal symptoms may be so mild that no medication is needed. MAW has costs above and beyond the direct financial implications. Failure to become alcohol-free reinforces the belief that abstinence is not possible, and each episode of MAW sensitises the body to withdrawal, a phenomenon called kindling. It follows that there should be good preparation to maximise the chances of MAW being successful.

Unplanned MAW may be necessary in some circumstances (e.g. an urgent hospital admission), but wherever possible MAW will be planned around readiness to change, for which the hallmark features are self-efficacy and positive outcome expectancy. In preparation for MAW the psychiatrist should involve the patient and their support network so that there is a shared understanding of the process and key points are reviewed:

- determining readiness for MAW and highlighting positive outcomes
- developing coping strategies other than pharmacotherapy for dealing with withdrawal symptoms
- identifying a support person and plan for the MAW period
- identifying a post MAW plan including a follow-up appointment
- revisiting learning points from previous episodes of MAW
- assessing risks

Most people prefer to be detoxified at home and often this can be arranged safely, even for an individual at high risk of a complicated withdrawal (such as having seizures) if they have appropriate support. However, an individual with a lower-risk profile but lacking support (i.e. homeless or socially isolated) will need a residential setting, though not necessarily in an acute medical or psychiatric bed. The indications for medical admission are:

- alcoholic delirium or seizures present at the time of assessment
- a history of seizures or alcoholic delirium and current high alcohol intake or high dose poly-drug use
- pyrexia greater than 38.5°C
- a history of recent head injury with loss of consciousness
- illnesses requiring medical or surgical treatment: liver decompensation, pneumonia, other infections, dehydration, malnutrition, cardiovascular failure, hypertension
- Wernicke's Encephalopathy
- conditions requiring psychiatric admission: suicidal intent, severe anxiety or depression, psychotic illness

The management of complicated MAW should be overseen by a suitably experienced doctor. The setting for MAW will depend upon an assessment of risks and the level of supervision required to manage the risks. There are three categories to consider:

(i)   *Severe withdrawal* symptoms and seizures or delirium are more likely with poly-drug use, high consumption levels, taking short-acting depressant medications, infection and poor health, and the presence of increased autonomic nervous system activity.

(ii)   The withdrawal syndrome increases the risk of *destabilising* pre-existing conditions such as diabetes, cardiovascular disorders, mental health disorders – in these cases, there is a need to lengthen the MAW period.

(iii) The process of MAW may make it difficult for an individual to provide child care or cover other carer roles, or support may be unavailable to an individual – for example, because of living in a remote location. Choosing a suitable *setting* for MAW requires judgement and discussion with patients, their family or friends.

The general method of MAW depends to some extent on the setting. There are three options:

(i)   *Front loading*: a set dose of the withdrawal medication, a long-acting benzodiazepine, is administered at regular intervals until the severity of withdrawal score falls below a predetermined level – at this point, no further medication is given. This method makes efficient use of staff time and significantly reduces the total amount of medication given. It requires skilled staff and is most suitable for inpatient care [17].

(ii)   *Fixed dose reduction*: a predetermined regimen is prescribed for a given severity of withdrawal – for example, one regimen for moderate and one for severe withdrawal. This method does not require experienced staff and can be used in any setting, but is insensitive to need and it is unlikely that complications will be picked up.

(iii) *Variable dose, symptom triggered reduction*: the dose of medication is determined by the severity of withdrawal and so it requires experienced and trained staff. It is the best method where the course of MAW is uncertain and complications are likely and where adequate monitoring is available.

The actual medication to be prescribed for MAW is well established and supported by guidelines [15].

Uncomplicated Withdrawal

Benzodiazepines are effective in reducing signs and symptoms of withdrawal and those with a longer half-life (such as chlordiazepoxide) may prevent delirium. Typical regimens for chlordiazepoxide are:

- severe withdrawal: 30 mg qds reducing over five days
- moderate withdrawal: 20 mg qds reducing over five days

If there is significant liver disease then oxazepam is the drug of choice. Carbamazepine has been shown to be equally efficacious to benzodiazepines but because of side effects is kept as a second-line drug.

Seizures and Delirium

Benzodiazepines, particularly diazepam, prevent *de novo* seizures. Anticonvulsants are as efficacious as benzodiazepines in seizure prevention, but there is no advantage when combined. To prevent delirium or a second seizure in the same withdrawal episode, lorazepam is the drug of choice: 30 mcg/kg, which for an average person is 1.5–2.5 mg, administered intramuscularly or by slow intravenous injection to be repeated six-hourly.

Clomethiazole is an option for very severe withdrawal where there is a history of seizures or delirium: two to four capsules on Day 1, six to eight on Day 2, reducing over nine days. This drug has a high dependence-forming potential, a risk of fatal respiratory depression if taken with alcohol and can quickly accumulate to toxic levels if there is liver damage, and so it should only be prescribed in inpatient settings.

Although the process of medically assisted withdrawal is straightforward, the skill is in getting the detail correct and being flexible in helping people who find themselves in difficult and disadvantageous circumstances. Sometimes patients, their families and friends, believe that if only somebody would offer them a MAW episode, everything else would sort itself out. Although MAW is generally not a good plan for someone who is clearly not ready to change, it may be expedient to go along with the request if it helps to engage the patient and their support network and unblocks progress in treatment. If there have been previous episodes of MAW it is always productive to review any learning points. The other side of this coin is when patients who are ready to change are refused MAW by a treatment service: heavy drinking is a high-risk activity in both the short and long term, especially if combined with other prescribed or illicit substance use. The greater the risk, the greater the urgency for MAW: delivering a timely episode of MAW that is going to work in the patient's situation may not be ideal but is better than doing nothing.

Psychosocial Interventions

The majority of people who go through a period of alcohol misuse recover without recourse to treatment or mutual aid groups – so-called *natural recovery*. It is normal for alcohol consumption, not necessarily misuse, to change throughout life in line with changing roles and responsibilities. People who do drink alcohol tend to drink more when young, and the majority of these become stable social drinkers as the responsibilities of family and work dominate their lifestyle. For people who do develop an alcohol problem, at whichever stage of their life, supportive relationships, spiritual involvement, new work responsibilities and friends who are social drinkers or abstainers can be routes out of problem drinking [18], whereas alcohol dependence tends to be more intractable and lead on to help seeking. Mental health problems, not wanting to seek help for reasons of embarrassment or social stigma, doubt about alcohol treatment services, time constraints, an absence of protective factors or plain failure to see any problem all make continued problem drinking more likely.

What Works?

The search for what works in the treatment of alcohol dependence has focused on the question of whether one treatment modality is better than another. Several large clinical trials have taken this approach and have produced manuals to optimise treatment protocol adherence. Well-delivered behavioural treatments are generally found to be as effective as each other, enabling the identification of common factors (behaviour change mechanisms), which are associated with good outcomes. These are: goal setting, a planned weekly routine based on agreed goals, active social support and role models for these goals, planning of activities that replace the drinking and are rewarding, coping skills training and strengthening self-efficacy [19]. The new behaviours should become as rewarding as the drinking had been. These principles are common across many behaviours which are discrete and measurable, and therefore they are generalisable to other disorders that the psychiatrist is likely to treat.

Something of a prerequisite to embarking on a structured treatment plan, as opposed to harm-reduction or solely motivational interventions, is a desire on the part of the patient to change. The way that the psychiatrist and other practitioners behave will influence whether a patient becomes motivated to change and engage in a sustained treatment programme. Research across effective treatments for alcohol dependence and other psychotherapeutic work has identified two key practitioner behaviours:

(i)   the communication of respect and concern by way of asking open questions that allow the patient to describe things from their own point of view

(ii) reflections that allow the practitioner to communicate to the patient that they understand the things that concern them as well as the dilemmas they face in trying to resolve the behaviour change challenge.

These are the building blocks of the therapeutic alliance, which emerges clearly as an agent of engagement, retention in treatment and of improved outcomes. Where there is a positive therapeutic alliance, patients talk about feeling listened to, being understood and having a sense of collaborative goal setting and treatment planning decisions [13].

If the practitioner is effective at building a therapeutic alliance and enhancing the patient's motivation then they will detect important shifts in what the patient says. First, talk of a desire to change or of a need to change will be expressed in much more specific terms – namely, a belief that change will bring about particular benefits. These new beliefs that life can be better must come from the patient. By the time patients seek help for an alcohol problem they have probably had enough of being told what they ought to do and what is good for them, but will be motivated to change when thoughts about what they should do are their own. Second, once the belief that life can be better is established, patients then need to express their own belief in their ability to change and this can be the most challenging part of treatment; however, it is also the part where treatment or offers of help have the greatest impact.

What else does the patient need to bring to the table that the practitioner can influence? The presence of at least one person who can provide positive support for a change in lifestyle is important. This person needs to be an individual who is trusted by the patient, concerned about the well-being of the patient, available to the patient and willing to undertake and support activities consistent with change in a friendly, unobtrusive manner. If family breakdown has occurred and there are scores to be settled, then the practitioner is best looking elsewhere for positive support. If the patient remains in a heavy drinking circle of family or friends, or where a partner is a heavy drinker, there is little chance of achieving a new way of life and giving up or reducing drinking [20] until a new social network is established.

Integrated Social Behaviour and Network Therapy (iSBNT) is a structured, manual-based treatment that was designed to pull together the evidence on 'what works' in order to provide a framework within which to deliver treatment. It combines a motivational interviewing style of dialogue with behavioural interventions delivered in a social network. Manuals improve the quality of treatment delivery by helping practitioners to adhere to the essential tenets of the particular intervention. They are best used as a resource containing guidelines for good practice, including directions on style of consultation and context, broad descriptions of session structure and content, and what to do in difficult situations. The most effective practitioners do not use treatment manuals in a rigid way; rather, they adapt the guidance to their own style and to suit the patient and their concerned others' circumstances and resources. Manuals are to be embraced as a helpful tool for improving treatment delivery and effectiveness.

Every treatment will have an active phase and should be followed by structured aftercare. Pharmacotherapies and some psychosocial interventions – contingency management, for example – are effective for as long as they are applied but do not facilitate new learning or the capacity to continue improvement after active treatment has finished. The requirement for structure in treatment is important because patients who adhere to their planned, time-limited appointments are likely to do better than those attending unstructured sessions, which typically amount to little more than having a chat and from which no additional benefit accrues. Attendance is not just a function of the patient's motivation, it is also a reflection of the practitioner's ability to build a therapeutic alliance. A planned duration of treatment conveys a strong message of belief in the patient's ability to change and in the treatment to work for them. iSBNT is designed to ensure that the support network, which will usually include a mutual aid group, will provide aftercare once active treatment ends. The role of the psychiatrist may not involve the delivery of structured psychosocial treatment, but the principles of network therapy can always be applied and interventions from assessment to harm reduction and prescribing can always be delivered using motivational dialogue [14].

Additional support for maintaining behaviour change can be found in mutual aid groups, fellowships of people sharing common goals and supporting each other. Such groups work well when they have a stable membership of people who have achieved abstinence and are helping others to achieve abstinence. Best known is Alcoholics Anonymous (AA), whose meetings occur in nearly every country in the world and in larger cities may take place several times a day, every day of the week. The premise for attending AA meetings is the desire to stop drinking, although people are unlikely to be admitted to a meeting if they are intoxicated. The related Al-Anon is made up of, and supports, family members of problem drinkers, usually when the latter have not modified their drinking. Another movement is SMART Recovery, also a mutual aid group, but with more obvious behavioural components and less reliance on belief in a 'higher power', which is an important part of AA. There are myriad local groups set up by recovered problem drinkers who want to do things differently to the existing groups. It is worth finding out about these from patients who have local knowledge. People who move on to attend self-help and mutual aid groups will more likely embark on lifestyle change and achieve longer lasting stable abstinence than those who revert to their former lifestyles.

Mental Health Comorbidity

The term *dual diagnosis* has been widely adopted without a consensus on its meaning. In the UK the Department of Health restricts policy and guidance on dual diagnosis to severe and enduring mental illness such as schizophrenia or bipolar disorder. Alcohol misuse is not only associated with these conditions but also intertwined with them, and the same might apply to personality disorders. For some the scope of *dual diagnosis* is far more extensive than severe and enduring psychiatric illness and includes alcohol-induced disorders where depressive and anxiety symptoms are prominent. Addiction psychiatrists are needed to manage these cases. Practice-based evidence suggests that people with a dual diagnosis are best treated by a single clinical team where this can be achieved and 'what works' applies as much to people with comorbidities as it does to those with alcohol use disorders alone.

However, modifications are usually made to the delivery of alcohol treatments and some general points should be kept in mind:

(i)   The first priority is to achieve abstinence or reasonable control of drinking.

(ii) Psychoactive drugs, particularly stimulants and hallucinogens, can mimic mental illness: a toxicology screen is a useful check.

(iii) Psychological distress, when caused by heavy drinking or dependence, can mimic mental illness, notably anxiety and depression.

(iv) Where the mental health problem is most likely to be alcohol-induced, dealing with the drinking first is the best approach. This is a judgement call and obvious exceptions to the rule include the Wernicke-Korsakoff Syndrome, safety concerns such as suicide risk and drinking used as self-medication.

(v)   Where a diagnosis of mental illness or personality disorder is established, then the usual treatment of these disorders may need to be modified:

- Thoughts and feelings, including the content of delusions and hallucinations, often have interwoven substance use references and this needs to be considered in therapeutic interactions.
- The burden of comorbidity can overwhelm an individual and so there is a need to make sense for the patient of what is going on and typically extend the treatment duration.
- The psychiatrist's knowledge of mental illness will dictate how to adapt treatment for particular disorders. For example, people with schizophrenia will have a reduced capacity to process information independently of their delusions, and people with bipolar disorder may not be responsive to alcohol treatment when either 'high' or 'low'.

Pharmacotherapies

A number of medications have been evaluated for use as relapse prevention agents, but only disulfiram, naltrexone, nalmefene and acamprosate are regularly prescribed. The anticonvulsant topiramate and the muscle relaxant baclofen, which is a central nervous system depressant, are promising alternatives. Relapse prevention pharmacotherapies have different mechanisms of action and, based on the evidence of their efficacy, different indications for clinical practice. A combination of pharmacotherapy and psychosocial interventions is usually more effective than either on their own.

Medications to Maintain Abstinence

Much of the evidence for naltrexone and acamprosate derives from studies where abstinence was the main outcome measure. The early trials consistently demonstrated small benefits from both medications while the largest trial, the COMBINE study [21], found no benefit from taking acamprosate and a modest benefit for naltrexone. Recent evidence supporting disulfiram shows statistically significant superiority over acamprosate and naltrexone: respectively a mean of 46.4, 17.6 and 22.0 days before a heavy drinking episode, and 6.3, 4.5 and 4.6 days' abstinence each week [22].

Disulfiram is a sensitising agent, meaning that it causes an unpleasant reaction if alcohol is consumed having taken it. Taking a sensitising agent alters the expectations of the consequences of drinking from something nice to something unpleasant. For many, these changed expectations are sufficient to prevent drinking; others will experiment to see what happens if they do drink and will experience a disulfiram-ethanol reaction. If they do not experience a reaction, the standard 200 mg dose can be doubled. It is important to set up supervision of the prescription and to do so in a way that all parties are comfortable with – once the medication has been taken, then drinking is unlikely and family, friends and workmates are able to feel relaxed and positive, creating a virtuous cycle of taking disulfiram and continued abstinence.

Disulfiram inhibits liver enzymes responsible for the breakdown of dopamine and of acetaldehyde, which is the principal metabolite of ethanol. Acetaldehyde is a toxic substance and it is the raised levels that are responsible for the disulfiram-ethanol reaction, which is characterised by flushing, tachycardia, sweating, nausea, vomiting, headache and raised blood pressure. There is considerable variation in sensitivity to acetaldehyde such that there may be no reaction. Disulfiram should be prescribed with caution in the presence of cardiovascular disorders and psychosis and is contraindicated in pregnancy. Hepatotoxicity is rare but is associated with a high mortality rate, and a protocol for monitoring liver enzymes should be agreed prior to commencing disulfiram treatment. An information leaflet for patients is useful and, given the possible side effects, formal consent is prudent. In choosing a relapse prevention medication for abstinence the risk of alcohol-related liver damage and mortality needs to be balanced against the possibility of disulfiram-related hepatitis. Prescribing naltrexone or acamprosate carries less risk, but neither is effective at securing a prolonged period of abstinence [23].

Medications for Attenuated Drinking

Nalmefene is the only medication marketed specifically to reduce alcohol consumption. The putative mechanism of action of both nalmefene and naltrexone is antagonism of endogenous opioid pathways. As these project into the substantia nigra and ventral tegmental area of the brain, known as the 'pleasure centre', the effect is to blunt the enjoyment of drinking. However, opioid pathways are only one way in which alcohol exerts its reinforcing effects, so the overall theoretical importance of blocking opioid systems is limited. Acamprosate is marketed as an anti-craving medication but its action on neurochemical systems is unclear. It is thought to enhance GABA, although not as a simple agonist as this would make it susceptible to the same problems of dependence as benzodiazepines, and it also inhibits the action of stimulant amino acids such as glutamate at the NMDA receptor.

The idea of using medication as a public health measure to reduce drinking is not generally accepted, albeit that the small reductions in consumption expected from these medications could be significant as a whole-population prevention measure. In choosing a medication to attenuate drinking, naltrexone is well suited to drinking prevention in high-risk situations: it is prescribed as a once-daily tablet which can be taken as and when there are perceived risks of drinking. An equivalent acamprosate prescription is two tablets three times daily, and repeated tablet taking has the disadvantage of reinforcing the idea that medication is a solution to alcohol misuse. Taking *total amount of alcohol* consumed as the outcome measure, naltrexone and acamprosate have been found to be ineffective as compared to nalmefene, topiramate or baclofen, which were significantly better than placebo [24]. However, secondary analyses of the COMBINE study raise the possibility that acamprosate is more effective for 'frequent drinkers' and not for 'pre-treatment abstainers' while naltrexone is best for 'very frequent drinkers' [25]. Most people seen by psychiatrists will have an abstinence goal and medications that are effective only for reduction in frequent drinking are not conducive to supporting psychosocial treatments. It is probable that polymorphism accounts for at least some of the differential response of individuals to acamprosate and naltrexone but clinically useful matching has yet to be elucidated.

Outcomes from Alcohol Use Disorders

Measuring the outcomes from a specific treatment episode is difficult because there are so many variables in play. Predictors of a good outcome are: female gender, employment, adequate income, religious involvement, motivation to change and self-efficacy; predictors of a poor outcome are: severity of dependence, frequency and intensity of drinking, mental health problems and neuropsychological impairment [26]. The predictive value of age, marital status, education, ethnicity and alcohol-related problems is inconsistently reported. In summary, it can be said that social stability and positivity about the future are associated with a good outcome, while severity of the drinking problems and mental health problems are associated with poor outcome. A good number of these are pre-treatment predictors which also underpin *natural recovery*.

Specific treatment modalities account for only a small slice of the outcome variance. This is partly because of the impact of pre-treatment variables but also because of therapist behaviours [27] and organisational constraints, which are not accounted for in treatment efficacy trials. For people who are alcohol dependent, life opportunities may realistically be limited regardless of socioeconomic status, and a prior bad experience of treatment can add to the pessimism [28]. Building an alliance is difficult and the effective practitioner will need to be imaginative rather than slavishly following guidelines or treatment protocols. Psychiatrists are capable of this, but are likely to find risk-averse substance misuse and mental health organisations to be antagonistic to practitioners going off-piste. The organisational constraints that fail people with high-risk drinking problems are concealed because organisations cite adherence to guidelines as a clinical governance necessity – a disingenuous interpretation of both good practice and of guidelines. Paradoxically there are many studies of specific treatments, accounting for a small percentage of the outcome variance, and few studies of the far more important practitioner characteristics and organisational constraints that have such a large influence on outcomes.

Looking at the bigger picture, a one year follow-up of people diagnosed as alcohol dependent found 25 per cent were still classified as dependent, 27.3 per cent were classified as being in partial remission, 11.8 per cent were asymptomatic drinkers at risk of relapse, 17.7 per cent were low-risk drinkers and 18.2 per cent were abstainers [18]. However, only 25 per cent ever received treatment. Heavy drinkers who score low on dependence see their drinking as an activity that brings benefits in several life areas: socialising, raising self-confidence, relaxation, coping with stress and meeting potential sexual partners. The drawbacks of drinking are also seen as related to socialising, notably relationship problems, rather than health worries as might have been expected [29]. What happens during treatment can predict outcomes up to three years after treatment. An analysis of three large treatment trials (Project MATCH and COMBINE in the United States and the UK Alcohol Treatment Trial) identified seven patterns of drinking based upon *percent days drinking (PDD)* and *drinks per drinking day (DDD)*:

(i)   18.7 per cent persistent heavy drinking: DDD=10.6, PDD=69 per cent
(ii) 9.6 per cent relapse to heavy drinking: DDD=11.9, PDD=25.2 per cent
(iii) 6.7 per cent heavy and low-risk drinking: DDD=5.5, PDD=49.2 per cent

(iv) 7.9 per cent heavy drinking: DDD=9.0, alternating with abstinence

(v) 6.8 per cent consistent low-risk drinking: DDD=2.9, PDD 49.4 per cent

(vi) 10.5 per cent abstinence to low-risk drinking: DDD=3.5, PDD=10.7 per cent

(vii) 39.8 per cent abstainers throughout

At 12 months there were no significant differences on general functioning and drinking consequences between abstainers and low-risk patterns, meaning a total of 57.1 per cent had a good outcome. Poor outcomes were predicted by severity of dependence, the number of drinkers in the social network and negative mood states [30].

Recovery has been defined by the Betty Ford Institute as 'a voluntarily maintained lifestyle characterised by sobriety, personal health, and citizenship' or, in plain language, it is the ideal lifestyle for someone getting over an addiction problem. It is a moot point as to when treatment ends and recovery begins. The Addiction Recovery Questionnaire (ARQ) is a PROM, derived from the views of service users and their families, to measure progression along the continuum of recovery [9]. Stable recovery builds over months and years and is an accumulation of lifestyle changes: having suitable accommodation; enough money; constructive activities, including personal and home care, work, hobbies or studying; moving out of drinking cultures; and feeling good about the future. There are many roads, including structured psychosocial interventions, that lead to recovery. Lasting change, including dealing with mental health problems, is unlikely to happen if readiness to change is not then converted into abstinence or, at the least, control over drinking.

In Summary

Alcohol misuse is a problem that affects all manner of groups in society. For some it releases artistic creativity, for others it is simply a social pleasure and for others it is a coping strategy. There is always a fascination about how people use alcohol and why some individuals lose control over its use, often with disastrous consequences. Psychiatrists are well qualified to rise to the intellectual challenges of making a diagnosis and piecing together a formulation for people with complex drinking problems. Effective practitioners will empathise with the limitations to life that go hand in hand with alcohol misuse and spawn high-risk, seemingly irrational behaviours. Empathy is the key to building a therapeutic alliance and delivering high-quality treatment, which in turn will deliver rewarding outcomes.

References

1 Weaver T., Madden P., Charles V., Timso GS., Renton A., Tyrer P. et al. Comorbidity of substance misuse and mental illness in community mental health and substance misuse services. *British Journal of Psychiatry*. 2003; **183**: 304–13.

2 Saitz R., Cheng D. M., Allensworth-Davies D., Winter M. R., Smith P. C. The ability of single screening questions for unhealthy alcohol and other drug use to identify substance dependence in primary care. *Journal of Studies on Alcohol and Drugs*. 2014; **75** (1): 153–7.

3 Conigrave K. M., Davies P., Haber P., Whitfield J. B. Traditional markers of excessive alcohol use. *Addiction*. 2003; **98** Suppl2: 31–43.

4 Oluyase A. O., Raistrick D., Abbasi Y., Dale V., Lloyd C. A study of the psychotropic prescriptions of people attending an addiction service in England. *Advances in Dual Diagnosis*. 2013; **6**.

5 Terwee C. B., Bot S. D., de Boer M. R., van der Windt D. A., Knol D. L., Dekker J. et al. Quality criteria were proposed for measurement properties of health status questionnaires. *Journal of Clinical Epidemiology*. 2007; **60** (1): 34–42.

6   Jacobson N. S., Truax P. Clinical significance: A statistical approach to defining meaningful change in psychotherapy research. *Journal of Consulting and Clinical Psychology.* 1991; **59** (1): 12–9.

7   Del Boca F. K., Noll J. A. Truth or consequences: The validity of self-report data in health services research on addictions. *Addiction.* 2000; **95** (11s3): 347–60.

8   Raistrick D. S., Tober G. W. A summary of selected scales, 2018 [Available from: www .result4addiction.net.]

9   Iveson-Brown K., Raistrick D. A brief Addiction Recovery Questionnaire derived from the views of service users and concerned others. *Drugs: Education, Prevention and Policy.* 2016; **23** (1): 41–7.

10 Raistrick D., Tober G., Sweetman J., Unsworth S., Crosby H., Evans T. Measuring clinically significant outcomes – LDQ, CORE-10 and SSQ as dimension measures of addiction. *Psychiatric Bulletin.* 2014; **38** (3): 112–5.

11 Najavits L. M., Weiss R. D. Variations in therapist effectiveness in the treatment of patients with substance use disorders: An empirical review. *Addiction.* 1994; **89** (6): 679–88.

12 Chafetz M. E., Blane H. T., Abram H. S., Golner J., Lacy E., McCourt W. F. et al. Establishing treatment relations with alcoholics. *The Journal of Nervous and Mental Disease.* 1962; **134** (5): 395–409.

13 Apodaca T. R., Longabaugh R. Mechanisms of change in motivational interviewing: A review and preliminary evaluation of the evidence. *Addiction.* 2009; **104** (5): 705–15.

14 Tober G., Raistrick D., eds. Motivational Dialogue: Preparing Addiction Professionals for Motivational Interviewing Practice. Abingdon: Routledge; 2007.

15 Lingford-Hughes A. R., Welch S., Peters L., Nutt D. J., Ball D., Buntwal N. et al. BAP updated guidelines. Evidence-based guidelines for the pharmacological management of substance abuse, harmful use, addiction and comorbidity:

Recommendations from BAP. *Journal of Psychopharmacology.* 2012; **26** (7): 899–952.

16 Sullivan J. T., Sykora K., Schneiderman J., Naranjo C. A., Sellers E. M. Assessment of alcohol withdrawal: The Revised Clinical Institute Withdrawal Assessment for Alcohol Scale (CIWA-Ar). *British Journal of Addiction.* 1989; **84**: 1353–7.

17 Day E., Patel J., Georgiou G. Evaluation of a symptom-triggered front-loading detoxification technique for alcohol dependence: A pilot study. *Psychiatric Bulletin.* 2004; **28**: 407–10.

18 Dawson D. A., Grant B. F., Stinson F. S., Chou P. S., Huang B., Ruan W. J. Recovery from DSM-IV alcohol dependence: United States, 2001–2002. *Addiction.* 2005; **100** (3): 281–92.

19 Moos R. H. Theory-based active ingredients of effective treatments for substance use disorders. *Drug and Alcohol Dependence.* 2007; **88** (2–3): 109–21.

20 McCrady B. S. To have but one true friend: Implications for practice of research on alcohol use disorders and social networks. *Psychology of Addictive Behaviors.* 2004; **18** (2): 113–21.

21 Anton R. F., O'Malley S. S., Ciraulo D. A., Cisler R. A., Couper D., Donovan D. M. et al. Combined pharmacotherapies and behavioral interventions for alcohol dependence. The COMBINE study: A randomized controlled trial. *JAMA.* 2006; **295** (17): 2003–17.

22 Laaksonen E., Koski-Jännes A., Salaspuro M., Ahtinen H., Alho H. A randomized, multicentre, open-label, comparative trial of disulfiram, naltrexone and acamprosate in the treatment of alcohol dependence. *Alcohol and Alcoholism.* 2008; **43**(1): 53–61.

23 Skinner M. D., Lahmek P., Pham H., Aubin H.-J. Disulfiram efficacy in the treatment of alcohol dependence: A meta-analysis. *PLOS ONE.* 2014; **9** (2): e87366.

24 Palpacuer C., Duprez R., Huneau A., Locher C., Boussageon R., Laviolle B. et al. Pharmacologically controlled drinking in the treatment of alcohol dependence or

alcohol use disorders: A systematic review with direct and network meta-analyses on nalmefene, naltrexone, acamprosate, baclofen and topiramate. *Addiction*. 2018; **113** (2): 220–37.

25 Gueorguieva R., Wu R., Fucito L. M., O'Malley S. S. Predictors of abstinence from heavy drinking during follow-up in COMBINE. *Journal of Studies on Alcohol and Drugs*. 2015; **76** (6): 935–41.

26 Adamson S. J., Sellman J. D., Framptom C. M. A. Patient predictors of alcohol treatment outcome: A systematic review. *Journal of Substance Abuse Treatment*. 2009; **36**: 75–86.

27 Moyers T. B., Miller W. R. Is low therapist empathy toxic? *Psychology of Addictive Behaviors*. 2013; **27** (3): 878–84.

28 Gilburt H., Drummond C., Sinclair J. Navigating the alcohol treatment pathway: A qualitative study from the service users' perspective. *Alcohol and Alcoholism*. 2015; **50** (4): 444–50.

29 Orford J., Dalton S., Hartney E., Ferrins-Brown M., Kerr C., Maslin J. How is excessive drinking maintained? Untreated heavy drinkers' experiences of the personal benefits and drawbacks of their drinking. *Addiction Research and Theory*. 2002; **10** (4): 347–72.

30 Witkiewitz K., Pearson M. R., Hallgren K. A., Maisto S. A., Roos C. R., Kirouac M. et al. Who achieves low risk drinking during alcohol treatment? An analysis of patients in three alcohol clinical trials. *Addiction*. 2017; **112** (12): 2112–21.

Psychological Approaches to Addiction

8

Rob Hill and Jennifer Harris

Introduction

Psychological theory and practice have a lot to offer in terms of understanding addictive patterns of behaviour, yet despite the theoretical advances that have occurred over the years, change at the individual level often remains slow and precarious. Motivation to change sometimes appears as a magical moment seemingly unrelated to the severity of symptoms, and when change does occur it often follows what Marlatt and his colleagues have called 'the rocky road to recovery'. White has acknowledged this problem and notes that while there have been many advances in our knowledge and treatment of addictions, not least in the field of cognitive behavioural therapy (CBT), there are still limitations in the efficacy of addictions treatment [1]. Thus, some clients, generally those whose substance use is part of a broader cluster of problems, quickly relapse after treatment. This finding has led to a call for a reorientation of treatment away from an acute care model to a recovery management model or what White calls 'focusing on the lived solution'. Put simply, tackling dependency, while an important first step in the process of change, is rarely sufficient to maintain change over time or indeed to necessarily create a better life. Thus, many self-help groups are increasingly focusing on what is known as 'recovery capital', which refers to the sum of resources necessary to initiate and sustain recovery from substance misuse. As such it conveys a more positive way of conveying to clients the reasons for ensuring a robust relapse prevention strategy.

Theories and Interventions for Addictive Behaviour

Psychoanalytic Theories of Addiction

Psychoanalysis, as conceived by Freud, is both a theory and a treatment which seeks to understand conflicting elements or parts that often remain hidden or inaccessible (unconscious) to an individual without treatment. Freud posited a structural model that combined the 'ego' (based in reality), a 'superego' (conscience) and an 'id' (immediate desire for pleasure and satisfaction, which includes the libido). The ideal outcome of treatment is considered to be a strengthening of the ego so that it is less in thrall to either the wayward id or the more rigid superego. Addiction in terms of this model is thought of as a form of defence against feelings of helplessness and hopelessness along with a failure to regulate powerful emotions stemming from early aversive childhood experiences. Addiction provides a temporary but all-enveloping reprieve from such feelings, along with positive feelings of being in control and all-powerful that are not based in reality. Other writers of a psychoanalytic slant focus on early experiences of deprivation or over-indulgence which result in unmet attachment needs, disturbances in the sense of self and difficulties with drive and affect, self-care, dependency and need satisfaction. Although psychoanalytic theories tend to be infrequently used as an individual treatment modality, the ideas remain influential, particularly in the areas of group psychotherapy and are therefore worth becoming acquainted with [2, 3]. It is also important to note that the roles of transference and counter-transference remain important considerations in any therapeutic relationship.

Learning Theories of Addiction

Classical Conditioning

Addiction from the perspective of classical conditioning notes that a specific stimulus (a neutral stimulus) causes a specific response, so that those factors that occur immediately prior to, or at the same time as, the learned stimulus (the substance) elicit some of the same responses as the substance itself. This is commonly reported by substance dependent clients, in that paraphernalia associated with using drugs such as needles or foil can elicit a desire to use substances. Other environmental triggers such as images of people drinking and smoking, the smell of alcohol or tobacco can trigger craving in an addicted individual as a conditioned reflex. Cravings often lead to giving in or indulging in the addicted behaviour unless the individual has learned skills to cope with this. Cue exposure is an intervention based on classical conditioning to reduce the conditioned response [4].

Operant Conditioning

While classical conditioning is almost entirely behavioural, operant conditioning seeks to understand how the consequences of a particular behaviour on an individual come to moderate the frequency of the behaviour. Behaviour can be increased through the removal of negative consequences (negative reinforcement) or by providing a reward (positive reinforcement). Behaviour can also be reduced through punishment or removal of rewards (extinction). Operant conditioning is useful to understand why the mood-altering consequences of substance use can reinforce continued use (positive reinforcement) and why substance dependent clients seek to avoid withdrawal through continued substance use (negative reinforcement). Contingency management uses the principle of positive reinforcement to change substance-using behaviour by reinforcing abstinence from a specified drug. This is done through the provision of a reward that has some meaning to a client.

Social Learning Theory

Bandura describes a third way in which learning takes place [5]. Cognitive processes such as anticipation, planning, expectancies, attributions, self-efficacy and decision making have been shown to be an integral part of learning. All of these factors have been shown to be involved in the development and maintenance of addictive behaviours. Bandura also noted that while we do learn by direct experience, we also learn indirectly by observing others around us. Through watching, making sense of and encoding how, for example, a parent uses alcohol to relax or socialise, we develop our own substance-related 'outcome expectancies'. Such expectancies can consciously or unconsciously mediate our own behaviour towards initiating and continuing substance use [6]. We are more likely to imitate behaviours coming from the same gender and those of higher status. We are also motivated to model behaviour we have previously been rewarded for, have observed being rewarded ('vicarious learning') or imagine will bring rewards ('incentives').

One can see how social learning theory supports such interventions as AA/NA as it highlights the importance of learning from and being exposed to others in recovery. Moreover, clients and professionals don't need to get over-invested in agreeing or disagreeing with the disease theory of alcoholism, for as Flanagan suggests [7]: 'AA works not because it is right or correct on many of its core principles, e.g. alcoholism is a disease, alcoholism involves loss of control, but rather that it works because it is a repository of collective wisdom about self-control and recovery.' Professionals should therefore facilitate client's access to mutual aid or self-help groups such as AA and attendance should be suggested as a matter of course at the beginning of any treatment journey or as part of routine information giving for individuals with substance misuse problems. Public Health England recommends a three-stage process for facilitating access to mutual aid: (i) introducing mutual aid; (ii) encouraging the client to engage with a mutual aid group; (iii) taking an interest in the client's experience of mutual aid groups [8].

Although a behavioural perspective on addiction focuses chiefly on an individual's responses, it is important not to ignore the social context. Initiation into substance use invariably happens in a social context and social factors often contribute to its maintenance. Culture and subcultures are often associated with the presence or absence of particular substance use. The social pressures resulting from expectations in certain settings for the use of substances can make it very difficult for an individual not to conform. Interventions that do not take into consideration this social context of substance use are likely to fail. The focus on high-risk situations within relapse prevention programmes targets precisely these issues. There are also times when addictive behaviours, particularly substance misuse, have been confined to a particular context and do not transpose themselves into different contexts. The work of Lee Robins and her colleagues with Vietnam veterans on heroin use highlights this. During the war heroin use was widespread and, out of those who were addicted, almost 50 per cent used heroin after their return home but only 12 per cent went on to be re-addicted [9]. This research has led some to argue that the concept of addiction itself is entirely socially constructed [10].

Jim Orford in his book *Excessive Appetites* describes 'how appetites that mostly give pleasure, delight, joy or harmless entertainment can sometimes become so excessive that they threaten to spoil our lives' [11] (p. 201). Using a Social-Behavioural-Cognitive-Moral model, Orford identifies two factors that predispose an individual to excess – namely, unconventionality and non-conformity. Most people will restrict their behaviour on the basis of social conformity or other similar deterring forces. Orford then highlights a number of factors that can tip the balance into noticeable excess, beginning with social change or transition, a deeper immersion into the world of substance use and a subsequent reduction in non-using social activities or as ICD-10 notes, the 'progressive neglect of alternative pleasures or interests because of psychoactive substance use, increased amount of time necessary to obtain or take the substance or to recover from its effects'. Orford also highlights the reduction in discrimination, so that restrictions and judgements about when, where and in what circumstances it is appropriate to use become less frequent, contributing to a normalisation process of the changed behaviour state.

Social deprivation has also perhaps not surprisingly been linked to substance misuse. Mental health problems and associated substance misuse in areas of social deprivation is well documented. Poverty linked to drink and drug culture is another example of the association of substance misuse and social deprivation [12]. In cultures where substance use is not acceptable, for religious or other reasons, there is a lower prevalence. Early maladjustment may also be detrimental to treatment success [13].

The Cognitive Approach to Addiction

Cognitive theory focuses on how an individual's beliefs shape addiction and can then be worked with to promote recovery. Since many high risk situations are internal or inevitable, cognitive therapy focuses on how individuals can identify and modify their belief systems. The cognitive theory of addiction proposes that individuals develop addictive beliefs alongside their beliefs about the self; these may reflect social learning processes and become activated in response to life stressors.

The cognitive theory of addiction suggests that beliefs are activated in a particular sequence starting with anticipatory beliefs about the expected effects from using drug/alcohol such as 'Drinking will help me to relax'. As the individual begins to rely on substances to cope with distress, they will also develop relief-oriented beliefs that have a more imperative quality (e.g. 'I need a drink to cope'); both sets of beliefs which are sometimes referred to under the term 'positive outcome expectancies' trigger cravings and are likely to be acted upon if they remain unchallenged. Furthermore, inhibitions about using/drinking are overcome by permission-giving beliefs that justify drinking/using or minimise harm ('I've worked hard this week, I deserve it'; 'Just one won't matter'), thereby allowing the individual to act on plans to seek out and use/drink.

Orford notes that while 'cognitive processes may operate outside or on the borders of consciousness', it is 'self-talk, self-statements and the use of self-instruction' that may both contribute to the development of and the solution to excessive behaviours [11] (p. 221). Dual system models focus on understanding addiction from the perspective of the joint operation of a controlled, reflective response system and an automatic, impulsive response system [43]. More recent work on non-reflective approaches to addiction includes the idea of implicit cognition which is seen as a default in human decision and as 'automatic, implicit and associative' [14] (p. 17). Implicit cognition suggests that 'influential cognitions are the ones that are spontaneously activated during critical decision points' [14](p. 1). It is thought that such activations occur due to associations in memory but remain below conscious awareness. This unconscious or automatic processing does not refer to the stimuli or content (i.e. the drug or drug-related cues), but refers to the process of activation itself, so that there is conscious awareness of the stimuli but unconscious awareness of the effects of the stimuli [14] (p. 2).

The Cognitive Behavioural Approach to Addiction

CBT focuses on the role of thinking biases in maintaining specific problematic emotions and behaviours. By using techniques to make these thoughts explicit and assisting clients to develop alternative, more useful and realistic thoughts, emotions can be changed and behaviours managed or brought under control. CBT generally focuses on difficulties that are manifest in the here and now. It is an explicit collaboration between therapist and client and aims to teach clients skills to self-manage their difficulties as well as maintain improvements. Formulations may be highly circumscribed by the model for a specific disorder, such as panic disorder, or may be idiosyncratic and individually tailored, but still within the broad cognitive and behavioural framework that links thoughts, emotions and behaviour within an environmental context. The formulation is used to plan and evaluate interventions and may be adapted on the basis of how the client responds to treatment.

As a therapist it is important to know and to be able to share with clients four particularly important assumptions underlying the CBT approach to treating addictive behaviour:

(1) Addiction is a learnt behaviour.
(2) Addiction emerges in an environmental context.
(3) Addiction is developed and maintained by particular thought patterns and processes.
(4) CBT can be integrated well with other approaches as different approaches tend towards similar outcomes [15].

Stages of Change and Motivation

Motivation to change is a central concern when addressing addiction, and motivational interviewing (MI) is a counselling style that focuses on the interplay of ambivalence and motivation [16]. Ambivalence is defined as being 'in two minds' or 'feeling strongly towards two incompatible choices'. As such it is a normal and expected feature of addiction and recovery. Three key concepts in MI are that: (i) client motivation is critical for change; (ii) motivation is a dynamic rather than a static trait; and (iii) motivation is influenced by external factors including therapists' behaviour. MI is directive in that it facilitates the expression, clarification and resolution of any ambivalence that may stop the client from making a decision or commitment to change. Confrontation is the implicit goal of MI, but confrontation is not direct because this increases resistance to change. Instead, MI attempts to elicit the reasons for change from the client rather than attempting to persuade them that change is necessary [16, 17].

MI sees motivation as a state that fluctuates in response to shifting personal, cognitive, behavioural and environmental determinants and requires harnessing before other techniques such as RP can be successful. Miller and Rollnick coined the phrase 'ready, willing and able' [16]. Discrepancy between present reality and future values is registered by the self-regulation system and creates a state of discomfort, 'ambivalence' or 'cognitive dissonance'. This may well result in the individual seeing the importance of change ('willing') and searching for options for positive change. However, the individual needs to feel confident of succeeding in their plans ('able'); if not they may well shift their thoughts ('my drinking isn't such a problem') to be in line with the problem behaviour (carry on drinking). Actions are only likely to be taken when the individual also feels that these are important now ('ready'). How do we know, though, if an individual is ready for change?

The Transtheoretical Model of Change [18] provides a simple heuristic model which suggests that most people move through five stages of change: *Pre-contemplation, Contemplation, Preparation, Action, Maintenance* (and *Relapse*). This model which has gone through a number of iterations is useful in helping to understand where an individual may be in conceptualising their addiction, thereby allowing interventions to be more effectively targeted. An individual who is in *Pre-contemplation* may not be aware that they have a problem with addiction or may have no intention to change. While others may see there is a problem, the individual may become defensive when pressure is placed on them to change. In *Contemplation*, the individual may begin to show some distress about the addiction and begin to consider the pros and cons of making a change. Those in *Preparation* are more clearly ready to change their attitudes and behaviour and with appropriate support can move into the *Action* stage which is marked by taking steps to change and learning skills to make these changes. During the *Maintenance* stage the individual is focused on sustaining and strengthening their recovery. Individuals can exit the cycle at any time and return to an earlier stage. Relapse prevention is most appropriate during the *Action* and *Maintenance* stages together with 12-step approaches and structured treatments.

Robert West has formulated an integrated model of motivation, called the PRIME theory of motivation [19]. PRIME is an acronym for *Plans, Responses, Impulses/inhibitory forces, Motives* and *Evaluations*. PRIME theory proposes that the motivational system operates at different levels of complexity from simple reflex responses to motives and evaluations. *Motives* allow us to consider the possible outcomes of our behaviour and manifest themselves in our conscious awareness as feelings such as 'want', 'desire' or 'need'. Past experience will influence the generation of these motives. When motives are in competition, avoidance behaviours may be used. *Evaluations* involve the world being represented in terms of 'beliefs', which through their influence on motives can indirectly affect our behaviour. Competing evaluations result in dissonance: an uncomfortable state that motivates us to suppress, change or add new beliefs to try and resolve the dissonance. *Plans* are formulated when we cannot act upon an evaluation immediately. Of particular importance are plans for lifestyle change (e.g. giving up drugs/alcohol). Such plans are internally dictated; lack discrete action sequences; can exist even when we are not acting in accordance with those plans; and are long term requiring a sustained level of commitment and motivation.

While this theory lacks the ability to make explicit predictions and recommendations, it does highlight some principles of key relevance for addiction and relapse prevention strategies. West suggests that any of these motivational levels can malfunction and an effective intervention needs to address the whole motivational system. However, many interventions, like motivational interviewing, assume 'rationality' as integral to their execution and target higher levels of the motivational system, such as *Evaluations*, while arguably neglecting lower-level processes, such as emotional forces, drives, habits and impulse control. He recommends that the full range of abnormalities need to be identified, including dysfunctional beliefs, feelings, impulses, sense of identity, propensity to self-control and habit. This requires different treatment elements to be combined, or if resources are limited the PRIME theory can help to determine which element of the motivational system is best to target in which cases.

Developing a Therapeutic Alliance to Enhance Motivation

Developing a therapeutic alliance with clients requires establishing both a therapeutic bond and collaborative agreement on what to work on. CBT emphasises collaboration and active participation. Therapy should be viewed as teamwork with joint decision making about what to work on in each session and what should be done between sessions. Connecting with your client and gaining their trust is an essential component of treatment. Without it, dropout rates and resistance to change will be high. While building an alliance, you will also be gathering information about your client, which is an important part of assessment and formulation.

Beck and colleagues stress the importance of the therapeutic relationship, noting that the 'most brilliantly conceived interventions will be reduced in effectiveness if the patient is not engaged in the process of treatment' [20] (p. 54). They go on to note a number of reasons

Table 8.1 Techniques for enhancing treatment commitment

1. *Agenda setting*
2. *Monitoring readiness to change*
3. *Examining the advantages and disadvantages of using substances*
4. *Examining the advantages and disadvantages of changing substance use*
5. *Reviewing clients past efforts to change*
6. *Building self-efficacy*
7. *Positive self-statements*
8. *Asking for feedback at the end of sessions*

why there might be a hostile relationship between client and therapist at the beginning of therapy:

(1) Clients do not always enter treatment on a voluntary basis.
(2) Understandably, anyone would be reticent about opening up to a stranger until they felt more able to trust that person and more confident that person knew what they were doing.
(3) Clients may find it difficult to believe that their therapist really cares about their problems, particularly when their life circumstances are markedly different.

It is therefore extremely important to establish rapport in order to start building a therapeutic alliance and maximise client engagement with therapy. The basic ingredients necessary in any counselling situation include warmth, empathy, caring, genuine regard and competence. The issue of confidentiality should be discussed from the very start, spelling out its nature and limits according to the requirements of your service. Clients often view the therapeutic space as wholly private and inviolable and although they may find the limits to confidentiality difficult to hear they will appreciate knowing this.

Using a Motivational Communication Style within CBT

The skill required when talking to clients about the why, how, what and when of behaviour change is about structuring a conversation in a useful way which encourages the client to take as much of the lead as possible in order to start to consider change. Rollnick et al. refer to this as a 'guiding style' as opposed to an exclusively 'directing' (taking charge) or 'following' (going along with) style [21]. This can be achieved by focusing on the four core counselling skills that lie at the heart of MI: (i) asking open questions; (ii) affirming your client's position; (iii) listening reflectively; and (iv) summarising. These counselling skills are also part of the basic principles that underlie CBT. Using these skills as a 'guiding' style in your interactions you are more likely to facilitate motivation to change and foster a therapeutic environment that maximises the success of the treatment intervention.

There are several established techniques common to MI and CBT that will enhance therapeutic alliance and commitment to treatment (see Table 8.1).

Mental Health, Neuropsychological Deficits and Addiction

Many substance dependent clients have comorbid mental health problems, particularly depression and anxiety disorders [22], and it is well established that mental health and substance misuse problems can precipitate and perpetuate each other [23]. Zimberg identifies three different types of dual diagnosis [24]. Type 1 is a primary mental health problem where substances are used as a means of self-medication for that disorder – that is, an adaptive attempt to heal, self-repair and self-care. Type 2 is defined as a primary substance misuse problem with substance-induced mental health problems. This might be thought of as a 'toxicity' hypothesis; the substance may directly or indirectly contribute to the development of mental health difficulties, cognitive impairment and sometimes perceived personality disorder. A Type 3 problem is a coexisting mental health problem and/or personality disorder together with substance misuse. Such comorbidity might reflect shared predisposing factors that may underlie both the mental health and addiction presentations. Evans, Lamb and White offer a useful description of possible shared predisposing factors, including those relating to demographics, family (modelling of substance use, mental health, disrupted attachments), social factors and environment (earlier trauma, poverty, isolation), genetics (foetal alcohol syndrome, assortative mating), neurobiology and personality characteristics (e.g. unstable personality disorder, antisocial personality disorder) [25]. Dual diagnosis adds complexity to the individual's needs and if left unaddressed can contribute to difficulty engaging in and adhering to treatment.

Levels of personality disorder are high in addiction services and working with the interplay between the two problems is essential. Pickard and Pearce suggest that clients are able to regulate their consumption of drugs and that therefore the idea that drug use is a compulsive act should be questioned [26]. They argue that addicts can respond to pretty 'ordinary incentives' provided that comorbid psychiatric problems and dysfunctional backgrounds are also targeted. They identify five areas for clinical intervention and targeting: (i) strength of desire and habit; (ii) willpower; (iii) motivation; (iv) functional role; and (v) decision and resolve. They argue that by targeting these five factors, enhanced choice, improved control and augmented agency should follow. As they note 'we cannot help addicts unless we treat them as agents, capable of choice and control, and responsible for their behaviour'.

It has been suggested that a 'stepped care' approach is best in tackling underlying psychological issues in addicted individuals. Instead of attempting insight-orientated work at the first instance, a more targeted approach may be advocated. Depending on how stable an individual is from a biopsychosocial perspective, different psychological interventions ranging from behavioural (e.g. Contingency Management) to insight-orientated psychotherapy could be used to help that individual. This type of pragmatic approach has recently been adapted for all psychosocial work in a Psychosocial Toolkit approach produced by Public Health England [27].

It is estimated that around half of all clients entering treatment for alcohol dependence have some cognitive impairment [28]. Neuropsychological approaches to addiction tend to focus on deficits that make self-regulation of behaviour and emotions more difficult and thereby contribute to the development and maintenance of addictive behaviours. Executive functioning (EF) is particularly important in this respect due to its role as a mediator of self-regulation. Neuroanatomically, EF is often used to refer to the frontal lobes or prefrontal cortex due to its role in planning, rule switching, inhibition, working memory and self-regulation more generally [29]. EF also supports other neuropsychological processes such as intellectual functioning, working and prospective memory [30]. Given the importance for recovery of forming and sustaining goals and plans, maintaining motivation and altering plans and goals in response to new information, any deficit in EF and memory will, it could be argued, have a huge effect on the ability to pursue substance regulation and treatment goals. Indeed damage to any of the components of the memory system as well as frontal executive type difficulties have both been shown to be associated with poorer outcomes among those with substance use disorders [30, 31].

Despite a renewed interest in neuropsychological deficits and functioning, treatment approaches in addiction have tended to adopt either a knowledge deficit model or more recently a psychological/emotional regulation deficit model in which the role of psychological factors in the initiation and maintenance of addictive behaviours is given more prominence than cognitive deficits. The result is that deficits associated with mild to moderate neuropsychological impairments in alcohol dependence are rarely incorporated into current treatment modalities. At its most extreme this can result in an overemphasis on rationality as the primary vehicle for change, so that education becomes the route to successful change. Even where this is moderated through attention to motivational and psychological factors, many of the neuropsychological difficulties associated with dependence, such as reduced attention, poor executive self-control and poor memory, tend to be ignored.

Relapse Prevention

Lapse and relapse are still the rule rather than the exception [32] and risk is greatest during the first two to three months after treatment. Relapse prevention (RP) which is a theory, a model and an intervention aims to reduce such a risk.

There are many definitions of RP:

Relapse Prevention (RP) is a self-control programme designed to teach individuals who are trying to change their behaviour how to anticipate and cope with the problem of relapse. In a very general sense, relapse refers to a breakdown or failure in a person's attempt to change or modify any target behaviour. [33]

Relapse prevention can be conceptualized as essentially a problem-solving process and a reorientation of life attitudes and values. [34]

Relapse prevention is a generic term that refers to a wide range of cognitive and behavioural strategies designed to prevent relapse in the area of addictive behaviours and that focus on the crucial issues of helping people who are changing their behaviour to maintain the gains that they have made during the course of treatment of self-change. [35]

Marlatt and Gordon's original model of RP in 1985 introduced an important conceptual shift in viewing relapse not as a spontaneous event but rather the last step in a series of events [36]. The model noted that when individuals encounter high-risk situations (HRS) craving/urges to use/drink are triggered. Where individuals have prepared a positive coping response, they reduce their likelihood of relapse and increase their self-efficacy. However, failure to cope with a HRS is likely to reduce self-efficacy and via such cognitive processes as positive outcome expectancies and rule-violation effect, the chances of a lapse leading into a relapse are increased. Therefore RP aims to teach individuals to anticipate, recognise and cope with the possibility of relapse through identifying and coping with HRS, enhancing self-efficacy, lapse management and cognitive restructuring. Drink/drug diaries, the Inventory of Drinking Situations, the Inventory of Drug-Taking situations and the Situational Confidence Questionnaire all offer useful tools for identifying such high risk situations.

The global part of the model focuses on supporting longer-term change through identifying and coping with covert determinants of relapse such as lifestyle imbalance, craving and cognitive and behavioural processes that set up lapse by a series of decisions over time (e.g. seeking immediate gratification, denial, justification and seemingly irrelevant decisions or SIDs). RP focuses on promoting lifestyle balance so that the 'shoulds' of life do not outweigh the 'wants' and result in a desire for indulgence. Hence RP also entails working on balanced lifestyle, stimulus control, urge management and individualised relapse road maps. Clients' longer-term maintenance is likely to be maximised by timely access to additional resources that support lifestyle balance and learning skills to promote well-being, meaningful relationships and life purpose. Lapses are viewed within the model as temporary setbacks ('a fork in the road') that offer opportunities for therapeutic intervention and learning, thus offering a flexible and more optimistic view of behaviour change. It also offers a framework to intervene in this process to prevent and manage relapse. Indeed, alongside motivational interviewing [37] and Prochaska and DiClemente's Transtheoretical Model, relapse prevention has had the greatest influence in the addictions field over the last 20 years.

A number of research studies have investigated the reliability of the RP model. The Relapse Prevention and Extension Project (RPEP) supported the overall model of the relapse process – for example, finding that relapse was predicted by coping and not simply by exposure to high-risk situations [38]. The study supported other findings that many relapse episodes involve situations with negative emotional states and the role of the rule-violation effect in precipitating a relapse, specifically in those who had a greater belief in the disease model and higher commitment to abstinence [39].

Although RP does not seem to be associated with higher long-term abstinence rates than other active treatments, studies do support the effectiveness of RP interventions in reducing the frequency and severity of relapses, and also in positively impacting on mental health. Carroll suggests that there is a delayed emergence effect, with better longer-term outcomes in the maintenance phase – that is, one-year follow-up, as clients come to learn and establish skills [40]. A meta-analysis found that RP is equally efficacious across inpatient and outpatient settings, and individual and group delivery [41]. There is some evidence that while RP offers benefit for all substances, it is most effective for reducing alcohol and poly-substance use and least effective for tobacco and cocaine use [41]. This would point to the need to tailor RP approaches for tobacco and cocaine treatments. Review studies indicated the value of combining RP with pharmacotherapy for alcohol treatment [41] and smoking cessation programmes [42].

While the original relapse model offered a useful framework and set of techniques, it was criticised for being rather a static, linear, two-dimensional model that did not adequately account for negative emotional states, craving and withdrawal, motivation, cultural differences and social support. Clients, clinicians and researchers observed how a seemingly insignificant shift in one factor can kindle a downward spiral in other factors that result in relapse. Marlatt and Witkiewitz looked to explain the observed fluctuations in abstinence and relapse [43], and found this to fit well with catastrophe theory, the study of sudden discontinuous changes in behaviour resulting from slight continuous changes in system parameters. They therefore developed their thinking to account for these criticisms and new research findings to put forward their dynamic model of relapse [44]. This model presents relapse as a complex system of multiple elements that interact dynamically within a high-risk situation to maintain the status quo or tip the balance towards changes in substance use.

While relapse prevention remains a proficient tool for recovery, it has been suggested that it overemphasises the deliberate, conscious, controlled processes of behaviour and overlooks the automatic, habitual processes of addiction. Alan Marlatt's personal discovery of the benefits of transcendental meditation in the 1970s influenced his professional practice. In the early days of RP, Marlatt included the Buddhist practice of Vipassana ('seeing things as they really are') to develop lifestyle balance among high-risk drinkers. This ultimately laid the foundation for mindfulness-based relapse prevention (MBRP) [45]. It is patterned after/on mindfulness-based stress reduction, mindfulness-based cognitive therapy and Daley and Marlatt's relapse prevention protocol [46]. MBRP has been shown to result in improved abstinence rates, reduced drug and alcohol use, reduced relapse rates, and to be effective for individuals with dual diagnoses [47]. Mindfulness appears to target some of the automatic processes of addiction – for example, countering attentional bias by enhancing attention and countering avoidance by nurturing acceptance [48]. The accepting attitude of mindfulness towards present moment experience without seeking to change or avoid it can lead to a reduction in use. Neuroimaging has allowed us to examine how brain areas associated with craving and negative affect are positively affected by mindfulness training and overall it seems that mindfulness meditation may affect neural responses to negative affect, and may reverse, repair or compensate for neuro-adaptive changes associated with addiction [36].

MBRP has been shown to be associated with reduced drug/ alcohol use and improved abstinence rates [40, 41]. It also outperformed a 'treatment as usual' group receiving standard outpatient aftercare using a 12-step process-oriented format, bringing significantly lower rates of substance use [45]. The authors found that craving was mediated by acceptance, awareness and non-judgement. Brewer et al. [51] found that cocaine and alcohol users randomly assigned to the MBRP group showed lower psychological and physiological responses to stress in comparison to those assigned to the CBT treatment group. Treatment acceptability is good, although MBRP requires intensive participation and is best suited to highly motivated clients.

Borland presents a dual process theory of hard-to-maintain behaviours and hard-to-sustain behaviours [49]. He identifies existing theories of addiction as being 'limited in either scope or conceptualisation of the central problem' (p.5). Borland highlights three theories: (i) biologically focused theories which focus on biological mechanisms and learning; (ii) expectancy-value theories which look at the rational appraisal on a cost-benefit basis; and (iii) social determinant models which locate individual problems within imperfect social structures. Borland critiques the explanatory power of such theories on the basis that they are not able to explain individual differences and responses to the same set of circumstances.

Borland's central concern is on hard-to-maintain behaviour (HTM) changes and notes that what is required for initial behaviour change is not the same as what is needed to maintain such behaviour change. Borland notes that all behaviour change occurs within a particular individual and external context and that this then interacts with two internal processes, the operational and executive. Borland names his theory CEOS, which is a combination of social context, an adaptive operating system (OS), which controls responses on a moment to moment basis and controls the means by which we act on the world, and an executive system (ES), which is essentially linguistic and logical and is involved in self-regulation and determining preferential future courses of action. While the OS operates automatically and is the locus of action, the function of the ES is to monitor this, particularly in situations that are novel and/or complex and to override this automaticity. Indeed, novel situations require the use of the ES in order to be dealt with appropriately. Where addiction and dependence occur they can be thought of as becoming part of the OS and initial change requires the use of the ES in order to overcome automatic responses such as craving states. However, in order for behaviour change to be sustained, the OS needs to take over the function of the ES, so that the newly changed behaviour operates on a more automatic basis. In essence therefore the focus of Borland's work is on the relative unimportance of rationality once behaviour change has been instigated. If CEOS is correct, and it does at least appear plausible, then it has implications for relapse prevention treatment and gives some additional theoretical support for mindfulness, acceptance and commitment therapy, along with lifestyle balance programmes more generally. It also allows a more productive discourse to take place with clients who continually re-present to services with high levels of motivation and knowledge about the importance of integrated unconscious behavioural patterns. Where things get trickier is where an individual's neuropsychological functioning has been compromised so that executive functioning and memory systems destabilise effective ES functioning. While the OS can be assumed to take control in such circumstances, this should not underestimate the amount of time and skill-based cognitive remediation and restructuring that may need to take place.

Neuropsychological and Associated Difficulties When Undertaking Relapse Prevention

While RP recognises that an individual's motivational state can change over time, it tends to assume a level playing field with regard to their abilities. In some respects it is an empty vessel model in which the client needs to be filled up with RP information and strategies. It also assumes that individuals are essentially equal in being able to access the strategies they need when they need them. While this is an ideal situation, it does neglect the issue of differential capabilities and the damage caused by substance use to self-regulating capacities and memory systems. This is a complex area that requires a great deal of work to deal with adequately. Aside from the fact that some individuals may have specific learning or sensory difficulties, which always need to be taken into account when teaching, there are four main components which need to be taken into consideration when delivering RP:

(i)   current cognitive functioning and literacy levels
(ii) attentional ability
(iii) memory
(iv) executive functioning

Attention is very much the building block of any learning strategy and if an individual has poor attention then any subsequent failure of RP may be more to do with this than anything else. Attention is, of course, not a unitary construct. Thus we can measure sustained attention (keeping on task for a long period of time), focused attention (attending to the specific relevant information and excluding that which is extraneous) and divided attention (attending to more than one thing at a time). Difficulties in any of these areas will require an adaptation of the RP approach.

If attention is the ability to attend to information in the first place, memory is the ability to register that information into some form of short- or long-term storage, and then being able to access this information when needed. There are many different forms of memory, but arguably one of the most important is prospective memory, which is the ability to remember to do something in the future. RP essentially is also about remembering to do *x* instead of *y* in the future and to recall what that entails. Disruption to this often means that someone fails to sustain change not because their strategies fail, but because they fail to remember to use such strategies. Individuals also differ in the extent to which they can freely recall information and their ability to recognise information given a suitable cue. Recognition memory tends to be better for most people than free recall and this should therefore be built into the way RP is taught. One also needs to consider executive functioning (EF). EF is a 'multifaceted neuropsychological construct that can be defined as (a) forming, (b) maintaining, and (c) shifting mental sets, corresponding to the abilities to (a) reason and generate goals and plans, (b) maintain focus and motivation to follow through with goals and plans, and (c) flexibly alter goals and plans in response to changing contingencies' [50]. All of these skills have a huge effect on the ability to pursue treatment goals and remain abstinent.

For some individuals building RP into their change programme will be sufficient for them to prevent further lapses or relapses through the operation of learnt strategies. The individual may have made some overall changes to their lifestyle or implemented strategies to prevent lapses and relapse. This is the gold standard of treatment, the delivery of an intervention resulting in long-term behavioural change. However, in addiction services it is a minority of individuals who will experience successful change immediately without either lapsing or relapsing.

What about RP where a client's goal is not total abstinence? An obvious example in the UK is the increasing number of people, particularly younger sections of the population, who are engaged in periodic but regular binge drinking. Here the goal may not be abstinence but harm reduction or drinking in moderation. Does RP have anything particular to offer with regard to such groups? Generally, where people are still using drugs or alcohol but are seeking behavioural change, they are either looking to minimise, reduce or control their use of the target substance or they are looking to deal with some form of causal outcome from such use, such as reducing cocaine use after excessive drinking or trying to reduce their anger after drinking. RP can have a role in such scenarios provided that the model is adapted slightly, particularly that the wording of strategies is made relevant to a goal of moderation, and also that the target behaviour to be changed is clearly specified. Such goals might focus on drinking days, quantities consumed or on other social consequences such as absences from work. Developing strategies to manage such changes, promoting self-efficacy and drawing on global interventions to address covert antecedents is where RP can play a significant role.

Clinical Considerations and Conclusions

This chapter has been primarily about psychological models and theories of addiction. As will hopefully have become apparent there is a great deal of crossover between seemingly different theories. Thus while psychodynamic models and implicit cognition may be quite different, both highlight the importance of sub-threshold awareness within addiction. This idea may also to some extent, relate to the impact of neuropsychological deficits. Thus, one might conclude that our current state of knowledge regarding the psychology of addiction would best acknowledge processes occurring both at the conscious level, such as self-efficacy and contingency management, as well as those occurring unconsciously and more implicitly. This has implications for treatment approaches, and the role of lifestyle balance, recovery and mindfulness-based approaches is a positive movement towards this understanding. The chapter has also touched on the some of the other significant factors that influence addiction, such as social, economic and cultural determinants. It is important to note their importance for addiction and acknowledge that psychological understanding always operates in a particular context and that certainly as far as long-term treatment outcome goes, it is both the external as well as the internal world of clients that matters.

References

1 White W. L. *Recovery Management and Recovery-Oriented Systems of Care: Scientific Rationale and Promising Practices.* Pittsburgh, PA: Northeast Addiction Technology Transfer Center; 2008.

2 Flores P. J. *Group Psychotherapy with Addicted Populations: An Integration of Twelve-Step and Psychodynamic Theory.* Binghamston, NY: The Haworth Press; 1997.

3 Weegman M. Psychodynamics in groups or psychodynamic groups? In: Hill R., Harris J., eds. *Principles and Practice of Group Work in Addictions.* Hove: Routledge; 2011.

4 Drummond D. C. Theories of drug craving, ancient and modern. *Addiction.* 2001; **96**: 33–46.

5 Bandura A. Self-efficacy: Toward a unifying theory of behavioral change. *Psychological Review.* 1977; **84** (2): 191–215.

6 Brown S. A. Drug effect expectancies and addictive behavior change. *Experimental and Clinical Psychopharmacology.* 1993; **1** (1–4): 55–67.

7 Flanagan O. Phenomenal authority: The epistemic authority of Alcoholics Anonymous. In: Levy N., ed. *Addiction and Self-Control Perspectives from Philosophy, Psychology and Neuroscience.* Oxford: Oxford University Press; 2013. p. 67–93.

8. Public Health England. *Facilitating Access to Mutual Aid Three essential stages for helping clients access appropriate mutual aid support.* London: PHE; 2013.

9 Robins L. N. Vietnam veterans' rapid recovery from heroin addiction: A fluke or normal expectation? *Addiction.* 1993; **88**: 1041–54.

10 Peele S. *The Meaning of Addiction: An Unconventional View.* San Francisco: Jossey-Bass Inc.; 1998.

11 Orford J. *Excessive Appetites.* Chichester: John Wiley & Sons; 2001.

12 Baklien B., Samarasinghe D. *Alcohol and Poverty in Sri Lanka.* Colombo: Forut; 2003.

13 Hill R. G., Moran P., Cooper W., Bearn J. Early childhood maladjustment and adherence with inpatient drug detoxification treatment. *Journal of Substance Use.* 2006; **10** (6): 1–7.

14 Stacy A. W., Wiers R. W. Implicit cognition and addiction: A tool for explaining paradoxical behavior. *Annual Review of Clinical Psychology.* 2010; **6** (1): 551–75.

15 Kadden R. M., Carroll K., Donovan D., Cooney N., Monti P. M., Abrams D. et al., eds. *Cognitive-Behavioral Coping Skills Therapy Manual: A Clinical Research Guide for Therapists Treating Individuals With Alcohol Abuse and Dependence.* Rockville, MD: National Institute on Alcohol Abuse and Alcoholism; 2003.

16 Miller W. R., Rollnick S. *Motivational Interviewing: Helping People Change.* 3rd edn. New York: The Guildford Press; 2013.

17 Tober G., Raistrick D., eds. *Motivational Dialogue: Preparing Addiction Professionals for Motivational Interviewing Practice.* Abingdon: Routledge; 2007.

18 Prochaska J. O., DiClemente C. C. *The Transtheoretical Approach: Crossing the Traditional Boundaries of Therapy.* Melbourne, FL: Krieger Publishing Company; 1984.

19 West R. *Theory of Addiction*. Oxford: Blackwell Publishing; 2006.

20 Beck A. T., Wright F. D., Newman C. F., Liese L. Cognitive Therapy of Substance Abuse. London: Guilford Press; 1993.

21 Rollnick S., Miller W. R. *Motivational Interviewing in Health Care: Helping Patients Change Behavior*. New York: Guilford Press; 2008.

22 Weaver T., Madden P., Charles V., Timso G. S., Renton A., Tyrer P. et al. Comorbidity of Substance Misuse and Mental Illness in Community Mental Health and Substance Misuse Services. *British Journal of Psychiatry*. 2003; **183**: 304–13.

23 Tiet Q. Q., Mausbach B. Treatments for Patients with Dual Diagnosis: A Review. *Alcoholism: Clinical and Experimental Research*. 2007; **31** (4): 513–36.

24 Zimberg S. A dual diagnosis typology to improve diagnosis and treatment of dual disorder patients. *Journal of Psychoactive Drugs*. 1999; **31** (1): 47–51.

25 Evans A. C., Lamb R., White W. L. *Promoting Intergenerational Resilience and Recovery: Policy, Clinical, and Recovery Support Strategies to Alter the Intergenerational Transmission of Alcohol, Drug, and Related Problems*. Philadelphia: Department of Behavioral Health and Intellectual Disability Services; 2014.

26 Pickard H., Pearce S. Addiction in context: Philosophical lessons from a personality disorder clinic. In: Levy N., ed. *Addiction and Self-Control: Lessons from Philosophy, Psychology and Neuroscience*. New York: Oxford University Press; 2013. p. 165–89.

27 Day E. *Routes to Recovery via the Community*. London: Public Health England; 2013.

28 Maillard A., Cabe N., Viader F., Pitel A. L. Neuropsychological deficits in alcohol use disorder: impact on treatment. In: Verdejo-Garcia A, ed. *Cognition and Addiction: A Researcher's Guide from Mechanisms Towards Interventions*. London: Academic Press; 2020. p. 103–28.

29 Barkley R. A. *Executive Functions: What They Are, How They Work, and Why They Evolved*. London: Guilford Press; 2012.

30 Griffiths A., Hill R., Morgan C., Rendell P. G., Karimi K., Wanagaratne S. et al. Prospective memory and future event simulation in individuals with alcohol dependence. *Addiction*. 2012; **107** (10): 1809–16.

31 Manning V., Wanigaratne S., Best D., Hill R. G., Reed L. J., Ball D. et al. Changes in Neuropsychological Functioning during Alcohol Detoxification. *European Addiction Research*. 2008; **14** (4): 226–33.

32 Witkiewitz K. A., Marlatt G. A., eds. *Practical Resources for the Mental Health Professional: Therapist's Guide to Evidence-Based Relapse Prevention*. Burlington, MA: Elsevier Academic Press; 2007.

33 Marlatt G. A., George W. H. Relapse prevention: Introduction and overview of the model. *British Journal of Addiction*. 1984; **79** (3): 261–73.

34 Giannetti V. J. Brief relapse prevention with substance abusers. In: Wells R. A., Giannetti V. J., eds. *Applied Clinical Psychology Casebook of the Brief Psychotherapies*. New York: Plenum Press; 1993. p. 159–78.

35 Donovan D. M. Assessment of addictive behaviors for relapse prevention. In: Donovan D. M., Marlatt G. A., eds. *Assessment of Addictive Behaviors*. 2nd ed. New York: Guilford Press; 2005. p. 1–48.

36 Marlatt G. A., Gordon J. R. Relapse Prevention: Maintenance Strategies in the Treatment of Addictive Behaviors. New York: Guilford Press; 1985.

37 Miller W. R., Rollnick S. Motivational Interviewing: Preparing People to Change Addictive Behaviour. New York: Guildford; 1991.

38 Lowman C., Allen J., Stout R. L. Replication and extension of Marlatt's taxonomy of relapse precipitants: overview of procedures and results. The Relapse Research Group. *Addiction*. 1996; **91** Suppl: S51-71.

39 Larimer M. E., Palmer R. S., Marlatt G. A. Relapse prevention: An overview of

Marlatt's cognitive-behavioral model. *Alcohol Research and Health.* 1999; **23** (2): 151–60.

40 Carroll K. Relapse prevention as a psychosocial treatment: A review of controlled clinical trials. *Experimental and Clinical Psychopharmacology.* 1996; **4** (1): 46–54.

41 Irvin J. E., Bowers C. A., Dunn M. E., Wang M. C. Efficacy of relapse prevention: a meta-analytic review. *Journal of Consulting and Clinical Psychology.* 1999; **67** (4): 563–70.

42 Agboola S. A., Coleman T. J., Leonardi-Bee J. A., McEwen A., McNeill A. D. Provision of relapse prevention interventions in UK NHS Stop Smoking Services: A survey. *BMC Health Services Research.* 2010; **10** (1): 214.

43 Norman D. A., Shallice T. Attention to action: Willed and automatic control of behavior. In: Davidson R. J., Schwartz G. E., Shapiro D., eds. *Consciousness and self-regulation: Advances in research,* vol. **4**. New York: Plenum Press; 1986.

44 Witkiewitz K., Marlatt G. A. Relapse prevention for alcohol and drug problems – That was Zen, this is Tao. *American Psychologist.* 2004; **59** (4): 224–35.

45 Witkiewitz K., Bowen S., Douglas H., Hsu S. H. Mindfulness-based relapse prevention for substance craving. *Addictive behaviors.* 2013; **38** (2): 1563–71.

46 Daley D. C., Marlatt G. A. *Overcoming Your Alcohol or Drug Problem: Effective Recovery Strategies (Therapist Guide).* 2nd ed. Oxford: Oxford University Press; 2006.

47 Witkiewitz K., Bowen S. Depression, craving, and substance use following a randomized trial of mindfulness-based relapse prevention. *Journal of Consulting and Clinical Psychology.* 2010; **78** (3): 362–74.

48 Witkiewitz K., Lustyk M. K. B., Bowen S. Retraining the addicted brain: A review of hypothesized neurobiological mechanisms of mindfulness-based relapse prevention. *Psychology of Addictive Behaviors.* 2013; **27** (2): 351–65.

49 Borland R. Understanding Hard to Maintain Behaviour Change: A Dual Process Approach. Chichester: John Wiley & Sons; 2014.

50 Suchy Y. Executive functioning: Overview, assessment, and research issues for non-neuropsychologists. *Annals of Behavioral Medicine.* 2009; **37** (2): 106–16.

51 Brewer J. A., Sinha R., Chen J. A., Michalsen R. N., Babuscio T. A., Nich C., Grier A., Bergquist K. L., Reis D. L., Potenza M. N., Carroll K. M., Rounsaville B. J. Mindfulness training and stress reactivity in substance abuse: Results from a randomized, controlled stage I pilot study. *Substance Abuse.* 2009; **30** (4): 306–317.

Comorbid Substance Use and Mental Illness

Michael Kelleher and Luke Mitcheson

Introduction

The coexistence of problematic substance use and significant psychological distress is common in both addiction and psychiatric services. Unfortunately, the psychiatric diagnostic system has created an idea of discrete diseases instead of a single psychological entity – for example, separate diagnoses of alcohol dependence and generalised anxiety disorder in an alcohol dependent individual with underlying anxiety from their early teens. This false dichotomy has allowed the development of ideas and services that often serve to exclude those with the most complexity and greatest mortality or morbidity. In this chapter we will examine the scale of the problem, the consequences of this issue and some of the practical solutions.

A minor note on nomenclature: the phrase 'dual diagnosis' has been traditionally used about this group, but this term is also used in other settings beyond coexisting addiction and mental illness and may lead to confusion. Therefore, in this chapter it is replaced by the terms 'coexisting' or 'co-occurring' (addiction and mental illness) as used in recent NICE public health guidance [1] and Public Health England guidance [2].

The Scale of the Problem

Psychiatric disorders are much more prevalent in the population with substance use disorders than they are in the general population. The 1995 UK Household survey of psychiatric morbidity (surveying the population both in and out of treatment) showed that 45 per cent of the drug dependent population and 30 per cent of the alcohol dependent population had a co-occurring psychiatric illness [3]. The equivalent 2014 survey revealed that 27 per cent of men and 42 per cent of women with probable alcohol dependence were in receipt of some form of treatment for a mental or emotional problem [4]. More than half of those with probable drug dependence were in receipt of some form of treatment for an emotional or mental problem, when cannabis dependence was excluded, falling to 12 per cent for those with probable cannabis dependence. Globally, in general population surveys, the strongest associations are between substance use disorders and anxiety/depression [5]. Regarding the prevalence of co-occurrence within healthcare treatment populations, Weaver et al. [6] found that 44 per cent of the community mental health team sample had a substance misuse problem in the past year, and 75 per cent of the drug treatment population and 85 per cent of the alcohol treatment population had a mental health issue in the past year.

Studies of patients with schizophrenia across the UK, France and Germany have suggested that 35 per cent of the UK schizophrenia cohort may have co-occurring drug or alcohol dependence [7]. Those who were dependent were more likely to be younger men, with shorter clinical histories of psychosis, more severe symptoms, but fewer negative symptoms. They had poor functioning on psychosocial and quality of life scales.

Unsurprisingly, given the high rates of both historical and current substance use in incarcerated populations, levels of co-occurrence are high. One study of the English prison system suggested that 78 per cent of those in six English prisons with a severe mental illness (defined as a current episode of major depressive disorder, bipolar disorder or any form of psychosis) had a substance misuse issue [8]. The Bradley report in 2009 made it clear that co-occurring conditions were the norm rather than the exception among offenders [2]. Early data from police liaison and diversion schemes for mental health suggested that the 55 per cent of service users with mental health issues that had contact with these schemes also had problematic drug and/or alcohol use [2]. It has been estimated that between 58 and 65 per cent of the homeless population have co-occurring substance use disorder and mental illness [9]. Therefore the co-occurrence of mental illness and addiction is common in all diagnostic categories, and in some service populations it is the rule rather than the exception.

Association with Mortality and Morbidity

A large cohort study carried out in England suggested that the standardised mortality rate of an opioid dependent individual by suicide was 4.5. [10]. Another study in a south London opioid dependent population found that comorbid opioid and personality disorder was associated with increased mortality when compared to opioid dependence alone [11]. The National Confidential Inquiry into Suicide and Homicide by People with Mental Illness has found that 54 per cent of psychiatric patients in England and Wales that commit suicide are considered to be drug and/or alcohol dependent by their treating team at the time of death. The report goes on to note that only 11 per cent are receiving some form of addiction services at their time of death [12]. The standardised mortality rate of patients with schizophrenia from substance use–related issues in the Welsh population was found to be 8.2 [13].

Similar findings have been reported in other countries. In Australia, those released from prison with a co-occurring condition were at increased risk of being admitted to hospital with an injury when compared to those with a mental illness alone or no diagnosis (90 per cent of these admissions were not overdose related). Of the overdose-related events in this prison release cohort, 80 per cent were in the co-occurring group rather than the substance misuse only group [14].

Individuals with coexisting mental health and addictions conditions have increased levels of mortality above and beyond the increased mortality rates of those without cooccurrence. In an age of increasing life expectancy across the population as a whole this increased risk of death is worthy of greater focus and investment.

Aetiology of Co-Occurrence

There are many theories for why the co-occurrence of substance use disorder and mental illness is so common:

(1) The substance use disorder and psychiatric illness share a common root, be it social adversity in childhood, genetic or psychological vulnerability.

(2) Those who develop a substance use disorder are as a consequence biologically at risk of a mental illness, or suffer social and psychological adverse events due to the substance use that cause a psychiatric illness.

(3) Those with psychiatric illness turn to substances to alleviate negative mood states and reduce anxiety – in essence, a form of self-medication. This is exacerbated by the wide availability of alcohol and drugs in modern societies.

(4) Those who are socially isolated and stigmatised due to their mental illness engage with substance using networks due to their inclusivity.

The causes of co-occurrence are complex and multifactorial. It is important to understand both the external societal drivers of such conditions as well as internal psychological and biological factors. A common error in the current psychiatric epoch can be to focus largely or exclusively on individual factors, rather than recognising that patients swim in a social sea and are to a degree products of their past and present environment. For example, it is notable that the EuroSc study found that in the cohort with schizophrenia the rates of co-occurring substance dependence were much lower in France (19 per cent) and Germany (21 per cent) than the UK (35 per cent), even though rates of schizophrenia were similar [7].

Exclusion and Unmet Need

The Public Health England publication, *Better Care for People with Co-Occurring Mental Health and Alcohol/Drug Use Conditions* [2], sought the views of service users. It suggested that there is significant unmet need in this group and that drug and alcohol use can be used as a means of exclusion in mental health treatment services, and mental illness used as a means of exclusion in addiction services. It further noted that the Home Affairs Select Committee report on mental health and policing found that vital support could be withheld from those in crisis because alcohol or drug use was applied as an exclusion criteria. The Making Every Adult Matter (MEAM) coalition noted that addictions and mental health services often failed to work collaboratively on behalf of the most complex patients. For example, patients with anxiety disorders and a history of drug or alcohol dependence could be excluded from some Improving Access to Psychological Therapies (IAPT) services.

In practical terms, large amounts of time can be spent trying to decide primacy – that is, did the mental illness predate the addiction or vice versa? – and this can consume services and waste resources. Unfortunately, this question may have no meaningful or relevant answer, and more importantly it can serve to disillusion the patient about the availability and effectiveness of treatment and the friendliness of services. The service user may be consigned to seek treatment elsewhere in an unevidenced and widely derided sequential model of care.

Figures from the National Drug Treatment Monitoring System (NDTMS) suggest about 16 per cent of addiction patients in England were also receiving some form of treatment for a psychiatric condition. Such national figures are not available at the current time from the Mental Health Minimum Dataset.

Current Guidance in England

Until recently the main guide for co-occurring conditions in England was the 2002 Department of Health guidance, *Mental Health Policy Implementation Guide: Dual Diagnosis Good Practice Guide*, as part of the now-defunct NHS framework [10]. This document was aimed at specialist mental health services and focused on severe and enduring mental illness. An aim of the document was to create integrated addiction care of a high standard within psychiatric provision. While this was laudable, it has been patchily implemented across England. Although the themes contained within the 2002 guidance remain relevant, this guidance has now been superseded by more recent publications:

- From NICE: NG 58, 'Coexisting severe mental illness and substance misuse: community health and social care services' [1]
- From Public Health England: 'Better care for people with co-occurring mental health and alcohol/drug use conditions' [2] (produced as part of the Five Year Forward View for mental health)
- From NHS England: 'Achieving better access to 24/7 urgent and emergency mental health care' [11]

These three documents should form part of the basis of design of any services that deal with those with co-occurring mental illness and addiction. Given how common co-occurrence is, it is difficult to think of an addiction service or a mental health service to which at least one of these documents is not relevant.

The Public Health England document [2] is aimed at a strategic level towards both commissioners and providers of services; it does not provide clinical guidance. It has two key overarching principles for the provision of health services in this area.

1 No Wrong Door

The intention is that providers of mental health and addiction services should not turn a patient away because they consider that they are wrong for their service due to a co-occurring condition. Instead, they should offer assessment and if they think the individual patient is better placed in another part of the addiction and/or mental health treatment system they should facilitate the transfer of care to the appropriate part of the system in a collaborative fashion.

2 Everyone's Job

Given how common co-occurring conditions are and their association with increased mortality and morbidity, both mental health and addiction services need skills in identifying co-occurring conditions and need to be able, indeed have a responsibility, to work collaboratively with other agencies.

Collaborative Care

In addition to these key principles, guidance follows in relation to collaborative care. With co-occurring conditions, if a patient needs the care of both sets of agencies, addictions and mental health services should work in close collaboration centred on the needs of the individual patient. There should be a clear 'care plan' which is shared with the patient and all other agencies (provided appropriate consent is given). A lead agency should be nominated to coordinate the care. Such collaborative care can include fully integrated care in a single provider; however, on other occasions it may be more feasible for care to be provided in a collaborative fashion – for example, the patient in treatment for schizophrenia with a mental health team receiving methadone for their opioid dependence from an addiction service. What the guidance makes clear is that both commissioners and providers have a role and responsibility in creating the framework for such collaborative care to take place. It adds that there should be clear care pathways developed for such patients.

Specialist Dual Diagnosis Teams

The PHE guidance and indeed the NICE guidance (NG 58) both note that there is little evidence for specialist dual diagnosis teams. They state that this does not mean there should not be specialist dual diagnosis practitioners who can take on an advocacy and training role for those with co-occurring conditions. However, both pieces of guidance suggest that these conditions are so common that all staff and services need to be competent to respond to issues, rather than seeking a 'container' in which to place some of their most complex, stigmatised and disadvantaged patients.

Service Organisation and Delivery

At point of contact with treatment services, it is important to routinely ask about both mental health and substance misuse issues. In psychiatric services, screening tools such as the AUDIT [12] for alcohol and ASSIST [13] for alcohol, drugs and tobacco are useful validated screening tools that can help ascertain the level of need, although they are not a substitute for thorough, good-quality, clinical assessment.

Diagnosis of both addiction and psychiatric issues can help direct the treatment process. However, it is important not to be driven by statements such as 'drug induced psychosis' before there is strong evidence to support this, as this can serve to exclude a patient from suitable treatment. Needs should be identified, and efforts made to address these. Such needs can cross multiple domains including: physical health problems, social isolation, homelessness, adult and child safeguarding issues and involvement with criminal justice agencies. It is especially important to note the increased mortality from physical ill health including COPD, cancer, cirrhotic liver disease and blood-borne viruses and other infections. Levels of nicotine dependence are also high in this population. Services may need to advocate on behalf of patients with these conditions with allied health and social care agencies.

This patient group can face stigma and may find it difficult to access treatment services due to previous negative experiences. The first contact and offer of treatment should be as welcoming as possible. Patients and their carers should not feel passed off by services. Once a diagnosis is made of co-occurring mental illness and addiction, the patient should be referred to the appropriate secondary care mental health service and/or addiction service.

Severe Mental Illness and Addiction

Patients diagnosed with a severe mental illness should be referred to secondary care mental health as the lead agency for assessment and care planning. Guidance is clear that such patients should not be excluded from mental health services due to substance use and a person-centred approach as advocated by NICE (NG58) should be adopted [1]. This group includes not just those with psychosis, severe depression or dementia, but also those that present with repeated mental health crises such as self-injurious behaviour. Once accepted by mental health services, they should be provided with a care coordinator who will liaise with the patient and any carers, develop their care plan and coordinate with any other agencies involved.

Patients with Severe Addiction and Mild or Moderate Mental Illness

Those with significant addiction problems and mild to moderate mental illness may best have their care led by addiction services, coordinating with psychiatric services as needed.

Care Planning

The care planning process should involve patients and their family or carers (if the patient agrees) and should aim to meet the individual's needs. This process should provide the patient with information on what services are available and where they can access care. The care planning process should also involve workers from any other agencies involved, such as substance misuse, housing or physical healthcare. The care plan should be shared with the patient and any others involved in the patient's care (provided consent is given). As for all patients, any carers may have needs that also need to be assessed and potentially addressed. Care should be provided for the relevant psychiatric and addictions disorder, as set out in other relevant guidance.

Communication

Clear, regular and documented communication is important between all agencies involved. Where possible there should be agreement between the agencies and the patient that information will be shared appropriately. There should be agreement about who the lead agency is and a named professional to coordinate care (whether or not within the meaning of the Care Programme Approach). As the overarching coordinator of a patient's healthcare, their general practitioner should be included in communications.

Engagement in Services

As a group, patients with co-occurring mental health and substance use disorders often drift out of contact with services. There are a variety of ways of helping to sustain contact, including:

(1) Moving away from an exclusively abstinence-focused position (if the patient is unable or unwilling to achieve abstinence) and moving towards a harm minimisation one. This may involve tolerance of ongoing chaotic substance use.

(2) Having empathy for the individual and taking a non-judgmental or non-moralising position.

(3) Having consistent staff members that recognise that the patient may have had previous negative experiences in services that make them wary. Staff members need to avoid therapeutic nihilism with this group and recognise that quick fixes after brief episodes of treatment are often unsuccessful.

(4) Certain groups may avoid contact with services if they feel coerced or fear involvement with other agencies such as local authority child protection agencies. Another group that may struggle include the victims of intimate partner violence. Services should endeavour to adapt to become as welcoming and supportive as possible to these groups while at the same time being aware of their statutory responsibilities.

(5) The homeless have very high rates of co-occurring mental illness and addiction and service provision should endeavour to adapt to their needs.

(6) Asking patients about their view of the links between their substance use and mental illness allows them to communicate their view of the issues rather than one imposed by professionals.

(7) Taking an information-giving approach about the potential effects of substance use on psychological health can allow them to make an informed choice, and some patients may be able to self-limit their use.

(8) Coordinating care so that the patient does not feel passed between disparate, uncommunicative, fragmented services. A key element of this is avoiding the need for repeated assessments eliciting the same information.

(9) Having flexibility around a patient's work or family commitments that may impinge on their ability to attend at certain times.

(10) Endeavouring to re-engage patients repeatedly if they drop out of services prematurely. Such efforts may include telephone, text, paper or email contact, but consideration may also need to be given to contacting family members and home visits.

(11) If they are discharged in a planned or unplanned fashion, then the routes back into treatment must be made clear to the patient, any carers and their GP.

Crisis Planning

If relevant, patients should have a clear crisis plan that adapts to their ongoing needs. In the event of a crisis it is important that the presenting issue is addressed, rather than allowing substance intoxication, withdrawal or dependence to become the predominant focus of the crisis intervention. This is set out in part by NHS England in *Achieving Better Access to 24/7 Urgent and Emergency Mental Health Care* [11].

Broadly speaking crises fall into three domains:

(1) *Physical*: examples such as hepatic encephalopathy, synthetic cannabinoid-induced arrhythmia or opioid overdose are physical emergencies and should be transferred to A and E departments.

(2) *Psychiatric*: emergencies such as psychotic episodes or suicidality on a background of intoxication or withdrawal where the individual is considered a risk to themselves or others should be urgently transferred to emergency psychiatric care depending on local pathways. Such pathways include crisis care teams, A and E liaison psychiatry and 136 suites.

(3) *Social*: crises such as intimate partner violence on a background of substance use are issues for the local authority safeguarding services and/or the police.

Training and Support for Staff

As noted NICE, following an extensive evidence review, recommends adapting existing mental health services to the needs of this patient group rather than creating 'dual diagnosis services'. Consequently all staff need to be appropriately trained in the basics of alcohol and drug harm reduction/treatment interventions as set out in relevant NICE guidance and the 'orange guidelines' for the treatment of drug dependence [14]. Local substance misuse services should provide advice support and training where needed.

The professionals involved in the care of these patients should be appropriately supported and supervised. It is recognised that some staff in both addiction and mental health services may have negative attitudes towards this patient group and need support in overcoming such attitudes. At the same time, it should be noted that some patients with co-occurring conditions can present in repeated crises or with challenging behaviour which can prove difficult for staff members. Joint training and strong leadership can help to overcome these issues and foster good collaborative working relationships both with the patient and with other services.

There is a need for all addiction staff to have an ability to recognise psychiatric illness and understand locally agreed routes to psychiatric services, both for mental health crises and for ongoing psychiatric treatment. There is a need for psychiatric staff to be able to identify and provide addiction harm minimisation and recovery activities with relevant patients. Specialist interventions such as treatment in the community for opioid dependence or alcohol withdrawal, pharmacological treatment of psychosis or psychological treatment of depression usually belong in the relevant specialist service.

Interventions for Co-Occurring Mental Illness and Addiction

Problems of acute intoxication need to be separated from problems of dependence in those with mental illness. Much of the wider population is at risk of episodes of intoxication and the consequences are the same. As with the general population, the individual may only need a brief intervention if there is no evidence of systematic use.

Psychoeducation

Many (but not all) patients and their carers and families have limited knowledge of how psychoactive substances affect psychological health. During any intervention it is worthwhile discussing with patients how substances that are initially taken for pleasure can lead to depressed and anxious moods in the longer term and the most effective treatment for co-occurring depression or anxiety for some may be abstinence or possibly controlled use. If relevant for patients with psychotic features, it may be of benefit to discuss the role of stimulant drugs such as cocaine and methamphetamine in psychosis, and drugs such as GBL in causing psychosis in withdrawal.

Psychological Treatment for Psychiatric Illness for Those with Substance Dependence

NICE clinical guideline 51, *Drug Misuse: Psychosocial Interventions* [15], makes clear that substance using patients with mental health problems should have access to NICE-recommended psychological interventions. This includes treatment for depression and anxiety. It adds that there is no evidence that substance use by itself makes such interventions ineffective. This is echoed in a recent study which suggested that higher levels of alcohol use were not associated with worse outcomes in Improving Access to Psychological Therapies (IAPT) services, although it was associated with a higher dropout rate [16].

The IAPT positive practice guidance for working with people who use drugs and alcohol suggests that drug and alcohol use should not mean an automatic exclusion from psychological therapy services, but rather should prompt an assessment of the individual [17]. Most people who access psychological therapy services have relatively low levels of substance misuse which may require little more than a brief intervention, with a relatively small subset requiring addiction services.

Changes to the English specialist addiction treatment system, combined with a period of financial cuts, have meant that the level of expert psychology provision is very low in 2020. Often the only route that patients that use alcohol or drugs have to expert NICE-recommended psychological care is through services such as IAPT. In line with the guidance just quoted, psychological therapy services should work collaboratively with, for example, the patient who is alcohol dependent secondary to social anxiety. In this case the addiction service could provide the detoxification episode and the psychological therapy service the recommended cognitive behavioural intervention. A timely response from both services would be in the client's interests.

The positive practice guidance suggests that a patient who can control their alcohol and drug use, is motivated to change and attend sessions or is stable on opioid substitution therapy or abstinent should be assessed and may be suitable for psychological therapy. There is little evidence to support mandatory periods of abstinence prior to such therapy. A more collaborative approach would be to trust the patient's view of their illness, certainly in the initial stages of treatment, making a positive offer to the individual rather than offering exclusion. It may not be possible to engage chaotic drug and alcohol users in psychological therapy. In most cases it is unlikely they will attend but if they present to psychological therapy services in such a fashion they should be referred to local addiction services. Once stability is achieved they can be re-referred to psychological therapy. In those with severe mental illness Hunt and colleagues found little evidence to support the use of one psychological therapy such as CBT or MI over generic treatment as usual [18].

Use of Medication to Treat Mental Illness

Psychotropic medication including antidepressants and antipsychotics may be of use in this population. It is important to be aware of the risk that such medication may have side effects which interact with either prescribed drugs (such as the QT-prolonging effects of both methadone and citalopram) or illicit drugs (such as citalopram and cocaine). It is therefore important to check the interactions, as well as assessing the risk of over-sedation.

Any psychotropic medication has the potential to be abused; some such as benzodiazepines or the gabapentinoids have greater abuse potential than others. Prescribers should be aware of this risk and take appropriate measures to reduce risks of misuse and diversion if relevant. If psychiatric medication is prescribed it is important that it is reviewed on a regular basis by a suitably competent healthcare professional to ensure that benefit is being gained and that any side effects are minimised. The patient should be made aware of any potential side effects. If a psychiatric medication is stopped the prescriber should be aware of, and take steps to reduce/minimise, any withdrawal or discontinuation effects.

Antidepressants

Antidepressant use in the treatment of co-occurring depression in those with drug or alcohol dependence has a weak evidence base. The evidence that antidepressants reduce the severity of depression in people with alcohol dependence compared with placebo is weak, becoming non-significant once trials with a high risk of bias are excluded. There is slightly stronger evidence that antidepressants may have an effect on amount of alcohol consumed, but the clinical benefit is modest [19].

Antipsychotics

Clearly patients with psychosis often need evidence-based treatment with antipsychotic medication. There is little good-quality evidence to support the use of one antipsychotic over another in the co-occurring population and choice of medication may be driven by other factors [20].

Benzodiazepines, Z Drugs, Gabapentinoids and Allied Medication

Although such drugs have psychiatric indications they should be used with caution in this population, given the risks of dependence. If they are prescribed for reasons such as insomnia or anxiety, use should be confined to the recommended time frame and regularly reviewed.

Mutual Aid

Many patients find mutual aid groups such as 12-step fellowship meetings (e.g. AA or NA) or SMART Recovery extremely helpful. The process of natural recovery from addiction suggests that many patients achieve abstinence from substances without the involvement of formal treatment but rather with the support of mutual aid, family and friends. For patients in mental health services with addiction difficulties the option of mutual aid should be discussed.

Conclusion

The desire to experience an altered state of consciousness seems to be an intrinsic part of the human experience . . . . Drug taking remains one of the easiest and most immediate ways of altering psychological states . . . . Drug taking is here to stay and one way or another we must all learn to live with drugs. [21]

The use of substances is common throughout modern British society. As noted elsewhere in this book the problems associated with drug, alcohol and tobacco use are considerable. In 2018 the *New York Times* noted that life expectancy is declining in the United States for the first time in more than 50 years as a consequence of the opioid epidemic. As Gossop reminds us, the use of mind-altering substances is an intrinsic part for most of the human condition. It should not be a surprise that people with mental illness use psychoactive substances, and in doing so they achieve worse outcomes and become even more marginalised in society. The 2002 Department of Health guidance 'Mental health policy implementation guide: dual diagnosis good practice guide' was a good document that was poorly implemented. The latest guidance reworks much of this material: will the outcome be different?

This question can only be answered by professionals, service providers and commissioners. Reasons for disillusionment might include the poor track record of implementing such guidance previously and the funding environment as of 2020. There are, however, reasons for hope. The service user voice is now much stronger; there is a new generation of healthcare professionals that reject the false dichotomies of diagnosis rather seeing a total individual; and there are healthcare inspectorates in all parts of the United Kingdom tasked with ensuring guidance is implemented.

References

1   National Institute for Health and Care Excellence. *Coexisting Severe Mental Illness and Substance Misuse: Community Health and Social Care Services.* London: NICE; 2016.

2   Public Health England. Better Care for People with Co-Occurring Mental Health and Alcohol/Drug Use Conditions: A Guide for Commissioners and Service Providers. London: PHE; 2017.

3   Farrell M., Howes S., Bebbington P., Brugha T., Jenkins R., Lewis G. et al. Nicotine, alcohol and drug dependence and psychiatric comorbidity: Results of the national household survey. *British Journal of Psychiatry.* 2001; **179**: 432–7.

4   Drummond C., McBride O., Fear N., Fuller E. Alcohol Dependence (chapter 10). In: McManus S., Bebbington P., Jenkins R, Brugha T., eds. *Mental Health and Wellbeing in England: Adult Psychiatric Morbidity Survey 2014*. Leeds: NHS Digital; 2016. p. 238–64.

5   Lai H. M. X., Cleary M., Sitharthan T., Hunt G. E. Prevalence of comorbid substance use, anxiety and mood disorders in epidemiological surveys, 1990–2014: A systematic review and meta-analysis. *Drug and Alcohol Dependence*. 2015; **154**: 1–13.

6   Weaver T., Madden P., Charles V., Timso G. S., Renton A., Tyrer P. et al. Comorbidity of substance misuse and mental illness in community mental health and substance misuse services. *British Journal of Psychiatry*. 2003; **183**: 304–13.

7   Carrà G., Johnson S., Crocamo C., Angermeyer M. C., Brugha T., Azorin J. M. et al. Psychosocial functioning, quality of life and clinical correlates of comorbid alcohol and drug dependence syndromes in people with schizophrenia across Europe. *Psychiatry Research*. 2016; **239**: 301–7.

8   Senior J., Birmingham L., Harty M. A., Hassan L., Hayes A. J., Kendall K. et al. Identification and management of prisoners with severe psychiatric illness by specialist mental health services. *Psychological Medicine*. 2013; **43** (7): 1511–20.

9   Fazel S., Geddes J. R., Kushel M. The health of homeless people in high-income countries: Descriptive epidemiology, health consequences, and clinical and policy recommendations. *The Lancet*. 2014; **384** (9953): 1529–40.

10 Department of Health. *Mental Health Policy Implementation Guide: Dual Diagnosis Good Practice Guide*. London: Department of Health; April 2002.

11 NHS England, National Collaborating Centre for Mental Health, National Institute for Health and Care Excellence. Achieving Better Access to 24/7 Urgent and Emergency Mental Health Care. Part 2: Implementing the Evidence-based Treatment Pathway for Urgent and Emergency Liaison Mental Health Services for Adults and Older Adults: Guidance. 2016.

12 Saunders J. B., Aasland O. G., Babor T. F., De La Fuente J. R., Grant M. Development of the Alcohol Use Disorders Identification Test (AUDIT): WHO collaborative project on early detection of persons with harmful alcohol consumption – II. *Addiction*. 1993; 88 (6): 791–804.

13 WHO ASSIST Working Group. The Alcohol, Smoking and Substance Involvement Screening Test (ASSIST): development, reliability and feasibility. *Addiction*. 2002; **97**: 1183–94.

14 Independent Expert Working Group. *Drug Misuse and Dependence: UK Guidelines on Clinical Management*. London: Department of Health; 2017.

15 National Collaborating Centre for Mental Health. *Drug Misuse: Psychosocial Interventions*. London: British Psychological Society and The Royal College of Psychiatrists; 2008.

16 Buckman J. E. J., Naismith I., Saunders R., Morrison T., Linke S., Leibowitz J. et al. The impact of alcohol use on drop-out and psychological treatment outcomes in improving access to psychological therapies services: An audit. *Behavioural and Cognitive Psychotherapy*. 2018; **46** (5): 513–27.

17 Improving Access to Psychological Therapies. *IAPT positive practice guide for working with people who use drugs and alcohol*. London: IAPT, Drugscope, NTA; 2012.

18 Hunt G. E., Siegfried N., Morley K., Brooke-Sumner C., Cleary M. *Psychosocial Interventions for People with Both Severe Mental Illness and Substance Misuse*. *Cochrane Database of Systematic Reviews*. 2019(**12**).

19 Agabio R., Trogu E., Pani P. P. Antidepressants for the treatment of people with co-occurring depression and alcohol dependence. *Cochrane Database of Systematic Reviews*. 2018(4).

20 Temmingh H. S., Williams T., Siegfried N., Stein D. J. Risperidone versus other antipsychotics for people with severe mental illness and co-occurring substance misuse. *Cochrane Database of Systematic Reviews*. 2018(1).

21 Gossop M. *Living with Drugs*, 7th ed. Abingdon: Routledge: 2016.

Medical Aspects of Drug and Alcohol Use

David Pang and Mark Pucci

Alcohol

Alcohol is a water and lipid soluble molecule, allowing it and its metabolic by-products to affect every organ system in the body. Harmful alcohol use contributes to a wide range of adverse health outcomes, from risky behaviours such as drink driving and road traffic accidents to cardiovascular disease and cancer. Related to this, in 2016 the UK Chief Medical Officers published new safe limit guidelines recommending both men and women to not drink regularly more than 14 units per week, to keep health risks at a low level [1]. The definitions of hazardous, harmful, dependent and binge drinking are outlined in Table 10.1, as adapted from UK Government guidance over the past 10 years.

Cardiovascular System

There is some evidence to suggest that in small amounts, regular alcohol consumption has cardioprotective effects against the risk of ischaemic heart disease as well as hypertension. This is thought to be because of reduced platelet aggregation, increased levels of HDL cholesterol, inhibition of inflammation, fibrinolysis and the raising of plasma levels of adiponectin. On the other hand, heavy amounts of consumption and a binge pattern of drinking are linked to elevated relative risk of cardiovascular disease. This includes hypertension, ischaemic heart disease, stroke, heart failure and cardiomyopathy [2, 3].

There are various causes for this increased risk. Alcohol is directly toxic towards cardiac muscle, weakening it over time and it acts to increase blood pressure in a dose response fashion. Alcohol promotes the generation of reactive oxygen species or free radicals, small molecules which can damage proteins and DNA. It also interferes with the body's normal defence mechanisms which help protect against free radicals by reducing the levels of antioxidants. The outcome is a state known as oxidative stress which causes cell injury [4]. Furthermore, harmful alcohol use is often associated with other risk factors such as smoking and malnutrition with cumulative negative effects.

Alcohol may increase the risk of hypertension through increased activity of the sympathetic nervous system, causing constriction of blood vessels and possibly impairing the body's ability to regulate blood pressure through baroreceptors. Studies show a J-shaped relationship with regards to coronary artery disease and hypertension, with protective effects at lower levels (fewer than 2 units a day in men and women). Binge drinking is associated with an increased risk of myocardial infarction in the following 24 hours. Similarly, the same J-shaped relationship has been shown with regards to stroke incidence and mortality. Chronic heavy drinkers are at increased risk of all types of stroke (thromboembolic, haemorrhagic and subarachnoid haemorrhage).

Table 10.1 Definitions of hazardous, harmful, dependent and binge drinking

Term	Definition *(1 unit = 8 g of alcohol)*
Hazardous drinking	Drinking alcohol above recommended safe limits, either in terms of regular excessive consumption or less frequent sessions of heavy drinking. However, so far they have avoided significant alcohol-related problems. The current advice is defined in the current UK guidelines: • Men and women should not drink more than two units a day. • The safest approach in pregnancy or women planning to conceive is not to drink alcohol at all.
Harmful drinking	Drinking more than twice the recommended safe limits regularly which can lead to significant harm to physical and mental health or cause substantial harm to others. Examples include liver cirrhosis, pancreatitis, breakdown of relationships and loss of employment. Drinkers at the most risk of harm are women who regularly drink more than 35 units a week (or 6 units a day) and men who regularly drink more than 50 units a week (or more than 8 units a day).
Dependent drinking	This is when a person is unable to control their drinking, characterised by increased tolerance, withdrawal symptoms, use in larger amounts for longer periods than intended and persistent desire or unsuccessful efforts to cut down on alcohol use. Increasing amounts of time is spent obtaining alcohol or recovering from its effects, social, occupational and recreational pursuits are given up or reduced and drinking is continued despite knowledge of alcohol-related harm.
Binge drinking	Drinking too much alcohol over a short period of time, e.g. over the course of an evening. It is typically drinking that leads to drunkenness. It has immediate and short-term risks to the drinker and to those around them. People who become drunk are much more likely to be involved in an accident or be assaulted, be charged with a criminal offence, or contract a sexually transmitted disease. Women are more likely to have an unplanned pregnancy. Trends in binge drinking are usually identified in surveys by measuring those drinking more than 6 units a day for women or more than 8 units a day for men. In practice, many binge drinkers are drinking substantially more than this level, or drink this amount rapidly, which leads to the harm linked to drunkenness.

Recent studies suggest that not only the quantity, but also drinking patterns influence the relationship between alcohol and cardiomyopathy and subsequent congestive heart failure. Alcoholic cardiomyopathy is characterised by either left ventricular dilatation or hypertrophy. Possible benefits of moderate alcohol consumption have been suggested with a 59 per cent lower risk of heart failure in men as reported in The Framingham Heart Study. The Physicians' Health Study showed that US male physicians reporting seven or more drinks per week had a 38 per cent lower risk of heart failure [5].

Electrophysiological studies have shown that acute alcohol consumption induces tachyarrhythmias and heavy drinking increases the risk of sudden cardiac death. The likely mechanism is thought to be via heart muscle injury due to direct toxic effects producing delays in conduction, prolonged QT intervals as well as electrolyte abnormalities and impaired vagal heart rate control. It is seen most commonly in middle-aged men and is confounded by other factors such as smoking and social class. The term 'holiday heart syndrome' is defined as an acute cardiac arrhythmia or conduction disturbance, most commonly supraventricular tachyarrhythmia, associated with heavy alcohol consumption in a healthy individual without other clinical evidence of heart disease. The most common rhythm disorder seen is atrial fibrillation. Typically, the course is benign; it resolves spontaneously following abstinence, and specific antiarrhythmic medication is usually not indicated.

Respiratory System

Alcohol crosses from the bronchial circulation into the conducting airways of the lungs, and its negative effects are dependent on the concentration, duration and route of exposure. Chronic alcohol intoxication interferes with the body's innate immune response by reducing mucociliary clearance, one of the lungs' first lines of defence against pathogens. Chronic exposure reduces mucous secretion and inhibits pulmonary recruitment of neutrophils as well as the production of cytokines. The result is an increased susceptibility to infections such as community- and hospital-acquired pneumonia. Alcohol use, alcohol dosage and alcohol-related problems are associated with an increased risk of tuberculosis, thought to be associated with alcohol's influence on the immune system and the fact that alcohol consumption leads to presence in social environments that facilitate the spread of tuberculosis infection [6]. Aspiration pneumonia is a serious consequence of being under the influence of alcohol due to its muscle relaxant properties and reduced gag and cough reflexes.

High levels of intoxication lead to the depression of vital centres in the central nervous system which can ultimately lead to respiratory failure and stupor. In obstructive sleep apnoea, alcohol ingestion increases the duration and frequency of occlusive episodes and an increase in the degree of hypoxaemia. This is caused by alcohol-induced hypotonia of the upper airways and depression of arousal mechanisms. The toxic properties of alcohol expose the airways to oxidative stress from free radicals and depletion of antioxidants, resulting in cellular damage and lung injury. This is linked to a higher risk of the development of acute respiratory distress syndrome (ARDS) with higher rates of mortality when compared to non-drinkers. This is a condition characterised by widespread inflammation in the lung, surfactant dysfunction, activation of the innate immune response, impaired regulation of clotting and decreased oxygen and carbon dioxide exchange in the alveoli. There is substantial evidence to suggest that oxidative stress also plays an important role in the inflammatory responses seen in asthma and chronic obstructive pulmonary disease (COPD) [7].

Gastrointestinal System

Alcohol toxicity can cause stomatitis in the lips, glossitis in the tongue and inflammation of the oral mucosa. The risk is increased further in vitamin B and C deficiency, particularly relevant due to malnutrition in harmful alcohol users. Heavy drinking reduces the pressure of the lower oesophageal sphincter, slows motility and gastric emptying, thus facilitating the development of gastro-oesophageal reflux and oesophagitis. A reduction in salivary bicarbonate occurs and peripheral neuropathy affecting muscle contraction cause further issues with acid clearance. Barrett's oesophagus is a pre-malignant condition resulting from chronic exposure of the oesophageal epithelial mucosa to acid. Mallory-Weiss syndrome occurs due to frequent severe vomiting, which tears the mucosa at the junction of the stomach and oesophagus. It presents with haematemesis and the definitive diagnosis is made on endoscopy. Management includes cauterisation or injection of adrenaline to stop the bleeding and supportive measures to restore a haemodynamically stable state. Chronic alcohol consumption is associated with an increased risk of gastritis by enhancing gastric acid secretions and occurs in more than 80 per cent of dependent drinkers. This presents with upper abdominal pain, nausea, loss of appetite and heartburn. This may lead to the development of peptic or duodenal ulcers, and complications include heavy bleeding and perforation. There is increased intestinal permeability in alcoholics and autonomic neuropathy can cause malabsorption of nutrients and vitamins as well as diarrhoea due to decreased bacterial clearance from the gut.

Alcoholic liver disease covers a spectrum of conditions ranging from fatty liver (steatosis) to alcoholic hepatitis, liver fibrosis and cirrhosis. Chronic alcohol consumption results in oxidative stress, acetaldehyde toxicity and secretion of inflammatory cytokines. Steatosis develops following fatty acid and triglyceride accumulation in liver cells in approximately 90 per cent of heavy drinkers, but this is usually asymptomatic and resolves after four to six weeks of abstinence. In about 30–40 per cent of drinkers this progresses to alcoholic hepatitis where an inflammatory process destroys liver cells, leaving a diffuse fibrosis with nodules of regenerating liver cells. Cirrhosis is a late stage of liver disease eventually leading to liver failure. Liver cells are replaced with scar tissue and it develops in people with a long-standing history of heavy drinking for an average of 25 years [8]. Risk factors include obesity, malnutrition, being female, type 2 diabetes mellitus and hepatitis C.

Cirrhosis presents with a multitude of clinical signs and symptoms including right upper quadrant pain, spider naevi, an enlarged liver, jaundice, impaired production of coagulation factors, ascites, hepatic encephalopathy and portal hypertension (high pressure in the portal vein). Secondary complications of cirrhosis and portal hypertension include varices along the gastrointestinal tract (oesophageal, duodenal, colonic, rectal), which are abnormally dilated veins predisposed to heavy bleeding. The later stages of fibrosis and cirrhosis are irreversible and the only definitive treatment is liver transplant. Eligibility requirements include an extended period of abstinence, usually up to six months, a psychological evaluation and active engagement in rehabilitation (e.g. Alcoholics Anonymous) with an emphasis on motivation to make and sustain a change.

Acute pancreatitis is a well-recognised complication of heavy alcohol consumption with a dose-related toxic effect. Pancreatic enzymes are activated leading to inflammation, vascular injury and necrosis. The most common symptoms and signs include fever, epigastric pain radiating to the back, loss of appetite, tachycardia, respiratory distress and peritonitis. Chronic pancreatitis results in progressive replacement of pancreatic parenchyma with fibrotic tissue, manifesting in pancreatic enzyme insufficiency, malnutrition, insulin dependent diabetes mellitus, portal vein thrombosis, chronic pain, weight loss and steatorrhoea.

There are wide variations in the weekly upper limit drinking recommendations worldwide, such as in Spain (35 units in men), USA (24 units in men) and Japan (no recommendation in women). In the UK the Chief Medical Officers guidelines were revised in 2016 to 14 units a week in men and women in line with recent evidence of the risk of cancer. The current UK Government guidance is that there is no level of regular drinking that can be considered as completely safe in regards to cancer. Alcohol consumption is associated with cancers along the whole of the gastrointestinal tract. This includes cancers of the mouth, pharynx and larynx, oesophagus, liver, pancreas, colorectal and breast cancer in women. The mechanisms for this are proposed as direct toxic and carcinogenic effects of acetaldehyde, promotion of the generation of free radicals and then oxidative stress and cumulative cell injury and DNA damage. Other risk factors are cigarette smoking, particularly in cancers of the oral cavity; gastro-oesophageal reflux disease; malnutrition; inflammatory bowel disease, such as ulcerative colitis; chronic pancreatitis; and hepatitis B and C infections.

Haematological System

Chronic alcohol consumption is responsible for both direct and indirect effects on the system responsible for the production of bloods cells (haematopoiesis). The direct toxicity of alcohol affects the bone marrow, as well as platelets and red and white blood cells. On the other hand, malnutrition causes deficiency of vitamins and nutrients, indirectly impairing the production and function of blood cells. Abstinence from alcohol has been shown to reverse many of the detrimental effects on haematopoiesis and blood cell functioning [9].

Physicians used to consider cirrhosis to cause a hypocoagulable state, predisposing alcoholics to bleeding from oesophageal and gastric varices, ulcers in the stomach and duodenum and haemorrhagic stroke. However, research has shown that actually there is a hypercoagulability state despite thrombocytopenia and decreased levels of procoagulant factor synthesis, such as vitamin K–dependent clotting factors (II, VII, IX and X). A procoagulant imbalance occurs with increased thrombin generation and thus cirrhosis is associated with an increased risk of venous thromboembolism or portal vein thrombosis. Although quite controversial, there is now more evidence to suggest anticoagulation as a therapeutic option in patients with cirrhosis.

Vitamin B12 and folate deficiency impairs the progression of the blood cell cycle in the bone marrow from precursors to mature cells. Blood cells then continue to grow without division, leading to a raised mean corpuscular volume (MCV) and megaloblastic anaemia. Interestingly, alcoholism also causes macrocytosis, even in the absence of vitamin B12 or folate deficiency. Malabsorption and chronic pancreatitis in alcoholics further complicates nutritional deficiencies, particularly of thiamine which is an essential nutrient that must be obtained from the diet. Splenomegaly may result from the effects of portal hypertension, attenuating its normal functioning, leading to stasis and trapping of blood cells in the spleen. Macrophages may then attack and destroy red blood cells, causing a haemolytic anaemia.

Excessive alcohol consumption has long been associated with increased susceptibility to infections. Regarding white blood cells, there is reduced production of neutrophils in the bone marrow and diminished ability of neutrophils to reach the site of infection. Also, there is associated monocyte and macrophage dysfunction, with the resultant state known as leucopenia. This makes alcoholics less able to fight off bacterial infections, making them more susceptible to serious conditions such as sepsis, tuberculosis and pneumonia.

Endocrine and Reproductive System

Alcohol-induced dysregulation of the hypothalamic-pituitary-gonadal axis is associated with hyperprolactinaemia, with a range of adverse consequences. Women may experience irregular menstrual cycles, amenorrhoea, anovulation, early menopause and spontaneous abortions or miscarriages. The ovaries are subjected to injury from oxidative stress due to direct toxic effects of alcohol and the levels of prolactin and oestradiol may be elevated. Current UK guidance recommends pregnant women or those trying to conceive to not drink alcohol at all.

Studies have shown that in men, chronic alcohol abuse raises levels of follicle stimulating hormone (FSH) and luteinising hormone (LH), with a significant reduction in testosterone. Increased levels of circulating oestrogen secondary to liver failure may also contribute to the problem. In the long term this causes hypogonadism, testicular atrophy, subfertility, reduced libido, gynaecomastia and impotence. Dysfunctional spermatogenesis may occur with lower sperm volume, count, motility and numbers of structurally normal sperm.

Excessive glucocorticoid production may develop into an alcoholic pseudo-Cushing's syndrome with a typical rounded facial appearance, dorsocervical fat pad proximal muscle wasting, excessive bruising and abdominal striae. Alcohol interferes with the absorption of vitamin D and calcium and high levels of cortisol and parathyroid hormone lead to both decreased bone formation and increased bone breakdown. The cumulative result is an increased risk of osteoporosis, bone fractures and vertebral collapse. Glucose intolerance occurs in approximately 40 per cent of chronic drinkers and is associated with type 2 diabetes mellitus, although low alcohol consumption may have protective effects in a J-shaped dose response curve. Frequent episodes of hypoglycaemia may occur due to depleted liver stores of glycogen and altered glucocorticoid secretion [10].

Central and Peripheral Nervous System

Nutritional deficiencies develop in alcoholics for a variety of reasons. They neglect their diet and may instead gain a large proportion of their daily energy intake from the high calorific content that is typical of alcohol, particularly in cider and beers. For example, one pint of cider with 4.5 per cent ABV (alcohol by volume) contains a little more than 200 calories, the equivalent of a sugar donut. Of note is that alcohol contains 'empty calories' of no nutritional value. Drinking excessive amounts over a long period of time reduces the appetite and food intake and thus there is a gradual depletion of nutrients and vitamins, some of which can only be obtained from the diet. Furthermore, heavy drinkers may consciously or unconsciously reduce their food intake to help fund their addiction and then consume more alcohol to replace the missing calories in their diet. Nutritional deficiencies are further intensified via alcohol-induced malabsorption, liver and pancreatic damage.

The brain is dependent upon oxygen-mediated metabolism of glucose as its main energy source and for the synthesis of lipids and neurotransmitters. Normal glucose metabolism utilises vitamin B and therefore deficiency in these B vitamins, as well as the neurotoxic effects of alcohol intoxication or acute withdrawal such as hypoxia and electrolyte imbalances, combine to produce long term damage to the brain. Thiamine (vitamin B1) is essential to the normal functioning of the central and peripheral nervous system and the body does not produce endogenous thiamine; therefore, it must be obtained from the diet. Thiamine deficiency is known to cause wet beriberi, a form of cardiomyopathy which presents with tachycardia, sweating, lactic acidosis, orthopnoea and pulmonary and peripheral oedema. Dry beriberi presents with neurological deficits and a peripheral neuropathy typically in a glove and stocking distribution. The lower limbs are usually affected first with paraesthesia in the toes, a burning sensation in the feet and then distal sensory and motor neuropathy with muscle wasting. Paradoxically, Antabuse (disulfiram), used in patients trying to abstain from alcohol may also cause peripheral neuropathy as a well-known but relatively rare side effect. Beriberi was first recognised as a disorder due to nutritional deficiency in the 1890s, by Japanese naval doctor Kanehiro Takaki. He found that the incidence of beriberi reduced when Japanese sailors were given a more varied diet to include meat, milk and vegetables. Lower ranking crew members' diets consisted mainly of white rice and little else and he noticed that their rates of beriberi and mortality were much higher.

Carl Wernicke, a German neurologist, first described Wernicke's encephalopathy in 1881 and a few years later, Sergei Korsakoff, a Russian psychiatrist published his PhD dissertation on an amnesic condition occurring in chronic alcoholism. The link between the two conditions only occurred more than half a century later when thiamine deficiency was discovered as the common aetiology. Wernicke's encephalopathy is an acute neuropsychiatric condition due to thiamine deficiency and Korsakoff syndrome occurs as a consequence of chronic thiamine deficiency with profound impairment of the formation of new memories. Wernicke-Korsakoff syndrome is the combined presence of the acute disorder with progression to Korsakoff's psychosis.

Wernicke's encephalopathy is described with the classic triad of clouding of consciousness or acute confusion, ocular signs (nystagmus, opthalmoplegia) and ataxia. Of note, however, is that the triad of symptoms are only present together in fewer than 10 per cent of cases. There is also an associated diverse range of symptoms including impaired vision and hearing, apathy, irritability, psychomotor retardation, polyneuropathy, poor attention span and disorientation to time and place. Treatment and prevention are straightforward, but diagnosis may be missed as patients can present with vague symptoms such as irritability, fatigue and confusion that are associated with many other conditions. Therefore, it is important to have a high index of suspicion because if the patient is not promptly treated with parenteral thiamine, irreversible brain damage occurs and, in some cases, coma and death. Effective treatment and prophylaxis can only be achieved via parenteral thiamine as oral medication is not absorbed in significant amounts.

There is an estimated 20 per cent mortality rate, and in survivors of the condition up to 85 per cent progress to Korsakoff's syndrome [11]. This syndrome has been described by Victor et al. as 'an abnormal mental state in which memory and learning are affected out of all proportion to other cognitive functions in an otherwise alert and responsive patient' [12]. This characteristically presents with recent memory loss and confabulation but with relative preservation of other intellectual functions. Failure to make new memories leaves the patient only able to perform habitual routines or tasks with a limited level of independence, eventually requiring long-term institutionalisation. The brain lesions seen in Wernicke's encephalopathy have been observed in up to 2 per cent of cases in the general population, with a high proportion of them being undiagnosed, and in alcoholics, lesions are seen in up to 35 per cent [13].

Alcohol-induced blackouts occur during and after episodes of heavy consumption. The associated amnesia is primarily 'anterograde', meaning it affects the formation of new memories and is similar to transient global amnesia. Often, individuals are unable to recall any details whatsoever from events during the intoxication, although the episodes are not associated with impairment of consciousness and speech and behaviour may be normal. Alcohol withdrawal seizures typically occur 48–72 hours after last alcohol use, are generally tonic clonic in nature and the likelihood of them is increased with repeated detoxifications. Pre-existing epilepsy, brain damage due to trauma or other factors and illicit drug use are other predisposing factors in the context of alcoholics. Alcohol withdrawal seizures account for up to 25 per cent of cases of status epilepticus [14].

Swiss psychiatrist Paul Eugen Bleuler [26] described alcoholic hallucinosis as a rare but well-known complication of chronic alcohol abuse, and it is characterised by auditory hallucinations, delusions and mood disturbance. It can be easily confused with delirium tremens as they both occur after alcohol withdrawal, usually within 72 hours, but the differentiating features are that alcoholic hallucinosis occurs with clear consciousness and withdrawal symptoms are generally less pronounced. It usually responds well to treatment with antipsychotics with good resolution of symptoms and no residual psychopathology. Delirium tremens follows a period of severe alcohol withdrawal symptoms with fluctuating consciousness, agitation, impaired attention and cognition, persecutory delusions, visual or auditory hallucinations and autonomic symptoms (tremor, sweating, palpitations). Conservative management is the same as for any patient with delirium and involves treating the patient in a well-lit room, orientating them to time and place, trying to have consistent staffing and providing reassurance. Treatment with benzodiazepines, often high-dose is required and may be augmented with haloperidol to alleviate psychotic symptoms. Agitated patients may try to leave the ward and be generally uncooperative with treatment, necessitating the use of mental health legislation. There is a relatively high mortality rate due to medical sequalae and therefore management in a medical hospital rather than a psychiatric ward is recommended.

Cognitive impairment is common in chronic heavy drinkers with up to 80 per cent experiencing mild to severe cognitive deficits. Alcoholic liver disease, direct alcohol neurotoxicity, vitamin deficiencies, malnutrition, cerebrovascular events, traumatic brain injury and repeated episodes of intoxication and withdrawal all contribute to impairment in brain structure and function. Brain scans in alcoholics show loss of white and grey matter, particularly in the prefrontal cortex. Patients with alcohol-related brain damage (ARBD) exhibit difficulties with planning, organisation, memory, abstract thinking, learning of new information, lack of insight and in visuo-spatial coordination. Alcohol is also implicated as the primary cause in 10 per cent of dementia cases, necessitating further research, given the ageing population in the developed world and possible future upsurge of alcohol-related dementia [15]. Simple bedside tests such as verbal fluency have reasonable sensitivity to pick up on deficits in executive function, whereas these may be missed with basic screening tools such as the Mini-Mental State

Examination. Abstinence and adequate nutrition are the mainstay of management with cognitive deficits showing some improvement.

Traumatic brain injury is often a consequence of alcohol misuse due to falls, motor vehicle accidents and violent assaults. Outcomes range from full recovery or even death, to permanent disability with significant challenges to family life, work, social functioning and levels of independence. Frontal executive dysfunction, short-term memory, learning and speech and language may be impaired. Severe blunt head trauma leads to the development of acute subdural haematomas with some patients comatose at the time of injury and others remaining conscious, with a delayed deterioration as the haematoma expands. Chronic subdural haematomas can occur following minor head trauma and patients may develop symptoms after one to four weeks, with an insidious onset of symptoms such as headache, personality change, confusion, reduced consciousness, memory loss, difficulties with balance, motor deficits (e.g. hemiparesis) and aphasia.

Other rare neurological conditions associated with alcoholism and nutritional deficiencies include Marchiafava-Bignami syndrome, central pontine myelinolysis and alcohol amblyopia. Marchiafava-Bignami syndrome is characterised by necrosis and demyelination in the corpus collosum and may present with dementia, seizures, ataxia, hemiparesis, stupor and coma. Diagnosis is made via MRI and treatment is similar to that of Wernicke-Korsakoff syndrome with variable response. Central pontine myelinolysis is caused by rapid correction of chronic hyponatraemia, more common in beer drinkers due to large volumes of fluid consumed and leads to demyelination in the brainstem. Symptoms include dysarthria, dysphagia, catatonia and spastic quadriparesis. Treatment involves careful correction of electrolyte imbalances although prognosis is generally poor, and therefore prevention and early recognition is crucial. Alcohol amblyopia results from vitamin B deficiency in addition to optic neuropathy from the toxic effects of alcohol and presents with painless bilateral loss of vision that may eventually lead to blindness. This was more commonly seen in America during the prohibition era of the 1920s when 'moonshine' consumption was popular, a particularly strong spirit that was illegally distilled in peoples' homes.

Skin

Characteristic skin manifestations of spider naevi, palmar erythema and pruritis are due to the impairment of oestrogen and bilirubin metabolism from hepatic dysfunction. Caput medusae and haemorrhoids are caused by portal hypertension due to liver cirrhosis. There is a predisposition to fungal and bacterial skin infections, angular stomatitis and glossitis, attributable to vitamin deficiencies. There is also a distinct form of psoriasis that affects up to 15 per cent of chronic alcoholics. (For other physical signs of chronic alcohol misuse, see Table 10.2.)

Drugs

Drug addiction is increasingly becoming a major worldwide health problem that is prevalent in both Western societies and developing nations. Much akin to the prohibition era in America, the 'war on drugs' over the past few decades has failed, and has instead driven production and distribution into the hands of organised crime syndicates or the black market. Unlike the legal drugs, alcohol and tobacco, illicit drugs are unregulated, resulting in unscrupulous practices such as 'cutting', whereby additives

Table 10.2 Signs of chronic alcohol misuse on physical examination

General observation	• Agitation, restlessness • Sweating • Bruises
Face	• Fetor hepaticus (sweet, faecal smell of breath) • Parotid enlargement • Facial flushing • Icterus (yellow staining of sclera)
Hands & body	• Asterixis ('liver flap') • Peripheral oedema • Palmar erythema • Telangiectasia (small dilated blood vessels commonly on the face) • Dupuytren's contracture (one or more fingers bent into the palm) • Finger clubbing • Leuconychia (white discolouration of the nails) • Spider naevi • Loss of body hair • Gynaecomastia
Neurological	• Encephalopathy • Ophthalmoplegia • Nystagmus • Peripheral neuropathy and proximal muscle wasting
Cardiovascular	• Dysrhythmias • Hypertension
Abdomen	• Caput Medusae (prominent veins on abdominal wall) • Ascites • Hepatomegaly • Splenomegaly
Genitourinary	• Testicular Atrophy

are used either as bulking agents to increase profits (such as quinine or levamisole added to cocaine) or to increase potency (such as fentanyl added to heroin). This has had profound adverse consequences to the physical health of end users with drug poisoning deaths reaching record levels in England and Wales since comparable records began in 1993. In the United Kingdom, drug overdose has recently overtaken suicide as the leading cause of mortality in men aged 20 to 34. This section will cover the medical aspects of the various types of illicit drugs: opioids, cannabis, stimulants, depressants (such as GHB/GBL and benzodiazepines), hallucinogens and others (such as ketamine and nitrous oxide).

Opioids

Opiates are drugs naturally derived from the flowering opium poppy plant, whereas opioid is a broader term that refers to opiates and any synthetically produced drugs that bind to the brain's opioid receptors. Opioid abuse encompasses both illicit heroin and diverted prescription opioids such as oxycodone and codeine. In America, prescription opioid abuse has grown to epidemic proportions since the 1990s following aggressive marketing by drug companies, incentivising doctors to prescribe them, coupled with a belief during that period that they were not addictive. Americans constitute approximately 5 per cent of the world's population, but they have been consuming 80 per cent of global opioid supply, as well as two-thirds of the world's illicit drugs [16].

Opioids affect various bodily systems, but their abuse relates primarily to their effects on the central nervous system. Acute intoxication with opioids produces euphoria, an exaggerated state of well-being and freedom from anxiety and distress, both of which are commonly cited by users as triggers to continued opioid abuse. First time users may describe it as an unpleasant experience with nausea and vomiting but after repeated use, the pleasurable euphoria and floating sensation starts to prevail, and addicts begin to chase this experience. Following this, there is drowsiness and poor concentration, known as 'gauching', an appearance of semi-consciousness or nodding off to sleep. Opioid-induced analgesia changes both the perception and reaction to pain, with users having a raised pain threshold and an indifference towards it. There is inhibition of the brain-stem respiratory centre causing respiratory depression, with short and shallow breathing due to a reduced responsiveness to the accumulation of carbon dioxide. Users rapidly develop tolerance leading to physical dependence and a characteristic withdrawal syndrome due to an upsurge of adrenaline, which is described as very unpleasant. This presents typically with cold sweats, anxiety, low mood, muscle cramps, piloerection, nausea and vomiting, excessive yawning, diarrhoea and rhinorrhoea. This usually peaks after three to four days if use discontinues, but mild symptoms including insomnia may continue for several weeks.

Chronic opioid abuse predisposes users to several long-term physical health consequences, related not only to the effects of the drug, but also to the route of administration. Once dependent, seeking and maintaining a supply, and then using and recovering from its effects, becomes a full-time occupation, resulting in neglect of their physical health. There is opioid-induced immunosuppression with inhibitory effects on antibody and cellular immune responses, phagocytes and expression of cytokines. Coupled with malnutrition and nutritional deficiencies, there is an increased susceptibility to infections such as tuberculosis or pneumonia. Suppression of the respiratory centre and of the cough reflex can lead to the development of aspiration pneumonia. Opioid-induced endocrinopathy in men is associated with decreased libido, depression and erectile dysfunction due to hypogonadism, resulting from reduced testosterone levels and adrenal androgens. On the other hand, women experience dysmenorrhoea, sexual dysfunction, subfertility and reduced bone mineral density, with implications particularly for postmenopausal women of an increased risk of osteoporosis and bone fractures.

Paradoxically, there may be opioid-induced hyperalgesia, an increased sensitivity to pain despite increasing doses of opioids, thought to be due to interactions with GABA and NMDA receptors, as well as abnormal pain perception. Opioid effects on mu receptors commonly leads to the development of constipation and potentially of haemorrhoid formation and bowel obstruction. On discontinuing opioids after chronic misuse, there may be rebound diarrhoea which can be difficult to treat with a significant effect on quality of life. Methadone, which is used as substitution therapy in opiate abuse patients, is associated with QTc prolongation, particularly at higher doses (i.e. 80 mg or above), and can result in ventricular tachycardia, ventricular fibrillation and sudden cardiac death.

Patients may also be on other drugs that prolong the QTc interval such as certain antibiotics (erythromycin, clarithromycin), antipsychotics (risperidone, quetiapine) or antidepressants (citalopram, amitriptyline). Therefore, it is good practice to consider routinely screening such patients with ECGs.

Routes of Use and Complications

Heroin is often 'smoked on the foil', also known as 'chasing the dragon'. The powder is heated usually in a spoon or on foil and the resulting vapour is inhaled using a tube. It can also be smoked with tobacco in a 'joint' or 'spliff'. As expected, inhalation causes damage to the lungs and upper airways and can lead to the development of a variety of respiratory disorders such as COPD and emphysema. Injecting heroin provides the user with a heightened effect relative to the amount taken, but repeated intravenous use can cause veins to collapse, abscesses, thromboembolism, infective endocarditis and infections such as hepatitis B, C and HIV from sharing needles.

Infective Endocarditis

Endocarditis is diagnosed in up to 20 per cent of intravenous drug users (IVDUs) and can present with persistent fever, septicaemia, chest pain, pleural effusions or abscesses, and haemoptysis. The estimated incidence is 1.5–3.3 cases per 1,000 IVDUs per year [17]. The commonest infective organism is *Staphylococcus aureus* and the tricuspid valve is affected in more than half of cases. Most patients can be treated medically with IV antibiotics, but a small minority may require surgery when there are complications such as recurrent septic emboli or severe regurgitation.

Skin

Unhygienic injecting practices, contaminated equipment and repeated use of injecting sites causes hyperpigmented 'tracks' along the path of veins, inflammation of the veins (thrombophlebitis) and abscesses. If signs of infection are neglected, there is the risk of developing necrotising fasciitis, with death of the soft tissue, erythema, swelling and gangrene. In its early stages it can appear similar to cellulitis, so there should be a raised index of suspicion in these patients as there is a high rate of mortality and amputation.

Thromboembolism

Deep vein thromboses (DVTs) are common in intravenous drug users, resulting from a combination of repeated blood vessel injury, infection, inflammation and irritation of vein walls by adulterants. The femoral vein in the groin area is often used and poses a serious risk of DVT. In some cases, users may commence injecting into the lower limbs in order to conceal injecting sites. The femoral vein is generally easy to locate for the user and may be one of the only sites remaining once all other veins have collapsed.

Blood-borne Viruses

The transmission of blood-borne viruses occurs through the sharing of infected or blood contaminated equipment and is the greatest public health concern related to intravenous drug use. In May 2016, the UK signed up to the World Health Organization (WHO) Global Health Sector Strategy (GHSS) on Viral Hepatitis, with the long-term aim of the elimination of hepatitis C (HCV) as a major public health threat by 2030.

Recent estimates suggest that 71 million people have chronic hepatitis C virus (HCV) infection worldwide, and in England there are an estimated 89,000 people living with chronic HCV. Primary prevention involves raising awareness of HCV infection among high-risk groups which includes people who inject drugs (PWID), those who are homeless, in prison and the South Asian population, followed by easy access to testing and then effective treatment and action to prevent further transmission of the virus. Intravenous drug use remains the most important risk factor for HCV, recorded in 90 per cent of all laboratory reports where risk factors have been disclosed. NHS England commissioning data shows an upward trend of significant increases in the number of people accessing treatment since 2014, with 11,756 people treated in the 2018–19 tax year, compared with approximately 6,031 in 2016 and 9,440 in the following tax year 2016–17 [18].

HCV is a single-stranded RNA virus with at least seven genotypes, 1a or 1b accounting for 70–80 per cent of cases in the USA and Europe. Hepatitis C is typically asymptomatic in the acute phase of infection and symptoms may not appear until the liver is severely damaged. Many individuals remain undiagnosed for years and therefore fail to access treatment. The virus can be cleared spontaneously by the immune system, usually within the first few months of infection, but approximately 50–80 per cent of hepatitis C infections become chronic with a slow and variable rate of progression, over 20 to 50 years.

Symptoms occurring commonly during the chronic stages of illness include fatigue, nausea, muscle aches, right upper quadrant pain and anorexia. Chronic infection causes progressive damage to the liver, resulting in cirrhosis in approximately 20–30 per cent of patients and the development of hepatocellular carcinoma in a minority, which can manifest 20 to 30 years after the acute phase of infection. Patients with end stage liver disease or hepatocellular carcinoma may require liver transplantation. Predictors of HCV disease progression include alcohol consumption with faster progression to cirrhosis in people who have consumed 50 units of alcohol or more per week over a five-year period, old age, male gender, the South Asian population, BMI above 25, smoking and the viral genotype which influences the course of the infection and sensitivity to treatment.

The treatment of hepatitis C has been revolutionised in recent years. Historically HCV was treated with pegylated-interferon alpha (PEG-IFN) plus ribavirin (RBV) which consisted of a demanding regime of self-injections three times a week and daily dosage of oral ribavirin. This combination produced mediocre sustained virological response (SVR) rates of 40–50 per cent and was associated with intolerable side effects such as flu-like symptoms, anaemia, lethargy, muscle aches and adverse psychiatric effects including depression and anxiety. Treatment also lasted 6 to 12 months, often with poor compliance and significant drop-out rates.

The past few years have seen a radical shift in HCV treatment following a breakthrough in 2011 with the approval of the first direct-acting antiviral drugs (DAA). These medications are oral once- or twice-daily treatments that are well-tolerated and able to produce SVR rates of greater than 90 per cent. Several well-tolerated, all-oral DAA regimens are now approved to treat patients with various HCV genotypes, comorbidities and stages of liver disease. DAA drugs have been responsible for the significant increases in the number of people accessing treatment, owing to its several advantages over previous HCV treatment including potency, tolerability, shorter duration of treatment and reducing barriers to engaging those high risk populations [19].

The prevalence of hepatitis B in the UK is between 0.1 and 0.5 per cent and it is usually acquired through sexual activity and injecting drug use. It can present with nausea and vomiting, fatigue, fever and may progress to jaundice. However, chronic infection may be asymptomatic and can lead to the development of cirrhosis after several years. Like hepatitis C, individuals are at an increased risk of developing hepatocellular carcinoma. Management is via prevention and vaccines are routinely given to infants and to adults in high-risk groups, such as healthcare professionals. Chronic infection may resolve spontaneously in adults; otherwise, it is treated with antivirals as above.

In 2015 there were an estimated 100,000 people living with human immunodeficiency virus (HIV) in the UK with 13 per cent unaware of their infection and their risk of transmission to others [20]. Again, sharing of infected equipment is one of the main causes, alongside unprotected sexual intercourse, with high rates among men who have sex with men. More effective antiretroviral treatment in the past few decades has led to increased survival rates and improved quality of life. Late diagnosis, however, progresses to acquired immunodeficiency syndrome (AIDS), where individuals are immunocompromised and may develop AIDS-defining illnesses such as Kaposi's sarcoma or *Pneumocystis jirovecii* pneumonia.

Overdose

Individuals are at an increased risk of opiate overdose after a period of abstinence due to reduced tolerance, if there is polydrug abuse, or due to impurities of a drug bought on the street. The risk is high immediately following discharge from prison when addicts may 'celebrate' by scoring and then using the same amount or dose as prior to entering prison. It is becoming increasingly common for heroin to be cut with fentanyl, which is between 30 and 50 times more potent than heroin. Opiate overdose presents with pin point pupils, respiratory depression, reduced levels of consciousness and ultimately coma and death. Naloxone is an effective antidote, rapidly reversing opiate effects and it is now common for users and family members to be trained in its administration.

Cannabis

Recreational cannabis use has risen sharply in the past few decades and its legalisation and decriminalisation in some countries has garnered more interest in its long-term physical health effects. Intoxication with cannabis produces a feeling of light-headedness, feelings of relaxation and increases the appetite, also known as 'the munchies'. There may be psycho-motor under- or overactivity, impaired memory and motor coordination, lethargy, dry mouth and congestion of the conjunctival blood vessels causing reddening of the eyes.

It is usually smoked with tobacco in 'spliffs' or 'joints', but it can also be inhaled through vaporising devices or ingested in 'space cakes' or tablet form. Chronic heavy cannabis smoking is linked to the development of chronic bronchitis and bullous lung disease in relatively young users, attributable in part to tobacco. Some studies have shown no significant additional lung cancer risk in tobacco users who also smoke cannabis [20]. Chronic consumption leads to the development of tachycardia and hypertension with an increased risk of arrhythmias, acute coronary syndrome and cerebrovascular accidents. After acute intoxication, impaired motor coordination coupled with poor judgement may lead to risky behaviours with an increased risk of road traffic accidents. Regular cannabis use can hinder brain development in adolescents and is associated with poor educational outcomes, diminished life satisfaction and decreased achievement [21]. Subtle short-term memory and attention deficits may persist after periods of chronic use.

Stimulants

Stimulants include illicit drugs such as cocaine, cathinones amphetamines, ecstasy (methylenedioxymethamphetamine or MDMA) and abused therapeutic medications such as methylphenidate. Acute intoxication leads to increased energy levels and attention, alertness and self-confidence, decreased fatigue and reduced appetite. With ecstasy there is a sense of euphoria, increased empathy towards others, dilated pupils and enhanced sensory perceptions, making it popular as a party drug. Stimulant users may also experience agitation, restlessness, sweating, tremors, tachycardia and tachypnoea. Withdrawal can present with feelings of depression, hopelessness, lethargy, depersonalisation and protracted insomnia, typically 24–36 hours after cessation of use, leading to the coining of the phrase 'suicide Tuesday'.

Cocaine may be 'dabbed' by rubbing it on the gums, but it is usually taken via the nasal route, constricting the blood flow to the septum. Repeated intranasal use causes a perforated septum, epistaxis, nasal obstruction and deformity. Smoking crack cocaine can anaesthetise the lungs, which impairs the cough reflex that would usually expel foreign bodies associated with its use, such as ash, pieces of metal gauze, water vapour and parts of plastic pipes. Crack lung is a form of hypersensitivity reaction that occurs up to 48 hours after heavy crack cocaine smoking and presents with dyspnoea, haemoptysis, chest pain and fever. Injecting cocaine or crack cocaine is linked with a higher acute risk of death, local infection and the transmission of blood-borne viruses.

Crack cocaine goes hand in hand with heroin use because heroin helps users 'come down' from the intense high of crack and they may be injected in combination, known as 'speedballing'. Cocaine is used alongside alcohol in up to two-thirds of individuals as alcohol prolongs cocaine's pleasurable or euphoric effects. The metabolite ethylbenzoylecgonine (more commonly known as cocaethylene) is formed following concurrent use of alcohol and cocaine, which raises the risk of cardiovascular complications such as stroke and it is particularly toxic to the liver.

Chronic use or large doses of stimulants are associated with significantly raised blood pressure, accelerated atherosclerosis, coronary artery spasm and chest pain, with increased risks of myocardial infarction, strokes and sudden death. Arrhythmias, aortic dissection and dilated or hypertrophic cardiomyopathy are other serious long-term complications. The anorectic effect may contribute to weight loss and malnutrition, and chronic use reduces libido and sexual performance, which is reversible on stopping use. Ecstasy related fatalities are mainly attributable to hyperthermia, hyponatraemia secondary to water intoxication or 'counterfeit ecstasy' containing paramethoxymethamphetamine (PMMA) or paramethoxyamphetamine (PMA). In 2008 Professor David Nutt, who was at the time chairman of the Advisory Council on the Misuse of Drugs (ACMD), caused controversy when he published an editorial in the *Journal of Psychopharmacology* comparing the risks associated with horse rising (1 serious adverse event every 350 exposures) to that of taking ecstasy (1 serious adverse event every 10,000 exposures) [22].

Depressants

These drugs act directly on the central nervous system to reduce arousal and stimulation, causing a sedating or calming effect. These include barbiturates, gamma-hydroxybutyrate (GHB), gamma-butyrolactone (GBL), benzodiazepines and other abused therapeutic medications such as zolpidem or quetiapine. Effects of acute intoxication with depressants include ataxia, sedation, cognitive impairment, muscle relaxation, hypotension, reduced respiratory and heart rate and even coma or death.

Barbiturate abuse was widespread in the 1970s as barbiturates were used therapeutically as anxiolytics and hypnotics, but it is now much less common as their medical use has been largely replaced by benzodiazepines. They are particularly toxic in overdose, with profound respiratory depression and high risk of cardiac arrest and it is because of these properties that they are still used in capital punishment by lethal injection.

Benzodiazepines are one of the most common prescription drugs used recreationally as they are effective anxiolytics and sedatives, with acute effects similar to alcohol intoxication. Chronic benzodiazepine abuse leads to the development of a high degree of tolerance and physical dependence with a withdrawal syndrome that some addicts anecdotally describe as worse than withdrawing from heroin. It is characterised by sleep disturbances, agitation, anxiety, tremors, confusion, mood and perceptual disturbances. Once dependent, users become more concerned with relief from the withdrawal symptoms, rather than the acute effects. In practice, users who have been on historically large-dose benzodiazepine prescriptions are extremely resistant to any suggestion of reducing or stopping. Therefore it is important these days to be mindful and state to patients at the outset that they are very addictive and indicated for short-term use only, up to six weeks. The pattern of intoxication and withdrawal symptoms are highly variable and depend on the half-life of the benzodiazepine involved. Other complications of long term use include worsening of pre-existing anxiety or depression, memory loss, cognitive impairment, sleep disturbance and acute withdrawal seizures. Benzodiazepines are often abused alongside other depressants such as opioids or alcohol, significantly increasing the risk of overdose and of drug-related deaths. Management of benzodiazepine dependence involves converting to equivalent doses of diazepam due to its longer half-life and then initiation of a reducing regime. Flumazenil is a competitive inhibitor at GABA receptors and is an effective antidote in benzodiazepine overdose but it is also used in Italy as treatment for high-dose benzodiazepine dependency [23].

Gamma-hydroxybutyrate (GHB) and gamma-butyrolactone (GBL) produce stimulant-like effects at low doses with euphoria, enhanced libido and disinhibition. There has been a dramatic rise in its abuse in England in the past decade, as it is one of the main drugs associated with the so-called chemsex scene. There is high dependence liability, requiring regular dosing throughout the day and evening to avoid withdrawal symptoms, in some cases as often as every one to three hours. The withdrawal syndrome can be severe, producing an acute delirium like state that may require hospitalisation and intensive care. The mainstay of management of withdrawal is supportive care and high dose benzodiazepines. Chronic GHB/GBL use is associated with neurotoxicity with various cognitive impairments on working memory and learning. There is a very narrow dosing range making it relatively easy for users to accidentally overdose. Large doses taken within a short period or polysubstance abuse with other depressants such as alcohol also increase the risks of overdose, which presents with respiratory depression, bradycardia and cardiac arrest. The priority in overdose is management of the airway and patients may require intubation for several hours until all the GHB/GBL has been metabolised.

Hallucinogens

Hallucinogens, also known as psychedelics, are a group of drugs that exert their effects mainly through serotonergic receptors and do not have direct effects on the dopaminergic system. As such, these substances do not lead to addiction or dependence and their use is not considered to be reinforcing. The more well-known hallucinogens include lysergic acid diethylamide (LSD), psilocybin (magic mushrooms), mescaline and dimethyltryptamine (DMT), although many others exist. Jaffe [27] defined them as follows: 'the feature that distinguishes the psychedelics from other classes of drug is their capacity reliably to induce states of altered perception, thought, and feeling that are not experienced otherwise, except in dreams or at times of religious exaltation.' They can be ingested, inhaled or injected, with the resulting experience or 'trip' lasting up to 12 hours in some cases.

LSD was synthesised in the 1930s by chemist Albert Hofmann and was used as a medicine to aid psychotherapy in the 1950s, until restrictive drug laws in the 1960s prohibited its research and use. Psilocybin is a naturally occurring psychedelic found in more than 200 species of mushroom and its use in religious ceremonies and rituals is thought to predate recorded history. Mescaline is a naturally occurring phenethylamine found in the peyote cactus that has been used by Native Americans in religious ceremonies for thousands of years. Aldous Huxley described his experience of mescaline in his philosophical essay, 'The Doors of Perception' (1954), in which he recalls his insights ranging from purely aesthetic to sacramental vision. DMT is a naturally occurring tryptamine molecule found in plants and animals, with short-lived effects of up to 15 minutes when taken, unless it is ingested alongside a monoamine oxidase inhibitor (MAOI), such as in ayahuasca tea used by Amazonian shamans.

Psychedelic use can lead to tachycardia, nausea, tremors, muscle weakness, increased blood pressure, profuse sweating and dilation of the pupils. Psychedelics alter the user's perception of their surroundings and feelings, produce feelings of euphoria, a distorted sense of time, visual hallucinations or distortions and synaesthesia (cross-sensory perception). High doses of psychedelics can lead to acute vasoconstriction with coronary artery spasm as this is mediated by the 5-HT serotonin receptors. From a medical point of view, classic serotonergic psychedelics are generally considered physiologically safe when compared with opiates or stimulants, although there have been very rare reports of rhabdomyolysis and acute renal failure [24].

Other Drugs of Abuse

Ketamine

Ketamine has a history of abuse in the operating room due to its easy access, as a street drug, and is now increasing in popularity as part of the 'rave' scene. Ketamine is a dissociative anaesthetic, a derivative of phencyclidine (PCP or 'angel dust'), although less potent. It can be classed as both a depressant and a hallucinogen due to its various effects. Sub-anaesthetic doses induce analgesia, sedation, amnesia and a psychedelic state of mind where users experience synaesthesia, depersonalisation and derealisation and distortions of images and sounds. At higher doses, users enter the 'K-hole' where there is pronounced detachment from themselves and their surroundings and altered perceptions of space and time.

Ketamine has a wide margin of safety with regards to acute physical health consequences, with few adverse reported outcomes in overdose when taken without other illicit drugs. In overdose, users present with unconsciousness, but their coughing and swallowing reflexes are spared; there is minimal effect on the gag reflex and they remain haemodynamically stable. Tolerance follows repeated use due to induction of liver enzymes, although there is no specific recognised withdrawal syndrome. It may be snorted, ingested or injected and in recreational use typically may be taken alongside alcohol and ecstasy.

Chronic use leads to cognitive impairment, with deficits in working memory and short- and long-term memory. There may be progressive damage to the bile duct and liver with the resulting phenomena known as 'K-cramps', which can present with either vague abdominal pain or intense, colicky abdominal pain. There has been a substantial rise in cases of what is known as 'ketamine bladder', where following chronic abuse, there is progressive scarring, inflammation and fibrosis of the bladder with an array of lower urinary tract symptoms such as haematuria, urgency and dysuria. The most effective treatment is cessation of ketamine use, but some damage is irreversible with residual bladder contraction, hydronephrosis and subsequent damage to the ureters and kidneys. Treatment with steroids and anticholinergics may be helpful in preventing further deterioration in these patients, but surgery may be the only option in more advanced cases [25].

Alkyl Nitrites

Also known as 'poppers', these are inhaled as a recreational drug, causing euphoria and smooth muscle relaxation and have historically been linked with sexual encounters. With acute intoxication there may be profound hypotension, tachycardia, flushing of the skin, nausea, headache and loss of consciousness. Long-term effects include the risks associated with unsafe sexual practices, sinusitis, anaemia and rashes or irritation around the mouth and nose. They are also renowned for causing methaemoglobinaemia, leading to shifting of the oxygen-haemoglobin dissociation curve to the left, tissue hypoxia, cyanosis, fatigue and shortness of breath. Death may be caused by direct oral consumption of nitrites which causes cyanosis and coma, losing consciousness and choking on vomit or 'sudden sniffing death syndrome' where fatality is caused by cardiac arrhythmias.

Solvents

Solvents or volatile substances cover a broad range of household or industrial chemicals that can be inhaled to produce effects similar to sedatives or hypnotics, ranging from intense euphoria to vivid hallucinations. Adverse effects of acute intoxication include impaired coordination, cold sweats, headache, confusion, tachycardia, palpitations, loss of consciousness and risk of accidental injury. With regular use, users may develop nasal or perioral sores, peripheral and central nervous system damage, liver toxicity and kidney failure. Death may occur due to cardiac arrhythmias, asphyxiation or accidents such as falls.

Nitrous oxide

Known as 'laughing gas', nitrous oxide is an anaesthetic used in medicine, as an aerosol propellant in whipped cream canisters and in rocket motors and combustion engines. The routine use of nitrous oxide in anaesthesia has been in decline, but its recreational use has become commonplace. Once inhaled, there is a rapid onset of action within seconds with behavioural disinhibition, impairment of motor coordination, disorientation, analgesia and euphoria, as well as hypoxaemia, increasing the risk of arrhythmias, seizures or cardio-respiratory arrest. Chronic abuse may lead to functional vitamin B12 deficiency with resulting peripheral neuropathy and subacute combined degeneration of the spinal cord.

Table 10.3 summarises the symptoms and signs of intoxication, while Table 10.4 summarises three common withdrawal syndromes.

Table 10.3 Symptoms and signs of intoxication

Opioids	Stimulants	Depressants
• Analgesia	• Excessive activity	• Relaxation
• Euphoria	• Perspiration	• Drowsiness and sleep
• Sedation	• Poor appetite	• Confusion
• Psychomotor retardation	• Limited or no sleep	• Blurred vision
• Impaired attention and judgement	• Anxiety	• Mild euphoria
• Disinhibition	• Hypervigilance	• Light headedness
• Interference with personal functioning	• Grandiose beliefs / actions	• Lack of facial expression or animation
• Respiratory depression and reduced cough reflex	• Impaired judgement	• Flat affect
• Decreased level of consciousness ('on the nod')	• Auditory, visual or tactile illusions	• Slurred speech
• Hypotension/ bradycardia	• Dilated pupils	• Motor incoordination
	• Bruxism (teeth grinding)	• Ataxia
	• Tachycardia	• Seizures
	• Increased blood pressure	
	• Repetitive stereotyped behaviours	

Cannabis	Hallucinogens	Ketamine
• Sedation/ relaxation	• Pupillary dilation	• Impaired attention
• Tachycardia	• Blurred vision	• Sedation
• Conjunctival injection	• Tremors	• Analgesia
• Dry mouth	• Motor incoordination	• Depersonalisation/ derealisation
• Increased appetite	• Palpitations	• 'K-Hole'
• Paranoia	• Distorted sense of time	• 'K-cramps'
• Impaired judgement	• Synaesthesia	• Ketamine bladder (lower urinary tract symptoms)
• Hallucinations	• Altered perceptions	
• Euphoria		
• Disinhibition		
• Anxiety		

Table 10.4 Withdrawal syndromes

Opioids	Stimulants	Benzodiazepines
• Hot flushes • Chills • Goosebumps • Confusion • Diarrhoea • Vomiting • Tremors • Irritability, restlessness • Loss of appetite • Insomnia • Runny nose and eyes • Repeated yawning • Abdominal cramps • Muscle and joint aches • Tachycardia & tachypnoea	• Lethargy and fatigue • Psychomotor retardation or agitation • Increased appetite • Protracted insomnia or hypersomnia • Exhaustion alternating with depression • 'Suicide Tuesday' • Vivid unpleasant dreams • Anxiety • Paranoia	• Tinnitus • Muscle spasms • Cognitive impairment • Agitation • Anxiety • Insomnia • Constipation/ diarrhoea • Nausea and vomiting • Palpitations • Loss of libido • Ataxia • Depersonalisation/ derealisation

References

1 Department of Health. *UK Chief Medical Officers' Alcohol Guidelines Review: Summary of the Proposed New Guidelines.* London: DH; 2016.

2 Day E., Rudd J. H. F. Alcohol use disorders and the heart. *Addiction.* 2019; **114** (9): 1670–8.

3 Piano M. R. Alcohol's effects on the cardiovascular system. *Alcohol Research.* 2017; **38** (2): 219–41.

4 Wu D., Cederbaum A. I. Alcohol, oxidative stress, and free radical damage. *Alcohol Research and Health.* 2003; **27** (4): 277–84.

5 Djoussé L., Gaziano J. M. Alcohol consumption and heart failure: A systematic review. *Current Atherosclerosis Reports.* 2008; **10** (2): 117–20.

6 Imtiaz S., Shield K. D., Roerecke M., Samokhvalov A. V., Lönnroth K., Rehm J. Alcohol consumption as a risk factor for tuberculosis: Meta-analyses and burden of disease. *European Respiratory Journal.* 2017; **50** (1): 1700216.

7 MacNee W. Oxidative stress and lung inflammation in airways disease. *European Journal of Pharmacology.* 2001; **429** (1–3): 195–207.

8 O'Shea R. S., Dasarathy S., McCullough A. J., Practice Guideline Committee of the American Association for the Study of Liver Diseases, Practice Parameters Committee of the American College of Gastroenterology. Alcoholic liver disease. *Hepatology.* 2010; **51**(1): 307–28.

9 Ballard H. S. The hematological complications of alcoholism. *Alcohol Health and Research World.* 1997; **21** (1): 42–52.

10 Rachdaoui N., Sarkar D. K. Effects of alcohol on the endocrine system. *Endocrinology and Metabolism Clinics of North America.* 2013; **42** (3): 593–615.

11 Cook C. C. H. Prevention and treatment of Wernicke-Korsakoff syndrome. *Alcohol and Alcoholism.* 2000; **35** (Suppl. 1): 19–20.

12 Victor M., Adams R. D., Collins G. H. *The Wernicke-Korsakoff Syndrome.* Plum F., McDowell F. H., eds. Philadelphia: F. A. Davis Company; 1971.

13 Thomson A. D., Marshall J. The treatment of patients at risk of developing Wernicke's Encephalopathy in the community. *Alcohol and Alcoholism.* 2006; **41**: 159–67.

14 Hillbom M., Pieninkeroinen I., Leone M. Seizures in alcohol dependent patients: Epidemiology, pathophysiology and management. *CNS Drugs.* 2003; **17** (12): 1–18.

15 Gupta S., Warner J. Alcohol-related dementia: A 21st-century silent epidemic? *British Journal of Psychiatry.* 2008; **193** (5): 351–3.

16 Manchikanti L., Singh A. Therapeutic opioids: A ten-year perspective on the complexities and complications of the escalating use, abuse, and nonmedical use of opioids. *Pain Physician.* 2008; **11** (2 Suppl): S63-88.

17 Contoreggi C., Rexroad V. E., Lange W. R. Current management of infectious complications in the injecting drug user. *Journal of Substance Abuse Treatment.* 1998; **15** (2): 95–106.

18 Public Health England. *Hepatitis C in England 2020: Working to eliminate hepatitis C as a major public health threat.* London: PHE; 2020.

19 Harris R. J., Martin N. K., Rand E., Mandal S., Mutimer D., Vickerman P. et al. New treatments for hepatitis C virus (HCV): Scope for preventing liver disease and HCV transmission in England. *Journal of Viral Hepatitis.* 2016; **23** (8): 631–43.

20 Zhang L. R., Morgenstern H., Greenland S., Chang S.-C., Lazarus P., Teare M. D. et al. Cannabis smoking and lung cancer risk: Pooled analysis in the International Lung Cancer Consortium. *International Journal of Cancer.* 2015; **136** (4): 894–903.

21 Volkow N. D., Baler R. D., Compton W. M., Weiss S. R. B. Adverse health effects of marijuana use. *The New England Journal of Medicine.* 2014; **370** (23): 2219–27.

22. Nutt D. Equasy – An overlooked addiction with implications for the current debate on drug harms. *Journal of Psychopharmacology.* 2009; **23** (1): 3–5.

23 Lugoboni F., Faccini M., Quaglio G., Casari R., Albiero A., Pajusco B. Agonist substitution for high-dose benzodiazepine-dependent patients: Let us not forget the importance of flumazenil. *Addiction.* 2011; **106** (4): 853.

24 Berrens Z., Lammers J., White C. Rhabdomyolysis after LSD ingestion. *Psychosomatics.* 2010; **51** (4): 356-.e3.

25 Chung S.-D., Wang C.-C., Kuo H.-C. Augmentation enterocystoplasty is effective in relieving refractory ketamine-related bladder pain. *Neurourology and Urodynamics.* 2014; **33** (8): 1207–11.

26 Bleuler, E. *Textbook of Psychiatry*, translated A. A. Brill. New York: Macmillan; 1916.

27 Jaffe J. H. Drug addiction and drug abuse. In: Goodman A. G., Rall T. W., Nies A. S., Taylor P., eds. *Goodman and Gilman's the Pharmacological Basis of Therapeutics*, 8th ed, pp 522–73. New York: McGraw Hill; 1990.

Organising Treatment Services for Drug and Alcohol Misusers

Emily Finch

The Development of Treatment Services in the UK

Historical Background: Services Pre-1996

Before the early 1970s there were almost no treatment services for users of illicit drugs [1]. The small number of addicts who needed pharmacological treatment were treated by private GPs, mainly in London. Treatment took the form of prescribed opiates, often in injectable form. The drugs were generally prescribed on a long-term basis, and there were several high profile cases of doctors who were prosecuted for overprescribing and selling prescriptions. In contrast, services for people with alcohol problems were provided in the context of general psychiatry, although specialist services were starting to be set up in some areas of the country from the 1950s onwards.

In 1968, following an increase in the prevalence of heroin and other drug use, the first drug dependence clinics (DDCs) were set up. These were mainly in London, and although treatment coverage was not national, some specialist inpatient services were started in other large cities. Initially DDC outpatient services were focused on prescribing for opiate and stimulant users, and in the early days the clinics prescribed diamorphine, methadone and even cocaine. However, within a few years the results from this prescribing and the rapidly increasing opiate epidemic meant the practice in the DDCs became more conservative. By the early 1980 the clinics were focused on methadone prescribing and were becoming overwhelmed by the number of patients presenting for treatment.

In 1985 a group of injecting drug users in Edinburgh were found to be positive for the newly discovered HIV virus. This discovery highlighted the need for a much more effective response to the injecting drug use problem in the UK. Needle exchange services, first set up in an accident and emergency department, were rapidly expanded through funding from a central government initiative. This same initiative funded the set-up of early community drug teams (CDTs). The Advisory Council on the Misuse of Drugs (ACMD) produced a report on harm reduction which allowed these services to prioritise the prevention of HIV transmission rather than focus on reducing drug misuse itself [2].

Developing a Comprehensive Treatment Model

By the mid-1990s there were specialist services across the UK, but there was no comprehensive coverage nationally, and service users were not offered an equitable service. From 2001 funding was increased rapidly. National and international evidence was by then showing that good-quality drug treatment was effective in reducing illegal drug misuse, improving the health of drug misusers, reducing drug-related offending, reducing the risk of death due to overdose or infections (including blood-borne virus infections) and improving social functioning [3, 4]. This made the case for the comprehensive treatment system set out in the document *Models of Care* [5], which was initially commissioned by the Department of Health and later finished by the newly formed National Treatment Agency (NTA).

Models of Care set out to define what a good drug and alcohol treatment system looked like, and laid out a structure for services which we now recognise as standard. This included a four-tiered model of commissioning, which defined the roles of tier 1 or universal services, such as emergency services and social care; tier 2 or non-structured substance misuse services; tier 3 structured treatment services (including prescribing and detoxification); and tier 4 residential detoxification and rehabilitation services (see Table 11.1). Local screening and assessment systems set the standards for brief and comprehensive assessments. Care planning and coordination of care were put at the heart of structured drug treatment, and services were encouraged to work with agencies in other tiers to develop local integrated care pathways. In practice what this meant was that a service user could have access to non-specialist services from health and social care at tier 1, harm reduction and low threshold services at tier 2 from a street agency, prescribing and structured psychological and social interventions from a community drug and alcohol team at tier 3 and residential detoxification and rehabilitation services at tier 4.

National Influence and Control

Drug and alcohol services have always been subject to more political control than other health services because of the perceived moral dimension to substance use. To counter this, those managing the sector as providers and commissioners have to repeatedly make the case about the value of treating and supporting individuals with drug and alcohol problems. They have done this by reiterating the evidence base for treatment effectiveness. The sector has also suffered more reorganisation than other health sectors (such as adult mental health) because of changes in political ideology around issues such as re-procurement. It has also meant a substantial amount of scrutiny and performance management. The NTA was created (in 2002) to oversee the increase in resources for the sector, but also to implement a rigorous performance management structure. The latter included targets for a range of outcomes for treatment services, including waiting time for treatment, retention in treatment and drug-free exits from services. One of the enablers for this was the development of the National Drug Treatment Monitoring System (NDTMS) and the embedded Treatment Outcome Profile (TOP) [6], which has resulted in drug and alcohol treatment having some of the best treatment process and outcome data in the UK.

In 2012 the Health and Social Care Act created Public Health England, abolished the NTA and moved substance misuse commissioning into local authorities. The funding was to be provided from the Public Health grant. This move had the advantage of enabling a public health approach to service provision, and developing a focus on prevention of drug and alcohol use. However, it has had the disadvantage of moving the sector away from integration with other health services. It has also resulted in approximately a 30 per cent reduction in funding for treatment services as the amount within the Public Health Grant has declined [7].

Table 11.1 Drug and alcohol services (tiers adapted from *Models of Care*, 2002) [5]
All interventions can be provided together in the same place by the same agency, or can be provided separately by different agencies.

Type of intervention	Service provided
Tier 1 Non-substance misuse specific and universal services	• Primary care • Housing and homelessness • Employment rehabilitation • Safeguarding • Sexual health • Hepatitis C treatment • Emergency medical care (A&E) • Mental health services • Drug and alcohol education
Tier 2 Open access, drop-in or self-referral services	• Needle and syringe exchange (pharmacy or within services) • Other harm reduction interventions such as take home naloxone • Outreach • Arrest referral • Hospital liaison services • Brief interventions and extended brief interventions • 12-step, i.e. AA and NA
Tier 3 Structured community treatment	• Key working and care planning • Opiate substitution • Community opiate detoxification • Community alcohol detoxifications and alcohol relapse prevention prescribing • Psychosocial interventions – individual • Psychosocial interventions – group • Support to attend AA and NA • Criminal justice treatment, e.g. drug rehabilitation requirements • Post treatment support
Tier 4 Inpatient and residential services	• Inpatient detoxification for drugs and alcohol (medically managed and medically monitored • Residential rehabilitation programmes

The Evolution of Commissioning

Services were commissioned by Primary Care Trusts (PCTs) until the 1995 National Drug Strategy created multi-agency partnerships called Drug Action Teams. DATs were responsible for coordinating local (usually in boroughs or counties) initiatives and programmes on drug and alcohol use, and reporting how these programmes supported the national strategy to public health agencies. Over time many of these evolved into Drug and Alcohol Action Teams and increasingly took a commissioning role. From the late 1990s joint commissioning became the norm. This was an acknowledgement that drug and alcohol treatment covered a range of interventions and outcomes which spanned the health, social care and criminal justice sector.

After 2012 commissioning moved out of health into public health and currently sits in local authorities with funding from the Public Health Grant. This has been criticised because it means that drug and alcohol services have been subject to significant funding cuts (both commissioning and service provision) and also have not been part of other initiatives to plan and modernise health services.

Role of Primary Care and Psychiatry

GPs have always had a significant role in treating drug and alcohol users although when the first drug clinics were set up in the early 1970s they were run by psychiatrists. From then the sub-speciality of Addiction Psychiatry grew up with its own speciality training endorsement and its section in the Royal College of Psychiatrists. When drug and alcohol services started to expand in the early 2000s many GPs were interested in providing care for drug and alcohol users. GPs have many of the skills necessary to manage the broad range of physical and mental health problems substance users experience and many were happy to learn the specific skills needed to manage dependence. The Royal College of General Practice promoted a model of General Practitioner with Special Interest (GPwSI) and set up short accredited courses to train GPs and other primary care staff in the management of drug and alcohol addiction.

There were always many different ways that GPs worked with addicted patients. Some worked in a traditional shared care model (where the GP prescribed medication alongside specialist workers leading on key working and psychosocial interventions), while others became de facto specialists, with some even working full time in drug and alcohol services. In order to clarify which medical professionals had the skills to manage drug and alcohol users the Royal Colleges of Psychiatry and General Practice wrote a joint report in 2005 which clarified the roles and responsibilities of doctors in the provision of treatment for drug and alcohol misusers. This report clarified the role of the addiction specialist and set out a pathway for GPs to qualify as one, although this was never actually implemented [8].

In practice, as funding for drug and alcohol services has declined and the opiate using population has reduced, fewer GPs have been employed in drug and alcohol services and contractual arrangements to treat drug users have become less attractive for GP practices. However, the rising level of physical health problems in drug users means that GPs will always have an important role in their care.

Types of Treatment Service

Harm Reduction Services

The *Models of Care* document made clear that harm reduction services were a crucial part of the treatment system [5]. In practice, this means needle and syringe exchange services, although other interventions such as programmes in clubs or festivals to reduce harm from party drug use or take-home naloxone are in this category. Early needle exchanges were 'stand-alone' and were provided in a shopfront-type service with open access. Service users received a warm welcome as well as clean needles and other health interventions such as sexual health and wound care. They were encouraged to consider formal treatment but this was by no means obligatory.

As treatment provision evolved, harm reduction services were incorporated into 'one-stop shop' type provision where service users would attend for all their needs. This created conflict for providers when services users apparently seeking abstinence also sought to collect clean needles. In some areas needle exchange was moved into community pharmacy services, where pharmacists were paid to give out packs containing needles, syringes and other paraphernalia. This model has worked well in many areas and pharmacists are also able to offer other health interventions to drug and alcohol users. However, harm reduction provision (especially needle exchange) has also seen declining levels of funding. There is always a risk that if levels of provision become too low then the desired population effect of reduction in blood-borne virus transmission may not be achieved.

The Rise and Fall and Rise of Opiate Substitution Treatment (OST)

The evidence base for the effectiveness of methadone maintenance treatment began to build in the USA from the 1960s [9]. However, apart from a brief period in the 1970s maintenance treatment was unpopular with politicians and the public in the UK, and services were unable to explicitly maintain heroin addicts on methadone for indefinite periods (although many did so in practice). The first clinical guidelines on the management of substance users were published (by the various departments of health across the UK) in 1991, then again in 1999, 2007 and 2017. These guidelines became known as the Orange Guidelines. It was only in 2007 that they were able to enthusiastically endorse methadone maintenance as the most effective treatment for opiate use [10]. This was supported by the production of a series of NICE guidelines, which acknowledged the effectiveness of opiate substitution treatment [11]. The emphasis on service users being offered high quality OST, where the dose was effective and enough ancillary support was provided, resulted in many more opiate users being offered methadone maintenance. Around that time buprenorphine was licensed for the maintenance treatment of opiate users, resulting in a genuine choice of medication for patients for the first time.

Despite this evidence of effectiveness, by 2011 there were many critics of the approach of using long-term methadone prescriptions, with the accusation that drug users were being 'parked on methadone' [12]. Further criticisms and calls for time-limited methadone in 2014 led to the Advisory Council for the Misuse of Drugs (ACMD) being asked to comment on the issue. They concluded that 'OST can be a very helpful part of treatment and recovery for those with heroin dependence, but it is unhelpful to focus on the medication alone and if heroin users are receiving "medication alone" without concomitant psychosocial interventions and recovery support' [13]. Since then services have been able to prescribe long term.

Recovery-Focused Services

The increasing unpopularity of opiate substitution coincided with a rise in the prominence of the concept of recovery in addiction services. For many this meant abstinence, although the definitions of recovery acknowledged the need for service users to make progress in treatment and to have the support to improve their lives. The concept of 'recovery capital', the elements of an individual's life that support their ability to recover, was also developed following the writings of William White and others in the USA [14]. Definitions of recovery varied, with some encompassing individuals who remained in opiate substitution and others individuals who were completely drug-free. All emphasised the individual nature of recovery.

For a period recovery was seen as the 'opposite' of conventional treatment, but more recently the debate has matured. The concepts of recovery communities and person-centred services have now reached the mainstream. The debate about the role of OST in recovery was summarised in a report about 'Medications in Recovery' published by an expert group in 2012 [15], which set out how OST needed to improve at a system, service and individual level. These improvements included:

- treatment systems and services having a clear and coherent vision and framework for recovery visible to people in treatment, owned by all staff and maintained by strong leadership.
- purposeful treatment interventions that are properly assessed, planned, measured, reviewed and adapted.
- 'phased and layered' interventions that reflect the different needs of people at different times.
- treatment that creates the therapeutic conditions and optimism through which people, and especially those with few internal and external resources, can meet the challenge of initiating and maintaining change.
- programmes that optimise the medication according to the evidence and guidance.
- measuring recovery by assessing and tracking improvements in severity, complexity and recovery capital, then using this information to tailor interventions and support that boost an individual's chances of recovering and promote progress towards that goal.
- treatment services that are not expected to deliver recovery on their own but are integrated with, and benefit from, other services such as mutual aid, employment support and housing.
- treatment that works alongside peers and families to give people direct access to, or signposts and facilitated support to, opportunities to reduce and stop their drug use, improve their physical and mental health, engage with others in recovery, improve relationships (including with their children), find meaningful work, build key life skills and secure housing.

Treatment and the Criminal Justice System

Substance users, particularly opiate and crack cocaine users, are frequently involved in acquisitive crime to fund their drug habits, and there is good evidence that treating drug use reduces crime. The advent of the NTA in 2002 saw the development of a range of interventions designed to ensure that drug users committing crime have access to treatment. These included:

- *Arrest referral*: This is where an individual is referred to a drug worker after arrest and seen immediately in a police station or at court. Testing on arrest means that those who are using drugs can be identified.
- *Court-mandated treatment*: In 1998 Drug Treatment and Testing Orders (DTTO) were piloted. This involved service users being mandated by the court to attend for treatment and regular testing. They were subsequently replaced by Drug Rehabilitation Requirements (DRR), and drug users can still be mandated to receive treatment. Results of these programmes have been positive and those mandated to treatment do as well as those who are not mandated.
- Prisons have a parallel treatment system (Integrated Drug Treatment System, IDTS) where service users can receive opiate substitution and other psychosocial interventions including group and individual work. There is also an emphasis on maintaining continuity with community treatment, although with financial cuts to services this has started to become compromised.

Organising Treatment Services

One-Stop Shop versus Separate Services? Alcohol versus Drugs?

Different elements of service such as harm reduction, OST and abstinence-based or recovery services were previously provided separately. In the last five years this has become uncommon as financial pressures mean that services tend to be provided together. This has the advantage of the services being more accessible and easier for local communities to access, but it does reduce service user choice and may result in a homogenous service where individualised treatment becomes more difficult to provide.

The biggest casualties of the one-stop shop approach are alcohol services. People with drug and alcohol use disorders have some elements in common but the treatments may be very different, with opiate users needing treatment for many years and alcohol users needing shorter, more intensive periods of treatment. While a service that integrates drug and alcohol services suits polydrug users it may not suit primary alcohol users who are often older and less involved in criminality than illicit drug users. This may result in a reduced number of alcohol users receiving the treatment they need. Approaches such as providing alcohol treatment in primary care or in acute hospitals may be used to mitigate this.

Residential Services

Inpatient and detoxification services are needed for substance users who present risks for treatment in the community or whose outcomes are likely to be poor. This specifically includes those using multiple substances and those with high levels of medical and psychiatric comorbidity. People with social problems such as homelessness may need inpatient treatment to stabilise their current condition or in some cases withdraw from drugs completely. Alcohol-dependent individuals who need to stop using alcohol are at high risk of seizures and other physical complications. Those who drink more than 30 units of alcohol per day, have a score of more than 30 on the Severity of Alcohol Dependence Questionnaire (SADQ), have a history of seizures or delirium tremens or need concurrent withdrawal from alcohol and benzodiazepines need medically assisted withdrawal in a setting that allows adequate monitoring [16]. These patients need access to inpatient units (IPU) with staff who have the skills and resources to meet their needs. In defining an IPU it is helpful to make a distinction between 'medically monitored' and 'medically managed' residential treatment:

- *Medically monitored treatment*: this can be provided in non-acute medical settings such as residential rehabilitation services, and is most appropriate for individuals with lower levels of dependence and without a range of associated medical and psychiatric problems.
- *Medically managed treatment*: this is typically provided in a hospital environment (i.e. NHS IPUs) [17].

As funding for substance misuse services has declined in England in the past 10 years, most NHS inpatient units have closed. There is provision in the voluntary sector but there are concerns about the quality of some of these services [18, 19].

Residential rehabilitation is usually provided by the voluntary sector and involves an extended stay in a residential therapeutic unit. The treatment goal is abstinence and attendance requires a high level of commitment from the patient. The therapeutic process underpinning residential rehabilitation units varies from a 12-step–based 'Minnesota Model' [20] to a formal Therapeutic Community structure [21], although most now offer a more eclectic series of interventions. Treatment is usually psychotherapeutic and delivered mainly in groups. Residential rehabilitation is usually funded as a social care provision, although budgets have been reduced and many services have closed over the past 10 years. For well-motivated service users periods of residential rehabilitation can be very successful and form the bedrock of a prolonged recovery.

Services for Special or Complex Groups

Some groups of service users have needs that are best met in services that are separate from mainstream drug and alcohol provision, or in special groups or clinics. The list below provides some examples:

- *Women* are in a minority in drug and alcohol services. They may be involved in sex working or be subject to domestic violence, and they also have specific health needs. Childcare and the relationship with social services may be an issue for some. Treatment services may provide women-only groups and programmes that consider their particular needs. The need to attract women into treatment can mean services being provided in different environments such as family centres.

- *Pregnant women*, particularly those dependent on opiates and/or alcohol, are best managed in environments where communication between drug and alcohol services, children's social care and maternity services is good. Pregnant women should be screened for substance use and non-dependent users should be provided with brief interventions.

- *Lesbian, gay, bisexual and transgendered individuals* may be using a different range of substances, including those traditionally called 'party drugs' such as mephadrone, GBL and methamphetamine. Some groups may use drugs in association with sexual activity, so-called chemsex. Services should therefore be provided in different environments such as sexual health clinics, although some may also be using opiates and alcohol and need to be retained in mainstream services.

- *Poor responders to treatment*: Some opiate users fail to respond to conventional OST treatment by continuing to use 'on top' of their prescription. There is good evidence that this group achieve better outcomes from prescription of injectable opiate treatment (IOT), usually diamorphine [22]. The evidence supports this being provided in supervised clinics where users attend every day, but these services are expensive to provide and only benefit a small number of individuals.

- *People with comorbid mental health problems*: The coexistence of substance misuse and mental health problems ('dual diagnosis') is very common, and managing these issues presents a challenge to treatment systems. Common patterns of coexistence include opiate- and alcohol-dependent users with mood disorders and non-dependent stimulant use in those with schizophrenia. In order to ensure that all service users can benefit from evidence-based treatment, opiate and alcohol users need access to psychological therapies for mood disorders (in practice this means access to mainstream psychological services) and those with schizophrenia need to be managed in psychiatric services who can provide harm reduction and motivational interventions. As outlined in Chapter 9, both mental health and addiction services need policies and procedures to ensure that service users do not fall into the gaps between them [23].

Peer-Led Services

One of the benefits of the recovery agenda has been the increase in service users participating in both planning and providing services. The 12-step fellowships, most commonly Narcotics Anonymous and Alcoholics Anonymous, are provided entirely by people with lived experience and are run independently of the treatment system (see Chapter 15). SMART Recovery is an alternative peer-led intervention which is based on the principles of cognitive behavioural therapy. Many treatment services employ people with living or lived experience in a variety of roles, including meeting and greeting service users, advocacy and delivering a range of interventions including distribution of take-home naloxone and running groups. Some local areas have set up independent service user organisations who represent them locally as well as providing some services.

Staffing Specialist Treatment Services

The majority of staff in substance misuse services are drug workers who come from a variety of professional backgrounds. Some have had their own experience of addiction, some have professional qualifications, and others will have learned their skills on the job. The Drug and Alcohol National Occupational Standards (DANOS) set out the skills and competencies needed by drug and alcohol workers [24]. Staff with nursing qualifications – generally Registered Mental Nurses (RMNs) but sometimes Registered General Nurses (RGNs) – were traditionally the main workforce in specialist drug and alcohol services, but their numbers have declined with reducing budgets and they have often been replaced by generic 'drug workers'. Nurses are now often highly qualified, working as non-medical prescribers as well as providing specialist roles such as focusing on blood-borne viruses or safeguarding children.

Addiction is a sub-speciality of general psychiatry, and since the creation of the Drug Dependence units in the late 1960s psychiatry has been the main route to specialist status. GPs have also had an important role (as already explained in this chapter), although usually within 'shared care' settings. However, as funding for specialist addiction services has been cut and the majority of treatment is provided in the voluntary/third sector, training posts in addiction psychiatry have been increasing hard to provide. This means fewer addiction psychiatrists are being trained, leading to an increasing problem with recruiting consultants and providing training in addiction to all psychiatrists.

Service Models

Since the Health and Social Care Act (2012) substance misuse services in England have been subject to competitive tendering and a culture of performance management, including pilot schemes testing payment by results. This has resulted in the provider of service in each local area changing every three to five years as part of a mechanism to dramatically reduce costs. Although this has produced more efficient services, it has had unintended consequences. These include a reduction in the ability of services to recruit and retain staff, and the possibility that reduced access to services has resulted in an increase in drug-related deaths [7].

Many services traditionally provided by the NHS have been transferred to voluntary sector providers. These providers are generally specialists in substance misuse and are skilled at providing services which can achieve a core set of outcomes. Many of them started as local services but consolidation of the market has now resulted in it being dominated by a few large providers with very little diversity of provision. The voluntary sector can provide good patient-focused services, but as they sit outside the local NHS systems there is often poor integration with local hospitals and health systems. This can result in problems providing healthcare to the most complex patients.

Services in England are usually provided as a single contracted system with one or more providers being in the contract. The NHS may have a role in providing the clinical or medical services, and this model can deliver the benefits of both voluntary sector and NHS provision. In other areas, the voluntary sector providers are responsible for delivering the full range of clinical interventions. Good services provide a range of high-quality interventions for substance users, which can be accessed in a timely manner. They also ensure that a full range of recovery interventions are provided either internally or by partners. Services need to be focused on outcomes which should be tailored to the individual – that is, abstinence for some but harm reduction for others.

At the time of writing, substance misuse services are still being subject to a reductions in funding as Local Authorities budgets are cut in England. Services are regularly re-tendered with the resultant loss of staff skills and continuity for patients, and risk becoming less integrated with other local health services. Failing to treat substance misusers properly risks putting pressure on the whole treatment and care system (including the criminal justice system), as well as depriving this vulnerable group of the treatment they need.

References

1   Connell P., Strang J. The origins of the new drug clinics of the 1960s: Clinical demand and the formation of policy. In: Strang J., Gossop M., eds. *Heroin Addiction and the British System: Volume 2 – Treatment and Policy Responses*. Abingdon: Routledge; 2005. p.17–27.

2   Advisory Council on the Misuse of Drugs. *AIDS and Drug Misuse*, Part 1. London: HMSO; 1988.

3   Department of Health. *Task Force to Review Services for Drug Misusers: Report of an Independent Review of Drug Treatment Services in England*. London: Department of Health; 1996.

4   Gossop M., Marsden J., Stewart D., Kidd T. The National Treatment Outcome Research Study (NTORS): 4–5 year follow-up results. *Addiction*. 2003; **98**: 291–303.

5   National Treatment Agency for Substance Misuse. *Models of Care for the Treatment of Drug Misusers*. London: National Treatment Agency for Substance Misuse; December 2002.

6   Marsden J., Farrell M., Bradbury C., Dale-Perera A., Eastwood B., Roxborough M. et al. Development of the Treatment Outcomes Profile. *Addiction*. 2008; **103** (9): 1450–60.

7   Advisory Council on the Misuse of Drugs. *Commissioning Impact on Drug Treatment*. London: ACMD; 2017.

8   Royal College of Psychiatrists and Royal College of General Practitioners. *Roles and Responsibilities of Doctors in the Provision of Treatment for Drug and Alcohol Misusers*. Council Report CR131. London: Royal College of Psychiatrists and Royal College of Physicians; 2005.

9   Dole V. P., Nyswander M. E. Methadone maintenance treatment: A ten-year perspective. *JAMA*. 1976; **235** (19): 2117–9.

10 Department of Health (England) and the Devolved Administrations. Drug Misuse and Dependence: UK Guidelines on Clinical Management. London: Department of Health (England), the Scottish Government, Welsh Assembly Government and Northern Ireland Executive; 2007.

11 Connock M., Juarez-Garcia A., Jowett S., Frew E., Liu Z., Fry-Smith A. et al. Methadone and buprenorphine for the management of opioid dependence:

A systematic review and economic evaluation. *Health Technology Assessment.* 2006; **11** (9): 1–171.

12 Gyngell K. *Breaking the Habit: Why the State Should Stop Dealing Drugs and Start Doing Rehab.* London: Centre for Policy Studies; 2011.

13 Advisory Council on the Misuse of Drugs. *Time Limiting Opioid Substitution Therapy.* London: ACMD; 2014.

14 White W., Cloud W. Recovery capital: A primer for addictions professionals. *Counselor.* 2008; **9** (5): 22–7.

15 Recovery Orientated Drug Treatment Expert Group. *Medications in Recovery: Re-Orientating Drug Dependence Treatment.* London: National Treatment Agency; 2012.

16 National Institute for Health and Clinical Excellence. *Alcohol-Use Disorders: Diagnosis, Assessment and Management of Harmful Drinking and Alcohol Dependence.* London: NICE; 2011.

17 SCAN Inpatient Treatment Working Party. *SCAN Consensus Project: Inpatient Treatment of Drug and Alcohol Misusers in the National Health Service.* London: Specialist Clinical Addiction Network; 2006.

18 Care Quality Commission. Briefing: Substance Misuse Services. 2017. [Available from: https://bit.ly/3fyfsBQ.]

19 Drummond C. The BMJ Opinion [Internet]. *BMJ.* 2017. [Available from: https://bit.ly/3sGmSXl.]

20 Cook C. C. H. The Minnesota model in the management of drug and alcohol dependency: miracle, method or myth? Part II – Evidence and conclusions. *British Journal of Addiction.* 1988; **83**: 735–48.

21 De Leon G. *The Therapeutic Community: Theory, Model and Method.* New York: Springer Publishing Co.; 2000.

22 Strang J., Groshkova T., Uchtenhagen A., van den Brink W., Haasen C., Schechter M. T. et al. Heroin on trial: Systematic review and meta-analysis of randomised trials of diamorphine-prescribing as treatment for refractory heroin addiction. *British Journal of Psychiatry.* 2015; **207** (1): 5–14.

23 Independent Expert Working Group. *Clinical Guidelines on Drug Misuse and Dependence Update 2017 – Drug Misuse and Dependence: UK Guidelines on Clinical Management.* London: Department of Health; 2017.

24 Skills for Health. Drug and Alcohol National Occupational Standards. 2014 [Available from: www.skillsforhealth.org.uk/resources/service-area/19-alcohol-drugs.]

Tobacco Use Disorders

Debbie Robson and Ann McNeill

Tobacco and Nicotine

Tobacco is used in different ways. Although there is no safe form of tobacco, combustible tobacco products (cigarettes, cigars, cigarillos, waterpipes) are considerably more harmful to the user than non-combustible products (snus, snuff, chewed tobacco). This chapter focuses on cigarette use, as it is the most common form of smoked tobacco, with a billion smokers worldwide. Dependence on tobacco (like most drug dependence) involves an interaction of pharmacological, genetic, behavioural, psychological, social and environmental factors, including tobacco product design and marketing.

What is in a Cigarette?

In addition to dried and fermented tobacco leaves, tobacco companies add several hundred ingredients to manufactured cigarettes and roll-your-own tobacco. Additives include humectants (moisturisers) to prolong shelf life; sugars and flavourings such as chocolate, vanilla and menthol to make the smoke more palatable and easier to inhale; and compounds such as ammonia to increase the speed and absorption of nicotine into systemic circulation. Additives are generally safe to consume in their natural form, but many are harmful when burned and inhaled in tobacco smoke. The burning of tobacco produces more than 7,000 toxic chemicals, 70 of which are carcinogenic (e.g. arsenic, benzene, heavy metals, hydrogen cyanide, formaldehyde and polycyclic hydrocarbons), alongside a range of other toxins [1].

Separating the Nicotine from Tobacco Smoke

As a drug, nicotine is widely misunderstood by smokers, clinicians and members of the public as it is often confused with the harm of tobacco. Such misunderstandings are a barrier to seeking and offering smokers appropriate support to quit. Nicotine is a naturally occurring alkaloid present in the leaves of the tobacco plant and the primary addictive component in tobacco products and cigarette smoke. It is one of the main reasons why people, once they start smoking, continue to smoke (and use other forms of tobacco). The dose and speed at which a drug reaches the brain influences its addictive potential. Cigarettes are deliberately engineered to deliver nicotine to the brain as fast as possible. When tobacco smoke is inhaled, the smoke particles carry the nicotine into the lungs, where it rapidly enters the circulation and moves into the brain within seconds. Nicotine delivered in tobacco smoke is absorbed much more quickly, and in higher doses than can be achieved by other routes of absorption, including intravenous injection [2]. It is the capacity to achieve rapid increases in systemic arterial blood levels through pulmonary absorption that makes tobacco smoking particularly addictive. In addition, monoamine oxidase inhibitors in tobacco smoke, substances added to tobacco such as sugars, flavourings, manipulation of the pH of tobacco smoke and design characteristics can all potentiate the addictiveness of nicotine [3].

Nicotine binds to nicotinic acetylcholine receptors in the ventral tegmental area of the midbrain, which has a knock-on effect of releasing dopamine in the nucleus accumbens. As with other drugs this acts as a neural teaching signal and the brain forms an association between the current situation and the impulse to engage in whatever action immediately preceded the release of dopamine. What this means for a smoker is that they get the urge to smoke in situations where smoking frequently occurs. These are referred to as cue-specific cravings.

Each manufactured cigarette has an average content of about 10 mg of nicotine. Although the dose of nicotine a smoker gets from a tobacco cigarette depends on many things (such as the brand of cigarette, frequency, size, depth of inhalation and puffing patterns), inhaling smoke from one cigarette will typically deliver 1–3 mg of nicotine to the smoker. A 20-pack-a-day smoker is believed to absorb around 20–40 mg of nicotine a day [4]. Nicotine has a short half-life (about two hours); regular smoking produces intermittent peaks and troughs of nicotine in the blood throughout the day, with an overall rise in nicotine levels over six to eight hours, with a slow decline overnight (providing a cigarette is not smoked). Regular puffing on cigarettes, with the subsequent rapid delivery of repeated high doses of nicotine to the brain, also plays a role in the addictive nature of cigarettes. Sustained use of nicotine is also reinforced by some of the co-stimuli of smoking and the pleasure experienced, such as the taste and sensation of tobacco in the throat, the smell and behaviours associated with smoking (e.g. smoking after a meal, with a cup of coffee or alcoholic drink or with friends who smoke). Even negative mood states can become conditioned cues for smoking, as a smoker learns that not having a cigarette causes irritability and poor concentration and that smoking provides relief; after repeated experiences, a smoker can sense irritability from any source as a cue for smoking [3]. Addictiveness and pleasure are likely to be intertwined and it can be hard to distinguish positive reward and relief from incipient withdrawal.

Nicotine alone carries minimal harm. Research on the safety of long-term nicotine use in humans without combustion products has found no association between sustained nicotine replacement therapy (NRT) use and the occurrence of cancer or cardiovascular disease [5, 6]. Animal research has suggested foetal exposure to very high doses of nicotine has adverse consequences that are maintained through to adolescence, but the relevance for humans is unclear. Indeed, it was recently reported that infants born to pregnant smokers who had used nicotine replacement therapies to stop smoking during pregnancy were less likely to have impaired development compared with those who used placebo, two years after birth [7].

Hence, nicotine sustains dependence on tobacco cigarettes, but the hazards of sustained nicotine use are negligible compared with sustained tobacco use. The harm of smoking is not caused by nicotine, but by other constituents of tobacco smoke. Professor Michael Russell, an addiction psychiatrist, was one of the pioneers of nicotine research and explained that over recent centuries 'no population has dispensed with one form of tobacco use without replacing it by another' and 'once experienced, nicotine use has continued in populations as it does in individuals'. He subsequently commented that 'people smoke for the nicotine, but die from the tar ' and that nicotine replacement products should be as acceptable and palatable as possible to compete with tobacco products [8].

As mentioned, misperceptions about nicotine impede smokers from seeking treatment. Among the general population of Great Britain, knowledge about the portion of harm of smoking attributable to nicotine is poor. In 2017, fewer than 1 in 10 adults (7.5 per cent) correctly answered that none (or a very small part) of the risk of smoking came from nicotine; 14 per cent thought that it was nearly all the risk and nearly a quarter (24.2 per cent) said they didn't know. Similarly, surveys have shown that around 40 per cent of smokers erroneously believe that nicotine is the chemical in cigarettes that causes most of the cancer [9]. These findings are supported by international data. Misperceptions about nicotine in tobacco likely underpin similar misperceptions about the relative harmfulness of nicotine replacement therapies and electronic cigarettes [9].

The safest thing is to never start smoking in the first place, and if you do, to stop using tobacco products completely. A later section of this chapter explains how to help smokers stop and the different types of support available. However, once tobacco smoking has a grip on you, it is hard to let go of. For those who cannot or do not want to give up nicotine, encouraging smokers to switch to a tobacco-free source of nicotine will improve their health and life expectancy. There is a continuum of harm of nicotine-containing products, from the high harm of combusted tobacco in cigarettes to minimal harms of non-combustible nicotine delivered in licenced NRT products and electronic cigarettes.

Prevalence of Tobacco Smoking

It is often argued that tobacco smoking is decreasing and that we should switch our attention to the prevention and treatment of other addictions. However, there is a strong counterargument for this. Worldwide, while the *proportion* of adults who smoke has declined over time, because of the growing population, the overall *number* of people who smoke and the number of cigarettes smoked has increased since 1980. Worldwide, there are an estimated 1.1 billion smokers, with 80 per cent of them living in low- and middle-income countries. The prevalence of cigarette smoking among the population in the UK has fallen since the 1970s, when 51 per cent of men and 41 per cent of women smoked. In 2019, 14.1 per cent of adults (16 per cent of men and 12.5 per cent of women) in the UK smoked, equating to approximately 6.9 million people [10]. The decrease in smoking prevalence masks huge disparities among the population. Smoking rates have remained relatively static among disadvantaged and vulnerable groups.

For those with a common mental disorder such as depression or anxiety, rates are almost twice as high when compared with those who are mentally well and three times greater for those with schizophrenia or bipolar disorder [11]. People with the highest smoking rates are those receiving treatment for a substance use disorder (SUD) [12]. Rates of smoking in these populations are akin to rates in the 1960s in the general population – in other words, these populations have generally been untouched by tobacco control interventions. An international systematic review of 54 papers involving 37,364 participants reported a smoking prevalence of 84 per cent in people receiving treatment for a SUD, compared with 31 per cent among a matched population; highest rates were consistently observed in opiate users compared with other illicit drugs or alcohol misuse [13]. As far back as the 1980s smoking among people receiving substance misuse treatment was described as a 'neglected problem', and three decades later it has been referred to as a 'neglected epidemic' [14]. Indeed, in England in 2010 it was estimated that 42 per cent of all cigarettes smoked were done so by people with a mental disorder and/or SUD [15], with similar estimates reported in the USA [16]. Smoking is highly prevalent among people in prison (~80 per cent) and up to 93 per cent of people who are homeless smoke [11], partly a reflection of the high rates of SUD and mental illness in these populations.

Harm from Smoking

We have known since the 1950s that smoking kills people prematurely. Half of all lifelong smokers lose around 10 years of life and they suffer diseases of old age around 10 years earlier compared with never-smokers [17]. Although smoking causes an extensive range of diseases, most smoking-related deaths are from cancers, respiratory diseases and cardiovascular diseases – that is, diseases that are highly prevalent in people with a SUD and/or mental illness. In England in 2016 there were 81,490 smoking-related deaths in people aged 35 and over, representing approximately 16 per cent of all registered deaths and the largest single cause of preventable death [18]. For comparison, in the same period there were 23,839 alcohol-related deaths in people of all ages, representing around 5 per cent of all deaths [19]. In England in 2016–17, there were 513,940 smoking-related hospital admissions in people aged 35 and over; this compares with 337,113 alcohol related hospital admissions in people of all ages [19, 20]. The Royal College Physicians [21] estimated that in 2015–16, current smoking cost the NHS in England £620 million in adult secondary care costs. The annual contribution to NHS costs from current smoking among people with a SUD and/or mental health disorder was £204 million in hospital care.

People with a SUD and/or mental health disorder smoke more heavily and intensely than people without these conditions. Their health and life expectancy are therefore disproportionally affected due to the greater exposure to toxins present in tobacco smoke. For example, cigarette smoking and alcohol independently increase the risk of cancer, though used together they synergistically act to damage health and greatly increase the risk of oral, laryngeal, oesophageal and liver cancer compared with either substance in isolation [22].

Tobacco smoking is associated with poorer outcomes for those in substance misuse and/or mental health treatment. An investigation of the effects of cigarette smoking during pharmacologically supported opioid detoxification found smoking during treatment was associated with increased opioid withdrawal discomfort, more intense opioid craving and lower detoxification completion rates compared with smokers who were not allowed to smoke and with non-smokers [23]. People with a mental health condition who smoke experience more severe symptoms of psychosis, depression and anxiety and have an increased risk of the onset of panic attacks; they spend longer periods in hospital and less time out of hospital and require higher doses of some psychotropic medicines [11]. There is also a growing body of evidence suggesting that cigarette smoking might be a risk factor for schizophrenia [24].

Health Service–Related Factors That Sustain High Rates of Smoking Prevalence

There are several factors that support continued smoking or interfere with efforts to quit in users of specialist substance misuse and/or mental health services. Historically, smoking has been viewed as a normative behaviour in these treatment settings and has neither been discouraged nor been a target of intervention. The health risks of smoking in these high-risk populations have frequently been viewed as less relevant than the perceived therapeutic benefits of smoking and staff rate tobacco-dependence treatment significantly less important than treatment of other substances [12]. Staff are often concerned that attempts to quit smoking will negatively impact treatment, undermine patients' abstinence from other drugs and that clients should not try and modify too many behaviours at once [25]. Clinicians, clients and carers often believe that smoking alleviates stress, regulates mood and cognition and is somehow therapeutic. This 'self-medication hypothesis', although popular, has very little empirical evidence to support it.

Staff are ambivalent about their role and responsibilities in providing smoking cessation support and many report a lack confidence and knowledge for addressing this clinical need [26]. Studies consistently find that staff who smoke are less likely to offer smoking cessation support to clients or see it as an important part of their role [26]. This is of particular importance as there are high rates of smoking among staff in mental health and addiction settings compared with staff who work in general health care settings [12].

Staff also underestimate the level of interest in quitting among clients. Around 70 per cent of smokers in the general population report that they want to stop smoking. Studies consistently show that a similar proportion of smokers with a comorbid substance use and/or a mental illness are interested in quitting, but they have limited access to smoking cessation treatment. In a study including 163 clients and 145 staff from community and residential addiction services in South London, 88 per cent of clients currently smoked and 79 per cent expressed a desire to quit, but only 15 per cent recalled they had been offered support to stop smoking during their current treatment episode [12].

The Benefits of Stopping Smoking

Stopping smoking at any age is beneficial compared with continuing to smoke. The risk of some smoking-related diseases reduces, and for others the risk is 'frozen' at the point when the smoker quits [27]. The excess risk of a smoking-related heart attack reduces by 50 per cent within 12 months of quitting. The rate of decline in lung function returns to the normal age-related decline. Quitting reduces the frequency of exacerbations in people with chronic obstructive pulmonary disease, and freezes the risk of smoking-related cancers at the level reached when stopping occurs [27]. People who have smoked for many years may believe that the damage has already been done and that there is no point of stopping. Health professionals can reassure people that it is never too late to stop smoking [28]:

- For the average smoker, if they have not contracted a smoking-related disease by the age of 30, stopping smoking may normalise life expectancy.
- Stopping before the age of 40 adds approximately nine years of life compared with continuing to smoke.
- Stopping at the age of 50 years adds approximately six years, while stopping at the age of 60 adds approximately three years.

People with a SUD and/or mental health condition have a lot to gain from stopping smoking. In addition to improved physical health and increased life expectancy, stopping smoking is associated with reduced depression, anxiety and stress, improved positive mood and quality of life [29]. In a systematic review and meta-analysis of 19 RCTs, including people in addiction treatment or recovery services, smoking cessation interventions provided during treatment were associated with a 25 per cent increased likelihood of long-term abstinence from alcohol and illicit drugs and increased long-term abstinence [30].

The first half of this chapter has outlined why tobacco dependence is a chronic relapsing medical condition that requires treatment. The second half will briefly describe population-level interventions to reduce tobacco use, followed by what clinicians can do to support people to quit smoking.

Population-Level Interventions

Effective population-level tobacco control interventions such as those in Box 12.1 prevent the uptake of smoking, increase the rate at which people who smoke make a quit attempt and increase cessation rates.

Although it is likely that population-level interventions influence smoking behaviour in people with SUD and/or mental health disorders, evidence specifically relating to these groups is scarce. However, literature about the impact of comprehensive smoke-free polices in mental health and addiction settings is available.

Comprehensive Smoke-Free Policies in Hospitals

The efforts to achieve a smoke-free National Health Service in the UK spans several decades, though it took until 2007 for smoking to be legally prohibited in acute hospital buildings and 2008 in mental health and SUD inpatient settings. Restricting smoking in hospital buildings was extended to the grounds of hospital settings in 2013 in England, Wales and Northern Ireland, with the publication of the NICE guidelines for 'Smoking: Acute, Maternity and Mental Health Services' [31]. NICE recommended that a comprehensive smoke-free policy covering buildings, grounds and vehicles and accessible tobacco-dependence treatment for all smokers is essential in order to provide a healthy environment and promote non-smoking as the norm for people using NHS services. The guidance applies to secondary care services (inpatient and community), including drug and alcohol services and emergency care settings; Table 12.1 describes the recommended changes. Although there are no current plans to legislate smoke-free NHS grounds in Scotland, the Health (Tobacco, Nicotine and Care) (Scotland) Act 2016 makes it

---

Box 12.1 Population level tobacco control interventions

Increasing the price (and taxation) of tobacco products

Controlling the illicit supply of tobacco (smuggling and illicit cross border shopping)

Advertisement bans and restrictions

Mandatory health warnings on tobacco products

Standardised packaging

Limiting the age of sale and enforcing restrictions on selling tobacco products to young people

Mass media and social marketing campaigns

Restricting access to cigarette vending machines

Smoke-free legislation to prohibit smoking in the workplace and public places

Comprehensive smoke-free policies to restrict smoking in healthcare settings and providing smokers with tobacco-dependence treatment support

Table 12.1 Recommendations in NICE guidelines for smoking: acute, maternity and mental health [31]

Changes to the treatment of tobacco dependence	Changes to the environment and staff behaviour
Provide clients with information for planned or anticipated use of secondary care, that smoking is prohibited in buildings and grounds and that support is available.	Develop and communicate smoke-free policies that include prohibiting smoking in grounds as well as buildings; removal of shelters or other designated outdoor smoking areas.
Provide advice for carers, family and visitors, that smoking is prohibited in buildings and grounds.	Do not allow smoking during work hours or when recognisable as an employee (e.g. when in uniform, or wearing identification, or handling hospital business).
Identify clients who smoke and offer help to stop.	Prohibit staff-supervised and staff-facilitated smoking breaks in secondary care.
Provide intensive support for people using acute, maternity, mental health and drug and alcohol services.	Support staff to stop smoking.
Make stop smoking pharmacotherapies available in hospital.	Provide stop smoking training for frontline staff.

an offence to smoke within 15 m of a hospital building. The implementation of such policies is associated with a positive effect on smoking behaviours and smoking-related motivation and beliefs [32] and may also have positive indirect effects such as a reduction in physical violence in inpatient settings [33, 34].

Individual-Level Interventions to Support Smoking Cessation and Harm Reduction

There are several evidence-based individual-level interventions to promote smoking cessation that apply to all smokers irrespective of their primary clinical condition or motivation to quit smoking. The initial step is the identification of smoking status, followed by the offer of support and the provision of pharmacological and behavioural support to quit or reduce tobacco use.

When Should Treatment for Tobacco Dependence Be Addressed?

For many years clinical lore suggested that quitting smoking at the same time as quitting both alcohol and/or illicit substances or when mentally unwell was too difficult and a quit attempt would undermine treatment outcomes. Staff and clients have different views about when smoking should be addressed. For example, in a survey of 145 health professionals and 163 clients across seven community and residential addictions services in London, UK, two-thirds of staff believed smoking should be addressed late in or after their primary addiction treatment, whereas 50 per cent of clients believed it should be addressed late in or after treatment [12]. The consensus of opinion is that people in treatment or in recovery from SUD and/or mental health disorder should be offered tobacco cessation interventions throughout their care pathway [35].

Very Brief Advice to Stop Smoking

Focusing on telling people who smoke about the harms caused by smoking and advising them to stop is not as effective as the *offer* of support to quit. Compared with no advice, the odds of quitting are 68 per cent higher if stop smoking medication is offered and 217 per cent higher with the offer of behavioural support [36]. Very brief advice (VBA) to stop smoking was originally designed to be used opportunistically by health professionals to trigger a quit attempt. Recently, this has been systematised in UK primary and secondary care settings through financially incentivising health care providers – that is, the Quality and Outcomes Framework (QOF) targets for GPs and Commissioning for Quality Improvement and Innovation (CQUIN) for NHS secondary acute, mental health and substance misuse services. Figure 12.1 shows the three elements of VBA.

Identifying and recording the smoking status of clients is an essential first step in encouraging people to quit. Confirming if someone is a smoker/tobacco user, should be followed up with brief advice about the best way to quit and an offer of support. Doctors and other health workers often say they don't have time to deliver brief interventions and are concerned that encouraging smokers to quit will annoy them. Most smokers know that smoking is detrimental to their health and those around them. They know they need to quit but often do not know how to. Asking a smoker if they are interested in stopping creates an

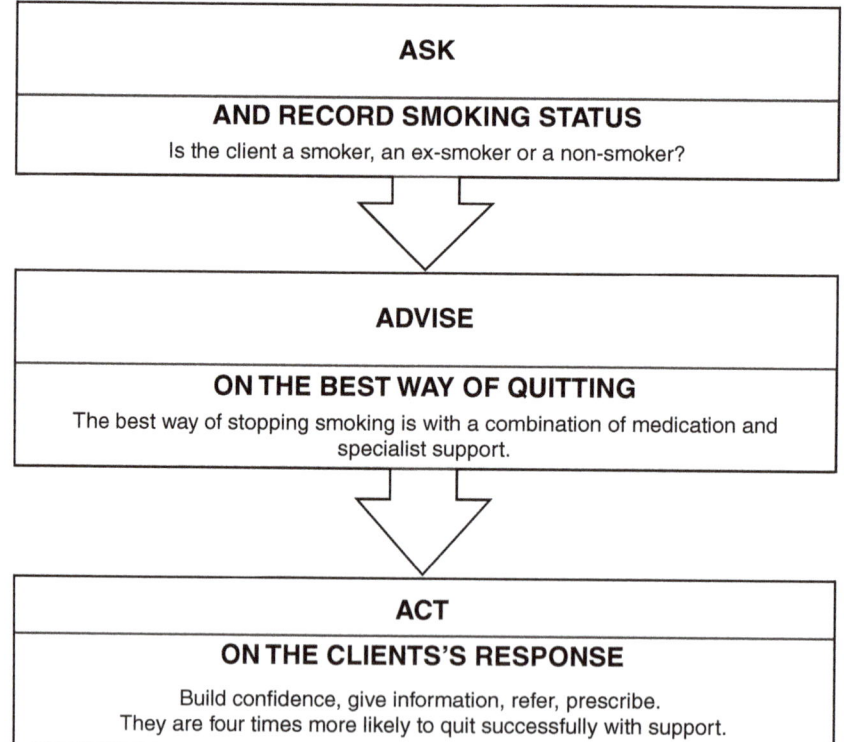

Figure 12.1 A summary of very brief advice (VBA) on smoking as described by the National Centre for Smoking Cessation and Training (NCSCT)

opportunity for the smoker to explain why it is not the right time, or that they have tried in the past but have been unsuccessful. The conversation usually stops and the opportunity to trigger a quit attempt is lost. It is unnecessary to ask people if they are ready to quit, when offering support (medication and/or a referral to a trained tobacco-dependence treatment advisor) avoids a lengthy conversation and is more effective than simply advising someone to quit [37].

Assessment of the Severity of Tobacco Dependence

The Fagerstrom test for cigarette dependence [38] is the most widely used assessment of tobacco dependence in cigarette smokers. The original scale was designed to measure physical dependence, but although the items remain relatively similar the name of the scale has evolved over time to take into account other factors associated with dependence, such as conditioning, the ritual of smoking and psychosocial functions. The Heaviness of Smoking index [39] (Box 12.2) is a shortened version of the original scale and uses only two questions; both questions are reliable over time and are important predictors of quitting.

Tobacco Withdrawal Symptoms and Cravings to Smoke

The first major hurdle in stopping smoking is managing the discomfort of tobacco withdrawal. Nicotine has a half-life of approximately two hours, therefore withdrawal symptoms can start very soon after finishing a cigarette (Table 12.2). Some smokers experience more severe withdrawal symptoms than others due to a variety of genetic, physiological and environmental factors and the pre-quitting level of nicotine intake. People with severe mental illness may be more sensitive to the effects of acute tobacco abstinence and experience tobacco withdrawal symptoms earlier and more intensely than those without a mental illness [40].

Cravings for cigarettes, or urges to smoke, can persist for much longer (many weeks or even months after stopping, albeit occurring far less frequent). Cravings for cigarettes manifests in two ways:

Box 12.2 Heaviness of Smoking index [39]		
How soon after waking do you have your first cigarette?	Within 5 minutes	3
	5–30 minutes	2
	31–60 minutes	1
	60+ minutes	0
How many cigarettes a day do you usually smoke?	10 or less	0
	11–20	1
	21–30	2
	31 or more	3
	SCORE =	

SCORING: 1–2 = very low dependence; 3–4 = low to moderate dependence; 5–6 = high dependence

Table 12.2 Tobacco withdrawal symptoms and signs

Symptom	Prevalence	Average Duration
Irritability	> 25%	< 4 weeks
Increased appetite	> 25%	> 10 weeks
Difficulty concentrating	> 25%	< 4 weeks
Restlessness	> 25%	< 4 weeks
Depressed mood	< 25%	< 4 weeks
Urges to smoke	> 25%	> 10 weeks but declines over time
Sleep disturbance	< 25%	<4 weeks
Increased appetite	< 25%	< 4 weeks
Sign	**Prevalence**	**Average Duration**
Cough/sore throat	< 25%	< 4 weeks
Mouth ulcers	< 25%	> 2 weeks
Constipation	< 25%	> 2 weeks
Weight gain	> 25%	permanent
Reduced heart rate	> 25%	permanent
Increased skin temperature	> 25%	permanent

(1) *Background or general cravings to smoke:* These occur as the body is deprived of tobacco and nicotine between each cigarette. They usually fluctuate over the course of the day, depending on how tobacco dependent the smoker is. If a person completely abstains from smoking these cravings will gradually disappear.

(2) *Cue-specific cravings or triggers to smoke:* These arise in response to being exposed to stimuli that may have become associated with smoking (e.g. certain places, seeing another person smoke, seeing a packet of cigarettes, talking about cigarettes, after a meal or with alcohol). These tend to have a fast onset, feel intense and are more short-lived than general cravings.

Any of these withdrawal symptoms during a quit attempt might drive someone back to smoking, though research suggests any association between withdrawal symptoms and relapse is inconsistent and weak; the main factors driving relapse appear to be cue-driven smoking urges and nicotine hunger [27].

Carbon Monoxide Assessment and Monitoring

Carbon monoxide (CO) is a colourless, odourless, tasteless and toxic gas. It enters the blood from the tobacco smoke in the lungs and combines with the red blood cells, lowering the body's ability to transport oxygen around the body. Reduced oxygen availability from CO exposure can lead to angina, congestive heart failure and chronic obstructive pulmonary disease. CO builds up in the body throughout the day with regular smoking and falls overnight (providing a cigarette is not smoked during the night). CO assessment and monitoring is a more valid measure of smoking status than self-reports and an effective motivational tool; it provides the smoker with immediate visual and verbal feedback about how much CO is in their lungs and an estimate of how much is in their blood. This information can then be used to have a conversation about the potential harmful effects of smoking. Regular monitoring and feedback can help the smoker track how well they are responding to treatment.

Tobacco-Dependence Treatment

It is vital for smokers to stop at the earliest possible opportunity, and for every quit attempt to have the best possible chance of success. Most smokers try to stop smoking without support. However, many relapse back to smoking, usually in the first week. Only about 4 per cent of smokers who try to quit on their own manage to stop and stay stopped. The UK has a national network of Stop Smoking Services and since 2000 they have supported an estimated 1 million smokers to quit for good. These services have been built around the principle of a universal offer of support available for all smokers. Typically, smokers are offered weekly sessions of either individual face-to-face or group support with a specialist stop smoking practitioner, averaging approximately 30–45 minutes over a 6–12 week period. Stopping in one step (abrupt cessation) with the support of pharmacotherapy and behavioural support from a trained tobacco-dependence treatment practitioner leads to the best chance of successfully quitting. An alternative method for people who have tried stopping in one go and have been unsuccessful, or they lack confidence in stopping in one step, is to gradually cut down their cigarettes before stopping with the help of nicotine replacement products.

Pharmacotherapy

When an individual wishes to make a quit attempt, there are three first-line medicines licensed in the UK that at least double the chance of successfully stopping smoking: nicotine replacement therapy (NRT), also licensed for temporary abstinence and reducing smoking; bupropion (Zyban); and varenicline (Champix). Although each medicine has a different mechanism of action, the underlying principles are generally the same (Box 12.3).

Nicotine Replacement Therapy (NRT)

All forms of NRT can be used for temporary abstinence, smoking reduction and to help those who want to quit or reduce smoking prior to quitting. In the UK it is licensed for people aged 12 and over who smoke and for pregnant and breastfeeding women making a quit attempt. All products are general sale medicines and can be bought over the counter. The aim of NRT in those making a quit attempt is to assist the transition from cigarette smoking to complete abstinence. This is achieved by temporarily replacing some of the

---

Box 12.3 Principles of pharmacological aids for smoking cessation

To alleviate the craving and withdrawal symptoms associated with stopping smoking

To reduce the pharmacological reward from smoking by indirectly disrupting dopamine release or by desensitising receptors

To deliver some positive reinforcement other than from a cigarette

nicotine obtained from tobacco cigarettes with nicotine from medicinal NRT products and minimising nicotine withdrawal symptoms and motivation to smoke. People who smoke can safely use NRT if they wish to continue using nicotine recreationally or to prevent relapse back to smoking.

In the UK there are eight different products to choose from:

- transdermal patch
- gum
- lozenge
- inhalator
- microtabs
- nasal spray
- mouth spray
- mouth strips

Regime

Smokers with a higher level of dependence need to start their NRT regime (Table 12.3) with the highest strength skin patch and oral NRT product. British National Formulary [41] guidelines recommend titrating down the dose of NRT over an 8–12-week period.

Table 12.3 Recommended regime for NRT [41]

Light smoker: smokes 1–10 cigarette a day and after 1 hour of waking	Moderate to heavy smoker: smokes more than 11 cigarettes a day or smokes within 30 minutes of waking
Patch 14 mg/24 hours for 6 weeks **then** 7 mg/24 hours for 2 weeks **OR** 15 mg/16 hours for 8 weeks **then** 10 mg/16 hours for 2 weeks	**Patch** 21 mg/24 hours for 6 weeks 14 mg/24 hours for 2 weeks 7 mg/24 hours for 2 weeks (Switch to 16 hour patch if client has side effects)
OR **(choose 1)** **Gum** 2 mg, max 15 a day **Lozenge** 1 mg/2 mg max 15 a day **Microtab** 2 mg/hour max 40 tabs/day **Inhaler** 2–4 cartridges a day **Mouth strips 2.5 mgs,** 1 x 1 an hour **Mouthspray 1 mg per spray** 1–2 sprays every hour (max 64 sprays a day) The nicotine from patches initially takes several hours to be absorbed. During the first 1–2 weeks, an oral product may also be needed	Combine with **(choose at least 1)** **Gum** 2 mg/4mg max 15 a day **Lozenge** 2 mg/4 mg max 15 a day **Microtab** 2/4 mg/hour max 40 tabs a day **Inhaler** 6 cartridges a day max **Nasal spray 500 mcg per spray** 2 sprays x twice an hour (up to 64 sprays a day) **Mouthspray** 1 mg per spray: 2 sprays every 30 mins–1 hour (up to 64 sprays a day) **Mouth strips 2.5 mg, Mouth strips 2.5 mg** 1 every 1–2 hours (strips are for clients who have their first cigarette of the day *more than 30 minutes* after waking up, but more dependent smokers may find them easy to use)

NRT is formulated for systemic absorption either through the skin in the case of patches, or the oral or nasal mucosa in the case of all the other products. This means that absorption of nicotine from NRT is much slower than nicotine from inhaling a tobacco cigarette and the risk of becoming addicted to NRT is minimal; a small proportion of people (~5 per cent) who use NRT continue to use it long term after stopping smoking and it appears to carry minimal or no risk to long-term users [42]. The nicotine from oral products has to be absorbed through the cheeks, gums and back of the lips. The correct technique is to chew the gum or suck the lozenge until the taste becomes strong and then rest it between the cheek and gum; when the taste starts to fade, it is advised to repeat this process for about 20–30 minutes. Drinking coffee and carbonated drinks may block the absorption of nicotine from oral nicotine products.

Effectiveness

NRT is the most studied medication for smoking cessation. There have been more than 150 trials, involving more than 50, 000 smokers. The odds ratio (OR) of abstinence for any form of NRT compared with placebo is 1.84 (95 per cent credible interval 1.71 to 1.99) [43]. There is no evidence that one product is more effective than another, therefore the choice of products should be guided by any contraindications and client preference. Studies have found that NRT bought over the counter from a shop, without any additional support, does not improve the chance of quitting [44]. Combining two NRT products (usually a nicotine patch plus one of the faster-acting products such as gum or mouth spray) is more effective than use of one product alone [44]. The mouth spray, nasal spray and 4 mg lozenge tend to act faster than other products and can be particularly helpful in addressing acute cravings.

NRT is effective in smokers with a severe mental illness, though there are no published studies of NRT compared with placebo. There is evidence from a systematic review of three RCTs involving 635 people that NRT is more effective than usual care at helping smokers with a SUD to quit for at least six months (RR 7.74 (95 per cent CI 3.00–19.94) [35].

Side Effects of NRT

Mild local reactions may occur at the beginning of NRT treatment (Box 12.4).

Box 12.4 NRT side effects

Preparation	Common side effects
Skin patches	Skin irritation. Sleep disturbance and insomnia may occur with 24-hour patches.
Nasal spray	Coughing, nasal irritation, epistaxis, sneezing and watery eyes.
Oral spray	Watery eyes and blurred vision, abdominal pain, flatulence and taste disturbance.
Lozenges and gum	Throat irritation, mouth soreness and hiccups.

Optimising Adherence

Better adherence to oral and transdermal NRT is associated with better quit rates. However, adherence to NRT is often undermined by misguided concerns of clinicians and clients, particularly around safety, efficacy and addictiveness. Underuse of NRT, incorrect use or stopping treatment early also undermine effectiveness. It is important that clients are given a realistic expectation of what stop smoking medications can do for them. They will not completely remove the urge to smoke but they can reduce these urges, alleviate most withdrawal symptoms and make temporary abstinence and quitting easier. As with all medications, their effectiveness partly depends on them being used as recommended and with the correct technique. Information should be regularly provided about how to use the NRT product correctly, what side effects and withdrawal symptoms to expect and how to manage them along with the importance of using the maximum dose and duration of use.

Varenicline – – Varenicline is a selective α4β2 nicotinic acetylcholine receptor partial agonist; it mimics the action of nicotine and causes a sustained release of dopamine in the mesolimbic pathway. It also blocks dopamine release resulting from subsequent nicotine intake. This means if taken as prescribed, any attempt to smoke a cigarette will be less pharmacologically rewarding and feel less satisfying to the smoker. Unlike NRT, varenicline does not contain nicotine and is a prescription only medicine licensed for smokers over the age of 18 who want to quit.

Regime

There are three options for taking varenicline. Smokers can choose a fixed quit date, a flexible quit date or gradually cut down the number of cigarettes they smoke and eventually quit. A fixed quit date is the most common way of taking varenicline as it fits in with the abrupt cessation (stopping in one go) model of Stop Smoking Services in the UK. Varenicline should be started while the client is still smoking and a quit date is usually set within the first two weeks of starting varenicline. The dose is titrated using the following schedule:

- days 1–3: 0.5 mg daily
- days 4–7: 0.5 mg twice a day
- days 8–: 1 mg twice a day

Clients who are unwilling or unable to set a target quit date within two weeks can start treatment and choose a more flexible quit date within five weeks of commencing varenicline. The dosing regime is the same as above. For clients who have successfully stopped smoking at the end of 12 weeks (with either a fixed or flexible quit date), an additional course of 12 weeks of treatment at 1 mg twice daily may be considered for the maintenance of abstinence.

Clients who are unable or unwilling to quit within one to five weeks can start varenilcline (using the same dosing regime as above) and gradually reduce the amount they smoke during the first 12 weeks of treatment and aim to quit completely by the end of 12 weeks. They should then continue to take varenicline for a further 12 weeks (i.e. 24 weeks in total). Consider tapering towards the end of treatment for clients with a high risk of relapse back to smoking. Figure 12.2 illustrates Varenicline treatment regimens that can be used with a fixed quit date, a flexible quit date or a gradual cessation of smoking.

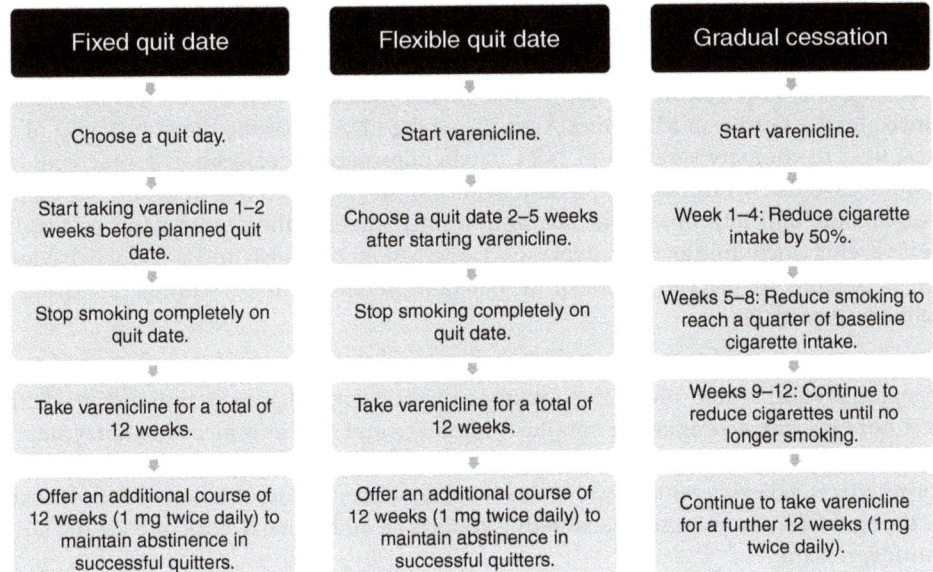

Fixed quit date	Flexible quit date	Gradual cessation
Choose a quit day.	Start varenicline.	Start varenicline.
Start taking varenicline 1–2 weeks before planned quit date.	Choose a quit date 2–5 weeks after starting varenicline.	Week 1–4: Reduce cigarette intake by 50%.
Stop smoking completely on quit date.	Stop smoking completely on quit date.	Weeks 5–8: Reduce smoking to reach a quarter of baseline cigarette intake.
Take varenicline for a total of 12 weeks.	Take varenicline for a total of 12 weeks.	Weeks 9–12: Continue to reduce cigarettes until no longer smoking.
Offer an additional course of 12 weeks (1 mg twice daily) to maintain abstinence in successful quitters.	Offer an additional course of 12 weeks (1 mg twice daily) to maintain abstinence in successful quitters.	Continue to take varenicline for a further 12 weeks (1mg twice daily).

Figure 12.2 Summary of treatment regimens using Varenicline

Effectiveness

A Cochrane review in 2016 found high-quality evidence that a standard dose of varenicline is more effective than placebo at helping smokers to quit for at least six months (RR 2.24, 95 per cent CI 2.06–2.43; 27 trials, 12,625 people) [45]. Low or variable doses of varenicline were also shown to be effective (RR 2.08; 95 per cent CI 1.56 to 2.78; 4 trials, 1,266 people) and reduced the number and severity of side effects. The review also found high-quality evidence that varenicline is more effective than bupropion at six months (RR 1.39; 95 per cent CI 1.25 to 1.54; 5 trials, 5,877 people) and moderate evidence that it is more effective than single NRT (RR 1.25; 95 per cent CI 1.14 to 1.37; 8 trials, 6,264 people).

Several trials of varenicline have been conducted in people with psychosis who smoke. When the results are pooled together, varenicline was found to improve the odds of quitting four- to fivefold compared with placebo [46, 47]. In the largest RCT to date, including 8,144 smokers with and without a history of psychiatric disorders who were randomised to receive either varenicline, bupropion, nicotine patch or placebo for 12 weeks and were followed for 24 weeks, varenicline was the most effective treatment for helping people with and without psychiatric disorders to quit [48]. A Cochrane systematic review identified four trials of varenicline to assess smoking cessation in people with a SUD. Two studies found it was more effective than placebo in methadone-maintained and alcohol-dependent smokers; one study found it more effective than NRT at three month follow-up in smokers receiving treatment for SUD, although another study did not find it increased quit rates at six month follow-up [35].

Side Effects, Contraindications and Cautions

Common side effects include nausea, strange dreams, insomnia and headache. Varenicline has no known interactions with psychotropic medication. For clients who are unable to tolerate side effects, consider temporarily or permanently reducing the dose to 0.5 mg twice daily.

Up until 2016 varenicline carried a black triangle symbol, indicating additional safety monitoring was required for people with a mental health condition. However, this was removed by the European Medicines Agency and the FDA following the publication of the largest RCT to compare varenicline, NRT patch, bupropion or placebo in people with and without a psychiatric disorder [48]. Anthenelli et al [48] reported that at six month follow-up varenicline and bupropion did not significantly increase the risk of neuropsychiatric adverse events (including anxiety, depression, aggression, psychosis and suicidal behaviour) when compared to placebo or nicotine patch in clients with or without a history of psychiatric disorders.

Bupropion

Bupropion is another non-nicotine-containing medication and prescription only medicine. It is a norepinephrine-dopamine reuptake inhibitor and is also a nicotinic antagonist; it mimics the effect of nicotine on dopamine and noradrenaline. It may work by blocking nicotine effects, relieving withdrawal or reducing depressed mood. It is licensed for smokers over the age of 18 who want to quit smoking and has an additional licence outside the UK as an antidepressant.

Regime

Bupropion should be started while the client is still smoking; a quit date is usually set within the first two weeks of starting the drug and taken for 8–12 weeks. The dose is titrated using the following schedule:

- days 1–6: 150 mg once daily
- days 7–49: 150 mg twice daily (with an interval of at least eight hours between doses)
- days 50–63: 150 mg bupropion twice daily (if the person has stopped smoking; discontinue if person has not quit)

Effectiveness

Evidence from a Cochrane review of 44 trials found that bupropion, compared with placebo or no pharmacotherapy, significantly increased smoking cessation (RR 1.62; 95 per cent CI 1.49 to 1.76, 44 trials, N = 13,728), and appears equally effective as single NRT but less effective than varenicline [49].

In smokers with severe mental illness, bupropion improves the odds of quitting fourfold compared with placebo [12]. In a Cochrane review of smoking cessation interventions provided during substance abuse treatment or recovery, six studies were identified that assessed bupropion on its own or combined with nicotine patches and/or counselling compared with placebo or treatment as usual; only one study found a positive effect for bupropion relative to treatment as usual in clients dependent on stimulants [35].

Side Effects, Contraindications and Cautions

Common side effects include dizziness, taste changes, gastrointestinal disturbance and insomnia, which can be reduced by avoiding a dose close to bedtime. Bupropion is contraindicated for people with seizure disorders, eating disorders and when withdrawing from alcohol or benzodiazepines. Clinicians should be cautious of the potential for manic switch in clients with bipolar affective disorder. Unlike NRT and varenicline, bupropion is known to interact with psychotropic medicines. Bupropion is associated with a dose-related risk of seizures. At doses up to the maximum recommended daily dose (300 mg/day) the incidence of seizures is approximately 1 in 1,000. Caution should be taken when administering bupropion with other medicines that lower the seizure threshold (e.g. antipsychotics and antidepressants), antihistamines and with conditions that predispose clients to seizures (e.g. alcohol dependence, history of head trauma).

Bupropion is primarily metabolised by the liver enzyme CYP2B6. Therefore, the potential exists for drug interactions between bupropion and drugs that are inhibitors (e.g. valproate) or inducers (carbamazepine, phenytoin) of CYP2B6. Bupropion also inhibits the CYP2B6 pathway and therefore co-administration with medicines metabolised by this enzyme (e.g. risperidone, haloperidol) should be used cautiously. Bupropion has an amphetamine-like structure, so theoretically can interfere with the results of urine drug screens.

Behavioural Support

Minimising withdrawal symptoms with the use of medication is an important part of supporting people to quit. However, the additional challenge of the behavioural and psychological factors of tobacco dependence should be considered, such as the ritual and behavioural habituation of smoking. Behavioural support from a trained practitioner such as those in the national network of Stop Smoking Services in the UK can support motivation to resist the urge to smoke and develop an individual's capacity to implement their plans to avoid smoking. Behavioural support is usually provided during the early stages of a quit attempt, when smokers are most likely to relapse. Behaviour change techniques that have been associated with better quit rates in smokers who attend a smoking cessation service include:

- boosting motivation and self-efficacy
- strengthening ex-smoker identity
- measuring CO and providing feedback
- providing information on withdrawal symptoms
- advising on changing routines
- facilitating relapse prevention and coping

In smokers in the general population, behavioural interventions and pharmacotherapies independently contribute to successful quitting. However, the highest smoking cessation rates appear to be achieved using specialist face-to-face behavioural support together with either varenicline or dual form NRT [27]. Behavioural support or counselling alone does not appear to be effective when provided during substance abuse treatment or recovery, but does appear to be effective when combined with any pharmacotherapy [35].

Electronic Cigarettes

Electronic cigarettes (e-cigarettes) are battery-operated devices that are used to inhale an aerosol, which typically contains nicotine (though not always), flavourings and propylene glycol/glycerine. Unlike cigarettes there is no combustion (burning) involved in e-cigarettes, which means there is no smoke and no other harmful products of combustion such as tar and carbon monoxide. There are several hundred e-cigarette models available and they can be grouped into several categories (Box 12.5). Regardless of their design and appearance, these devices generally operate in a similar manner and are made of similar components.

Box 12.5 Types of e-cigarette

Types of e-cigarettes	E-cigarette components
(1) one-time, disposable products (often referred to as cigalikes) (2) reusable, rechargeable kits designed with replaceable cartridges or pods (3) reusable, rechargeable kits that are designed to be refilled with liquid by the user (often referred to as tanks) but there are also refillable pods available (3) reusable, rechargeable kits that allow users to customise their product (e.g. by regulating the power delivery from the batteries to the heating element, often referred to as mods)	A mouthpiece to inhale through. A cartridge, pod or reservoir that holds a liquid solution (e-liquid or e-juice). A heating element (atomiser). A power source (battery). Puffing on an e-cigarette activates the battery powered heating element, which then creates an aerosol (vapour), which the person inhales. E-cigarette use is called vaping as opposed to smoking.

Box 12.6 European regulations about e-cigarettes

Component	Maximum allowed
Tank capacity	2 ml
E-liquid refill container capacity	10 ml
Nicotine strength of e-liquid	20 mg/ml

Minimum standards for safety and quality

Child-resistant and tamper evident packaging

Protection against breakage and leakage

A mechanism for ensuring re-filling without leakage

Prohibition of certain additives such as colourings, caffeine and taurine

---

In the UK, e-cigarettes are regulated under the European Union Tobacco Products Directive and subject to minimum quality and safety standards, packaging and labelling requirements along with restrictions on advertising. These regulations also cover ingredients in e-liquid, limits on nicotine strength, the size of tanks and refills and child- and tamper-proof containers (Box 12.6). E-cigarette manufacturers can apply to the Medicines and Healthcare products Regulatory Agency (MHRA) for a medicinal licence. To date the MHRA has licensed one e-cigarette but the manufacturers have not made this available. This means at the time of writing no e-cigarette can be prescribed by the NHS in the UK.

As with a tobacco cigarette, the dose of nicotine an e-cigarette user extracts from an e-cigarette varies depending on the device used, the volume of e-liquid, other ingredients in the liquid and the frequency, size, and depth of inhalation. Similar to when switching from tobacco cigarettes to licenced NRT, the more dependant a smoker is the higher strength of nicotine in the e-liquid is recommended.

Prevalence of E-Cigarette Use

The use of e-cigarettes among smokers and ex-smokers varies widely according to international surveys (4–22 per cent among smokers and 0.1–5 per cent among ex-smokers), whereas a consistently low prevalence (<1 per cent) of e-cigarette use has been reported among never-smokers [9]. In 2018 in Great Britain, prevalence of e-cigarette use was approximately 6 per cent of the adult population. E-cigarette use among never-smokers in Great Britain remains very rare at less than 1 per cent, similar to the level of use of licensed NRT [9]. Prevalence of use and trial among smokers has plateaued while use and trial among ex-smokers has increased over time. Dual use (e-cigarette use and smoking) occurs at a similar rate for e-cigarette users and users of NRT. Surveys conducted in Great Britain in 2018 suggest that the majority of e-cigarette users are ex-smokers and the most common reason for their use was to stop smoking tobacco cigarettes [9]. Despite some experimentation among children, young people and adults, e-cigarettes are attracting very few people (children, young people and adults) who have never smoked into regular use and do not appear to be undermining the long-term decline in cigarette smoking among children, young people and adults [9].

Effectiveness

In England, e-cigarettes have been the most popular quitting aid since 2013 and have contributed to tens of thousands additional quitters. In 2019, 33 per cent of smokers reported using an e-cigarette in their most recent quit attempt compared with 20 per cent who bought NRT over the counter and 5.1 per cent who used prescribed NRT [9]. E-cigarette use alone, or in combination with licensed medication and behavioural support from a Stop Smoking Service, appears to be just as helpful in the short term as licensed medication and behavioural support [9]. However, fewer smokers use an e-cigarette as part of a quit attempt with a Stop Smoking Service compared with licensed medication, possibly because of misperceptions about nicotine (see the section, Separating the Nicotine from Tobacco Smoke). A Cochrane review reported that combined results from three studies showed that using e-cigarettes containing nicotine increased the chances of stopping smoking in the long term compared with those without nicotine, and they were also found to be more effective at helping people quit compared with NRT [50].

Four observational studies of community patients and inpatients with schizophrenia or bipolar disorder who were not motivated to stop smoking found that the use of e-cigarettes was helpful in reducing smoking, but few people quit [51]. Additionally, a secondary analysis of RCT data found that the use of an e-cigarette had a similar effectiveness to NRT in motivated smokers with mental illness. Similarly, studies including people with a SUD also found that e-cigarettes are effective for smoking reduction [52, 53].

Side Effects

The most common adverse effects reported in a Cochrane systematic review were cough, mouth and throat irritation [50]. Since May 2016, consumers and health professionals in the UK have been encouraged to report suspected adverse reactions and physical safety concerns associated with e-cigarettes, using the MHRA's Yellow Card Scheme. This is a public-facing scheme by which anyone can report to the Agency an adverse reaction which they suspect may have been caused by vaping. It is not, by itself, proof of a side effect or causal link between vaping and an adverse reaction. It therefore includes all spontaneous reports submitted to the MHRA by consumers and healthcare professionals as well as reports of adverse reactions received from e-cigarette manufacturers. The inclusion of a report in the Yellow Card Scheme database does not necessarily mean that the reactions reported were caused by an e-cigarette (or any licensed medicine for that matter), only that the person reporting the event had a suspicion it may have, or it had a close temporal relationship to its administration.

Safety

E-cigarette prevalence has only been at a measurable level since about 2011–12, not long enough to measure long-term impacts of vaping on health. There is also the issue that most users are former or current smokers, and smoking-related health risks can persist for a long time. Therefore assessment of harm/risk from e-cigarettes has to account for the possible damage related to current or past smoking. Most reviews of toxicological, clinical and epidemiological evidence indicate that the chemicals found in e-cigarettes, when used as intended, are far fewer and well below levels seen in cigarette smoke. Public Health England [9], The Royal College of Physicians [54], The British Medical Association [55] and The National Academy of Sciences, Engineering and Medicine [56] advise that e-cigarettes offer a much less harmful alternative to tobacco for dependent smokers and bystanders. They conclude that the constituents of e-cigarette vapour are not completely safe but the magnitude of these risks relative to those of sustained tobacco smoking is likely to be small. Hazard to health arising from long-term vapour inhalation from e-cigarettes is unlikely to exceed 5 per cent of the harm from smoking tobacco [54].

To conclude, rates of tobacco smoking in people who are in treatment or recovery for a SUD and/or mental health condition remain at epidemic proportions, have a negative impact on substance use and mental health outcomes and contribute to the shorter lifespan these groups experience. In this chapter we have discussed the importance of understanding the difference between tobacco smoke and nicotine, the impact of smoking on health and individual level interventions to help smokers to quit. Every contact with a client provides clinicians with an opportunity to help people to take control of their tobacco dependence and make an impact on this neglected epidemic.

References

1 World Health Organization International Agency for Research on Cancer (IARC). IARC Monographs on the Evaluation of Carcinogenic Risks to Humans, vol. 83: Tobacco Smoke and Involuntary Smoking. IARC; 2004.

2 Rose J. E., Behm F. M., Westman E. C., Coleman R. E. Arterial nicotine kinetics during cigarette smoking and intravenous nicotine administration: Implications for addiction. *Drug and Alcohol Dependence*. 1999; **56**: 99–107.

3 Benowitz N. Nicotine Addiction. *The New England Journal of Medicine*. 2010; **362**: 2295–303

4 Henningfield J. E., Stapleton J. M., Benowitz N. L., Grayson R. F., London E. D. et al. Higher levels of nicotine in arterial than in venous blood after cigarette smoking.

Drug and Alcohol Dependence. 1993, **33**: 23–9.

5 Murray R. P., Connett J. E., Zapawa L. M. Does nicotine replacement therapy cause cancer? Evidence from the Lung Health Study. *Nicotine and Tobacco Research*. 2009; **11**: 1076–82.

6 Mills E. J., Wu P., Lockhart I., Wilson K., Ebbert J. O. Adverse events associated with nicotine replacement therapy (NRT) for smoking cessation: A systematic review and meta-analysis of one hundred and twenty studies involving 177,390 individuals. *Tobacco Induced Diseases*. 2010; **8** (1): 8.

7 Cooper S., Lewis S., Thornton J. et al. The SNAP trial: A randomised placebo-controlled trial of nicotine replacement therapy in pregnancy – clinical effectiveness and safety until 2 years after delivery, with economic evaluation. *Health Technology Assessment*. 2014; **18** (54): 1–128

8   McNeill A., Robson D. A man before his time: Russell's insights into nicotine, smoking, treatment and curbing the smoking problem. *Addiction.* 2018; **113** (4): 759–63.

9   McNeill A., Brose L., Calder R., Bauld L., Robson D. Evidence review of e-cigarettes and heated tobacco products. Public Health England; 2018.

10 Office for National Statistics. *Statistical Bulletin: Adult Smoking Habits in 2019.* London: Office for National Statistics; 2020.

11 Royal College of Physicians, Royal College of Psychiatrists. *Smoking and Mental Health: Royal College of Psychiatrists Council Report CR178.* London: RCP; 2013.

12 Cookson C., Strang J., Ratschen E., Sutherland G., Finch E., McNeill A. Smoking and its treatment in addiction services: Clients' and staff behaviour and attitudes. *BMC Health Services Research.* 2014; **14** (1); 304.

13 Guydish J., Passalacqua E., Pagano A., Martínez C., Le T., Chun J. et al. An international systematic review of smoking prevalence in addiction treatment. *Addiction.* 2015; **111** (2): 220–30.

14 Schroeder S., Morris C. Confronting a neglected epidemic: Tobacco cessation for persons with mental illnesses and substance abuse problems. *Annual Review of Public Health.* 2010; **31** (1): 297–314.

15 McManus S. H. M., Campion J. *Cigarette Smoking and Mental Health in England: Data from the Adult Psychiatric Morbidity Survey 2007.* London: National Centre for Social Research; 2010.

16 Lasser K., Boyd J., Woolhandler S., Himmelstein D., McCormick D., Bor D. Smoking and Mental Illness. *JAMA.* 2000; **284** (20): 2606.

17 Jha P., Peto R. Global effects of smoking, of quitting, and of taxing tobacco. *New England Journal of Medicine.* 2014; **370** (1): 60–8.

18 Public Health England. Local Tobacco Control Profiles; 2018a. [Available from: https://fingertips.phe.org.uk].

19 Public Health England. Local Alcohol Profiles;2018b. [Available from: https://fingertips.phe.org.uk].

20 Public Health England. Public Health Profiles; 2018c. [Available from: https://fingertips.phe.org.uk].

21 Royal College of Physicians. *Hiding in Plain Sight: Treating Tobacco Dependency in the NHS.* London: RCP; 2018.

22 Pelucchi C., Gallus S., Garavello W . Cancer risk associated with alcohol and tobacco use: Focus on upper aero-digestive tract and liver. *Alcohol Research and Health.* 2007: **29**: 193–8.

23 Mannelli P., Wu L. T., Peindle K. S., Gorelick D. A. Smoking and opioid detoxification: Behavioural changes and response to treatment. *Nicotine and Tobacco Research.* 15 (10); 1705–13.

24 Gage S. H., Munafò M. R. Rethinking the association between smoking and schizophrenia. *Lancet Psychiatry.* 2015; **2**: 118–19

25 Richter K. P., Gibson C. A., Ahluwalia J. S., Schmelzle K. H. Tobacco use and quit attempts among methadone maintenance clients. *American Journal of Public Health.* 2001; **91** (2): 296–9.

26 Robson D., Haddad M., Gray R., Gournay K. Mental health nursing and physical health care: A cross-sectional study of nurses' attitudes, practice, and perceived training needs for the physical health care of people with severe mental illness. *International Journal of Mental Health Nursing.* 2012; **22** (5): 409–17.

27 West R. Tobacco smoking: Health impact, prevalence, correlates and interventions. *Psychology and Health.* 2017; **32** (8): 1018–36.

28 Doll R., Peto R., Boreham J., Sutherland I. Mortality in relation to smoking: 50 years' observations on male British doctors. *BMJ.* 2004; **328** (7455): 1519.

29 Taylor G., McNeill A., Girling A., Farley A., Lindson-Hawley N., Aveyard P. Change in mental health after smoking cessation: systematic review and meta-analysis. *BMJ.* 2014; **348**: g1151.

30 Prochaska J., Delucchi K., Hall S. A meta-analysis of smoking cessation interventions with individuals in substance abuse treatment or recovery. *Journal of Consulting and Clinical Psychology.* 2004; **72** (6): 1144–56.

31 National Institute for Health and Care Excellence. Smoking: Acute, Maternity and Mental Health Settings [Internet]. NICE; 2013. [Available from: https://www .nice.org.uk/guidance/ph48].

32 Stockings E., Bowman J., Prochaska J., Baker A., Clancy R., Knight J. et al. The impact of a smoke-free psychiatric hospitalization on patient smoking outcomes: A systematic review. *Australian and New Zealand Journal of Psychiatry.* 2014; **48** (7): 617–33.

33 Robson D., Spaducci G., McNeill A., Stewart D., Craig T., Yates M. et al. Effect of implementation of a smoke-free policy on physical violence in a psychiatric inpatient setting: an interrupted time series analysis. *The Lancet Psychiatry.* 2017; **4** (7): 540–6.

34 Spaducci G., Stubbs B., McNeill A., Stewart D., Robson D. Violence in mental health settings: A systematic review. *International Journal of Mental Health Nursing.* 2017; **27** (1): 33–45.

35 Apollonio D., Philipps R., Bero L. Interventions for tobacco use cessation in people in treatment for or recovery from substance use disorders. *Cochrane Database of Systematic Reviews.* 2016; 11: CD010274.

36 Aveyard P., Begh R., Parsons A., West R. Brief opportunistic smoking cessation interventions: A systematic review and meta-analysis to compare advice to quit and offer of assistance. *Addiction.* 2012; **107** (6): 1066–73.

37 National Centre for Smoking Cessation and Training: http://www.ncsct.co.uk.

38 Fagerström K. Determinants of tobacco use and renaming the FTND to the Fagerstrom test for cigarette dependence. *Nicotine and Tobacco Research.* 2012; **14** (1): 75–8.

39 Heatherton T. F., Kozlowski L. T., Frecker R. C., Rickert W. S., Robinson J. Measuring the heaviness of smoking using self-reported time to first cigarette of the day and number of cigarettes smoked per day. *British Journal of Addiction.* 1989; **84** (7): 791–9.

40 Tidey J., Colby S., Xavier E. Effects of smoking abstinence on cigarette craving, nicotine withdrawal, and nicotine reinforcement in smokers with and without schizophrenia. *Nicotine and Tobacco Research.* 2013; **16** (3): 326–34.

41 Joint Formulary Committee. *British National Formulary.* 75th ed. London: BMJ Group and Pharmaceutical Press; 2018.

42 Hajek P., McRobbie H., Gillison F. Dependence potential of nicotine replacement treatments: Effects of product type, patient characteristics, and cost to user. *Preventive Medicine.* 2007; **44** (3): 230–4.

43 Cahill K., Stevens S., Perera R., Lancaster T. Pharmacological interventions for smoking cessation: an overview and network meta-analysis. *Cochrane Database of Systematic Reviews.* 2013; 5: CD009329.

44 Kotz D., Brown J., & West R. 'Real-world' effectiveness of smoking cessation treatments: A population study. *Addiction.* 2014b; **109** (3): 491–9.

45 Cahill K., Lindson-Hawley N., Thomas K. H., Fanshawe T. R., Lancaster T. Nicotine receptor partial agonists for smoking cessation. *Cochrane Database of Systematic Reviews.* 2016; 5: CD006103.

46 Roberts E., Eden Evins A., McNeill A. et al. Efficacy and tolerability of pharmacotherapy for smoking cessation in adults with serious mental illness: A systematic review and network meta-analysis. *Addiction.* 2016; **111** (4): 599–612.

47 Wu Q., Gilbody S., Peckham E., Brabyn S., Parrott S. Varenicline for smoking cessation and reduction in people with severe mental illnesses: Systematic review and meta-analysis. *Addiction.* 2016; **111** (9): 1554–67.

48 Anthenelli R. M., Benowitz N. L., West R. et al. Neuropsychiatric safety and efficacy of varenicline, bupropion, and nicotine patch in smokers with and without psychiatric

disorders (EAGLES): A double-blind, randomised, placebo-controlled clinical trial. *Lancet*. 2016; **387**: 2507–20.

49 Hughes J. R., Stead L. F., Hartmann-Boyce J., Cahill K., Lancaster T. Antidepressants for smoking cessation. *Cochrane Database of Systematic Reviews*. 2014; 1: CD000031.

50 Hartmann-Boyce J., McRobbie H., Lindson N., Bullen C., Begh R., Theodoulou A., Notley C., Rigotti N. A., Turner T., Butler A. R., Hajek P. Electronic cigarettes for smoking cessation. *Cochrane Database of Systematic Reviews*. 2020; 10: CD010216.

51 McNeill A., Brose L. S., Calder R., Bauld L., Robson, D. *Vaping in England: An Evidence Update Including Mental Health and Pregnancy, March 2020. A report commissioned by Public Health England.* London: Public Health England; 2020.

52 Felicione N. J., Enlow P., Elswick D., Long D., Sullivan C. R., Blank M. D. A pilot investigation of the effect of electronic cigarettes on smoking behavior among opioid-dependent smokers. *Addictive Behaviors*. 2019; **91**: 45–50.

53 Bonevski B., Manning V., Wynne O., Gartner C., Borland R., Baker A. L., Segan C. J., Skelton E., Moore L., Bathish R., Chiu S., Guillaumier A., Lubman D. I. QuitNic: A pilot randomized controlled trial comparing nicotine vaping products with nicotine replacement therapy for smoking cessation following residential detoxification. *Nicotine and Tobacco Research*. 2021; **23** (3): 462–70.

54 Royal College of Physicians. *Nicotine without Smoke: Tobacco Harm Reduction.* London: RCP; 2016.

55 British Medical Association. *E-cigarettes: Balancing Risks and Opportunities.* London: BMA; 2017.

56 National Academies of Sciences, Engineering, and Medicine. *Public Health Consequences of E-Cigarettes.* Washington, DC: The National Academies Press; 2018.

Novel Psychoactive Substances and Club Drugs

Dima Abdulrahim and Owen Bowden-Jones

What Are Club Drugs and Novel Psychoactive Substances?

'Club drugs' is a short-hand term used for convenience to refer to a group of psychoactive substances typically used in dance venues, house parties, music festivals and sometimes in a sexual context. Club drugs include well-established substances such as MDMA (Ecstasy), cocaine and methamphetamine, as well as novel psychoactive substances (NPSs) such as mephedrone. The term NPS is used by the Home Office in the UK to refer to psychoactive drugs which are not prohibited by the United Nations Drug Conventions, but which may pose a public health threat comparable to that posed by substances listed in these conventions.

In many countries, large numbers of NPSs remain outside legal control, but the UK is one of the countries that have imposed a blanket ban on NPSs, with the introduction of the Psychoactive Substance Act (PSA) 2016. At the time of writing, all NPSs in the UK are controlled through the PSA or have been classified through the Misuse of Drugs Act 1971. A very large number of NPSs have been detected around the world, with a total of 803 different NPSs reported to the United Nations Office for Drugs and Crime from 2009 to 2017 [2]. In Europe, NPSs detected for the first time in 2017 were reported at the rate of one per week [3].

NPSs mimic the effects of existing, 'traditional' drugs, such as cocaine, cannabis, LSD and heroin. They are specifically manufactured to avoid legal control, often by altering chemical structures of existing illicit drugs so that the new structures sit outside regulatory frameworks. Although the structural changes can be small, NPSs often have marked differences in potency and subsequent harm when compared to the established drugs they are trying to mimic. Globally, the most commonly reported NPSs are stimulants, synthetic cannabinoid receptor agonists and hallucinogens. In recent years, there has been an increase in newly detected synthetic opioids. Although the numbers of new opioids is small in comparison to the other drug groups, the percentage of opiates has increase from 2 per cent of all NPSs detected in 2014 to 4 per cent in 2016. In the UK NPSs are currently sold on illicit markets, including by street dealers and the Internet (both 'clearnet' and 'darknet').

A Conceptual Framework for Categorising NPSs

With hundreds of new substances detected in the last decade and more likely to emerge, it is not possible for clinicians to develop expertise in each and every NPS. In order to understand the harms of NPSs and how to manage them, it is useful to be able to classify them into different categories.

Classification of NPSs could be achieved using a variety of approaches, including chemical structure or pharmacological effect. However, a useful method of categorising NPSs is according to their primary physical and psychiatric effects. A drug's primary effects can be considered through an approach that will be very familiar to frontline clinicians as:

- predominantly **depressant**
- predominantly **stimulant**
- predominantly **hallucinogenic**

It is suggested that **synthetic cannabinoid receptor agonists** (SCRAs) be classified as a fourth separate category, as they do not fit easily into the other groups. This is because they are such a chemically and pharmacologically diverse group that their specific harms and clinical management also vary widely.

Similarities between NPSs and Traditional Drugs

This classification will help clinicians place an unfamiliar NPS into a familiar category. Clinicians can then draw on their previous experience of managing other drugs in the category. For example, a clinician meeting with a patient using a previously unknown NPS stimulant can draw upon their experience of treating people using established stimulant drugs such as amphetamine or cocaine to begin to formulate an appropriate treatment plan for the NPS. This approach necessitates that clinicians establish the primary psychoactive effect of a new NPS, which can be achieved through careful history taking and clinical assessment. As with traditional drugs, some NPSs will have clinical features of more than one broad group, and display different properties at different doses.

This approach also allows for the use of existing guidelines, guidance and protocols for established drugs to be used as a starting point for developing a treatment plan. The clinical management of NPSs should therefore be based on the same principles outlined in the Clinical Guidelines on Drug Misuse and Dependence Update 2017 together with products produced by the National Institute for Health and Care Excellence (NICE), including technical appraisals, standards and national guidelines. For up-to-date information on the management of acute NPS toxicity it is recommended that clinicians refer to the National Poisons Information Service (NPIS) and its online toxicology database and telephone enquiry service TOXBASE®.

Differences between NPSs and Traditional Drugs

As mentioned above, many NPSs have been developed to mimic the effects of other more established drugs such as cannabis, cocaine, heroin and LSD. They are, however, not the same as the drugs they mimic. The toxic and long-term effects of NPSs have not been well studied, but many are expected to be similar to those of better understood drugs. However, there are differing pharmacological and pharmacokinetic properties associated with specific NPSs and these will determine the substances' onset and duration of psychoactive effect, potency and toxicity and possible differences in patterns of harmful use and dependence.

Challenges of NPS

There are a number of clinical and public health challenges that are specific to the various NPSs [4], which will be discussed in the sections below.

Lack of Analytical Techniques for Clinic Based Testing

The proliferation of NPSs has presented a challenge to analytical detection. Sophisticated mass spectrometry testing techniques are not available for many NPSs. Even when tests are available, the detection of NPSs is limited because of the absence in most clinical settings of routine, rapid clinic-based urine or serum testing. Even for traditional drugs (such as amphetamine or MDMA), rapid bedside testing is not readily available in most clinical settings. The clinical implication is that the diagnosis of acute toxicity will most likely be based on knowledge and assessment of the clinical toxidrome (group of symptoms that constitute the basis for a diagnosis of poisoning) and effects, rather than by analytical toxicology.

Unpredictability of Content of NPS Products Sold

Whereas the adulteration of illicit substances is an issue for traditional drugs, it is a particular challenge for NPSs. Users are often unaware of the content and the dosage of the psychoactive substance or substances contained in NPS products, exposing them to additional serious health risks. NPSs are sometimes mis-sold as traditional drugs or other NPSs (e.g. substitution of MDMA by PMA/PMMA, or fentanyl substituted for heroin). There is also evidence that NPS preparations and products can include a combination of different NPS and/or traditional drugs. Evidence from test purchasing and analysis of products suggests that they can contain a mixture of two or three different active chemical compounds. The psychoactive constituents of branded NPS products are variable and can change regularly. Branded products of the same name can contain different active compounds, depending on time, place and batch purchased.

Club Drug and NPS User Populations

NPSs are used by various groups of people, including groups who do not typically present to drug treatment services, which are often perceived as focusing on heroin and crack cocaine users. These groups include 'clubbers', 'psychonauts', gay men and other people who often believe that existing drug services do not understand the drugs they use or their needs. For example, a treatment services may not be able to respond to gay men presenting with problems associated with 'chemsex'[1] unless staff are trained in LGBTQ+ cultural competence and management of problematic drug-induced sexual enhancement [5].

Some NPSs, on the other hand, are associated with a demographic more similar in profile to the 'traditional' problem drug users presenting to drug treatment services. For example, SCRAs are often used by vulnerable people with complex needs, including homeless people and those in custodial settings. SCRA users in these groups often have previous heroin, crack cocaine and alcohol problems. SCRAs now pose a serious problem in prisons and a wider public health challenge. The emergence of synthetic opioids, including fentanyl and its analogues, has also resulted in deaths, mainly among people who use heroin. Although it is currently a 'low use' substance in the UK, they are 'high-risk/harm' substances and vigilance is required.

---

[1] *Chemsex* is a short-hand term used to describe sexual activity carried out while under the influence of drugs and typically involving several sexual partners. At the current time in the UK, the most commonly used drugs in a chemsex context are methamphetamine, mephedrone and GHB/GBL.

Stimulant NPSs and Club Drugs

Introduction and Brief Pharmacology

Stimulants in general form one of the largest groups of drugs used for recreational purposes and the largest group of NPSs are stimulant drugs. They include:

(a) substances that have been established in the UK for many decades (e.g. amphetamine, cocaine, MDMA/Ecstasy)

(b) drugs, such as methamphetamine that have been well established in other parts of the world but have only appeared in the UK in recent years

(c) a range of recently detected stimulant NPSs. NPS stimulants detected globally from 2009 to 2017 include 148 synthetic cathinones and 136 new phenethylamines.

The desired effects of stimulants include increased energy, mood enhancement, euphoria, elation, mental clarity, improved concentration, improved sociability, increased talkativeness, empathy-inducing effects and amplification of sound and colour. The pro-sexual effects of some stimulants, in particular methamphetamine and mephedrone, have also been associated with their use in a sexual context, including chemsex parties.

Stimulant drugs in general belong to a variety of different chemical groups. They stimulate the central nervous system (CNS) by increasing the activity of key neurotransmitters, such as noradrenaline, dopamine and serotonin. The extent to which a specific drug elevates the levels of noradrenaline, dopamine and serotonin differentially will determine the effect:

- Stimulants that increase *dopamine* will induce significantly greater reward including pleasure and/or euphoria. They are also likely to increase a desire to re-dose.
- Stimulants that elevate *noradrenaline* will be less euphoric and more stimulatory, increasing alertness and potentially causing anxiety. They also have cardio-toxic effects.
- Drugs that elevate *serotonin* can increase emotions and behaviour related to sociability and empathy ('empathogens'). They can also have hallucinogenic effects, especially at high doses.

Acute Toxic Effects and Management of Stimulant NPS and Club Drugs

Predominantly stimulant drugs inhibit monoamine re-uptake (especially dopamine) and are associated with a sympathomimetic toxidrome. Some stimulants produce predominantly serotinergic toxic effects, and the release of large amounts of serotonin can lead to serotonin syndrome. People who have used NPSs or other stimulant club drugs may present to hospital with the following symptoms associated with the syndrome of stimulant intoxication: agitation, bruxism, sweating, dilated pupils, psychosis, tachycardia, hypertension, chest pain, seizures, arrhythmias and hyperthermia.

Physiological Acute Effects of Stimulant NPS

Acute effects include:

- *Cardiac effects*: Stimulants, including stimulant NPSs, are associated with sympathomimetic cardiac effects. These drugs are associated with chest pain, shortness of breath, tachycardia, hypertension and ventricular fibrillation. There is a risk that their use can induce strokes and heart attacks.

- *Hyperthermia* is a potential acute physiological consequence of stimulant drugs, and can be linked to fatal complications, including rhabdomyolysis, acute renal failure, disseminated intravascular coagulation, multiple organ failure and acidosis.
- *Hyponatraemia* has been reported in cases of MDMA use in particular, often associated with excess drinking of liquids over a short period of time.
- *Serotonin syndrome* (see Box 13.1): This is a potentially life-threatening adverse reaction to the use of stimulant drugs or the interaction between drugs. The simultaneous use of multiple serotonergic substances – both illicit (e.g. MDMA/Ecstasy) and prescribed (e.g. SSRIs) – increases the risk of serotonin syndrome.

Neurological and Mental Health Problems

Anxiety and panic are common reasons for hospital presentations among the users of the range of stimulants. Other features of intoxication associated with stimulant use include agitation, aggression, depression, dysphoria, lack of motivation, anhedonia, visual and auditory hallucinations, paranoid delusions, intensification of sensory experiences, transient mania and transient psychosis. The use of stimulants can be associated with bruxism, headache, dizziness/light-headedness, tinnitus, seizures, nystagmus, mydriasis, blurred vision, numbness, blue/cold extremities, fever, paraesthesia, confusion, amnesia and reduced consciousness.

Repeated use (even over a short period) can lead to paranoia, even psychosis. It will impact on mood and can precipitate depression and other mental health problems. Clinicians should be aware that depressive symptoms of varying severity may occur during or after withdrawal and there may be risk of suicide. Some people using stimulant NPSs, and methamphetamine in particular, will suffer from stimulant-induced psychosis. The likelihood and severity of effects is in part associated with the type of stimulant use, as well as other vulnerabilities, with some stimulants significantly more likely to be associated with higher levels of psychosis. Whereas MDMA does occasionally act as a stressor that precipitates acute psychosis, it does so at a much lower rate than amphetamine and

---

Box 13.1 Clinical symptoms of the serotonin syndrome

The clinical manifestations of serotonin syndrome range from the barely perceptible to the lethal. Signs of excess serotonin range from tremor and diarrhoea to neuromuscular rigidity and hyperthermia.

Mild: Patients can be afebrile. Tachycardia possible, shivering, diaphoresis, mydriasis.

Moderate: Tachycardia, hypertension, hyperthermia (40°C is common), mydriasis, hyperactive bowel sounds, diaphoresis, hyperreflexia and clonus (considerably greater in lower extremities than upper). Patient may exhibit horizontal ocular clonus; mild agitation or hypervigilance, slightly pressured speech; repetitive rotation of the head with the neck held in moderate extension.

Severe: Severe hypertension and tachycardia that might deteriorate abruptly into frank shock. The patient may have agitated delirium, muscle rigidity and hypertonicity (considerably greater in lower extremities than upper). Muscle hyperactivity may produce a core temperature of more than 41°C in some cases. Associated problems include metabolic acidosis, rhabdomyolysis, elevated levels of serum aminotransferase and creatinine, seizures, renal failure and disseminated intravascular coagulopathy.

methamphetamine. Psychosis has been linked to amphetamine and methamphetamine use in particular [6], but also to synthetic cathinones such as mephedrone.

A minority of people who use these stimulants will develop a psychotic episode that requires care from emergency departments or psychiatric units. Common symptoms include paranoid and/or persecutory delusions, as well as auditory and visual hallucinations, with extreme agitation. Symptoms of methamphetamine-induced psychosis usually remit after acute intoxication. However some individuals may develop psychosis in the weeks or months after stopping methamphetamine.

Stress can precipitate spontaneous psychosis in former methamphetamine users who are abstinent. Psychotic symptoms may recur rapidly, where there is new exposure to the drug. The resolution of symptoms among those who experience methamphetamine-induced psychosis usually occurs with abstinence, although it may be incomplete, thus increasing risks of relapse. In some individuals, psychosis may prove to be refractory to antipsychotic medication. There are reports of methamphetamine psychosis persisting for weeks or even months after cessation of methamphetamine use. For these individuals, treatment with standard antipsychotic drugs may not produce good outcomes, as many patients, even when receiving appropriate antipsychotic treatment, may remain clinically psychotic after many months of treatment.

Methamphetamine-induced psychosis has mainly been observed among users with vulnerability to mental health problems. Nonetheless, it has been reported in methamphetamine dependent people, with no prior diagnosis of schizophrenia, or other psychotic disorders. There is some evidence that serious psychiatric disorders may emerge or worsen as a result of methamphetamine use. This includes an increased risk of suicide. There is a well-established association with other mental health problems, including persistent anxiety, paranoia, insomnia, auditory hallucinations, delusion, psychotic or violent behaviour and suicidal or homicidal thinking. Some of the symptoms can resemble those of paranoid schizophrenia.

Harmful Use and Stimulant Dependence

Daily use of NPS stimulants or club drugs is considered to be the most harmful pattern and is associated with adverse effects on the health and psychosocial functioning of the user. However, even use on an occasional basis can be associated with adverse effects. Stimulants have a dependence liability, which is typically psychological rather than physiological. There are differences between the various stimulants in terms of their dependence liability. MDMA (Ecstasy) and its analogues are generally considered to have some potential for dependence and some users develop problematic chronic use patterns, have concerns about their use and seek treatment. However, most users will not do so and, compared with other stimulants, their dependence potential is thought to be relatively weak.

In contrast, stimulant NPSs, such as mephedrone and other synthetic cathinones, may have a higher potential for dependence than MDMA. They have been associated with strong and repeated compulsion to use, with 'wanting more' and with craving. There are user reports that tolerance to mephedrone can develop quickly. Mephedrone withdrawal symptoms have been reported. They include tiredness, insomnia, nasal congestion, impaired concentration concentration, depression, anxiety, increased appetite, irritability, unusual sweat odours and urge or craving to use. Methamphetamine in particular is associated with high levels of severe dependence and withdrawal syndrome, which is characterised by psychological and psychiatric symptoms, rather than physical symptoms. Methamphetamine withdrawal symptoms include sleep and appetite disturbances, akathisia/restless legs fatigue, depression, irritability, craving, severe dysphoria, depression, anxiety and agitation and paranoia. Intensity of post-binge dysphoria as well as withdrawal can lead to suicidal ideation and attempts. Longer-term withdrawal symptoms can last up to 12 months and include anhedonia, impaired social functioning, craving, hyper-arousal, vegetative symptoms, anxiety-related symptoms, severe dysphoria, mood volatility, irritability and sleep pattern disruption.

Management of Stimulant Dependence

At present, the most effective treatments for stimulant dependence are psychosocial interventions (PSI) and behavioural therapies, including cognitive behavioural therapy (CBT) and contingency management (CM). There are currently no approved pharmacotherapies for stimulant dependence and withdrawal management, or to support abstinence. The management of psychiatric and physical comorbidity and symptomatic prescribing (e.g. for anxiety, insomnia) may be required on a short-term basis. Ongoing psychosocial support may be required, including for the prevention of relapse.

Other Associated Reported Effects

Injecting Harms

Injecting stimulants such as methamphetamine or mephedrone is associated with an increased risk to physical and psychiatric health, including the risk of dependence. Mephedrone has been associated with compulsive and frequent injecting and with high-risk injecting practices, such as reusing and sharing of injecting equipment. It may also be linked to elevated rates of blood-borne infections and injecting site infections. There is emerging evidence of a greater risk of suicide attempts among those who inject methamphetamine than those who do not inject the drug, even after taking into account a wide range of potential confounders.

High-Risk Sexual Behaviours

Some stimulants have a disinhibiting and pro-sexual effect and their use in a sexual context has been linked to high-risk sexual behaviours, including condomless sex. Mephedrone and methamphetamine in particular have been associated with chemsex.

Management of Adverse Health Effects

The specific risks of injecting stimulants such as methamphetamine (see Case Study, Methamphetamine psychosis) and synthetic cathinones should be addressed with public health and harm reduction interventions.

The management of harmful and dependent use of mephedrone and other synthetic cathinones is similar to the management of other stimulants, and should take place within a structured plan of care [6]. Psychosocial interventions remain the best treatment option for the management of stimulant dependence including stimulant NPSs. Ongoing support may be required to prevent relapse. The use of mephedrone in a sexual context (e.g. by men who have sex with men) should also be addressed by the use of appropriate psychosexual interventions where relevant.

Case Study Methamphetamine psychosis

Jack is a 32-year-old gay man working at an IT company. He presented to drug services asking for help with a what he describes as a three-year history of escalating methamphetamine use. Initially Jack smoked methamphetamine using a pipe to enhance his sexual performance and pleasure, but rapidly moved to injecting ('slamming') after someone at a sex party showed him how to inject. For two years, Jack attended sex parties twice a month and would use methamphetamine for a period of around 48 hours. It would take him a few days to recover and he occasionally missed work. Over the last year, he has noticed a significant escalation in his use and at presentation he is using four days each week. He now uses alone, commenting that he needs methamphetamine 'just to get going'. He has received his second warning from work due to deterioration in his performance.

In the last two weeks Jack has stopped attending work. He has become concerned that he is under surveillance, but is not sure by whom or why. Jack keeps his curtains closed at all times to avoid being observed, and reports hearing 'scratching noises' at night which he thinks are an attempt to frighten him. Jack has stopped using his computer and mobile telephone as he believes they are being used to track him and feels too overwhelmed to leave his flat until after dark when he believes he can move around unobserved.

At assessment Jack acknowledged that his methamphetamine use could possibly be the cause of his symptoms but was not sure.

Following treatment, which included motivational enhancement, relapse prevention, harm reduction interventions, psychosexual therapy and mindfulness, Jack managed to stop using methamphetamine entirely and his psychotic symptoms resolved completely after a few weeks. Although he continued to experience cravings for methamphetamine, with support he was able to cope with these. He has not attended any more sex parties and is now significantly isolated. He is working on building a social network of people who do not use drugs but is finding this challenging. He is well engaged with local recovery services, something which is a highlight of his week.

Synthetic Cannabinoid Receptor Agonists (SCRAs)

Introduction and Brief Pharmacology

Synthetic cannabinoid receptor agonists (SCRAs) are one of the largest and fastest growing groups of NPSs around the world. They are a chemically diverse group of molecules and large numbers of different SCRAs have been identified: more than 251 different SCRAs were reported to the UN between 2008 and 2017. SCRAs used for recreational purposes are typically made by spraying an inert herbal product with SCRAs to produce a product which can be smoked in a similar way to natural cannabis. Products are generally smoked by mixing with tobacco, although oral and injectable SCRA preparations are also available. SCRAs are also used by 'vaping', using electronic cigarettes. There are reports that SCRAs are sometimes sprayed on letters or photos and smuggled into prisons for use by inmates [7].

SCRAs are often sold under different brand names. Products sold under the same brand will not necessarily contain the same SCRA, even when selected from the same batch. Branded products often include a number of different SCRAs, with unknown potential for interaction. SCRAs are sometimes referred to in the UK as 'Spice' or 'Mamba', which are two of the many branded products sold on the illicit market. From the perspective of clinical management, and particularly for acute harms, the use of terms like Spice can be misleading, as it implies a uniformity of effects regardless of the SCRA used. In practice, the effects of different SCRAs can be substantially and clinically significantly different.

Currently in the UK, the use of SCRAs appears to be concentrated among homeless people (rough sleepers in particular) and among prisoners. SCRAs in general have some similarity to delta-9-tetrahydrocannabinol (THC) and other phytocannabinoids, but there are important pharmacological and pharmacokinetic differences between natural cannabis and SCRAs. Both SCRAs and natural cannabis bind to CB1 receptors, but SCRAs typically have a higher affinity for CB1 than natural cannabinoids and so produce a stronger clinical effect and have higher potency. Some SCRA compounds are structurally similar to serotonin and may be associated with significant activation of serotonin receptors. SCRAs can act across a range of different receptors leading to their unpredictable effects.

SCRAs also differ from natural cannabis by the fact that they tend not to contain cannabidiol (CBD), a compound with anxiolytic, antipsychotic and anti-craving properties found in natural cannabis. There are also marked differences between the various SCRAs. The half-life and length of the effect of different SCRA compounds varies. There are reports that the duration of action and length of effects of SCRAs can range from one to two hours to up to six to eight hours. Some SCRAs also appear to have significantly stronger effects than others. The potency of different SCRAs can range from approximately 30 times more potent than THC, to those that are 100–800 times more potent.

Adverse Effects

Acute Toxicity

Negative mood changes are common and typify intoxication associated with SCRAs (in contrast to natural cannabis). There are reports of SCRA use leading to unpredictable effects ranging from profound sedation to intense agitation and psychosis. The risks associated with SCRA use are generally different and often more severe than those of natural cannabis. SCRA use is associated with a higher prevalence of adverse experiences, and SCRAs have a higher potential for overdose due to their neurotoxicity and cardiotoxicity and often a longer half-life. It is possible that they may be more likely to be associated with emergency hospital presentations compared to natural cannabis [8, 9].

Acute Physiological Effects

It cannot be assumed that the risks associated with SCRA use will be comparable to those of natural cannabis. There are concerns that they may have a greater potential to cause harm and have cardio-toxic effects and damaging effects on other organs (e.g. kidney). Different SCRAs will have different toxic effects, but overall SCRA toxicity is characterised by not only cannabis-like effects, but potentially also sympathomimetic effects including seizures, tachycardia, hypertension, diaphoresis, hyperthermia, agitation and aggression. New SCRAs are constantly being produced, and the latest generation (including MDMB-CHMICA, FUBIMINA and FUBIMINA analogues) are particularly linked to acute toxicity and adverse effects include fatalities. SCRAs also appear to be associated with altered mental states described as 'zombie-like' behaviours, including intermittent groaning and slow mechanical movements of the arms and legs. Catatonic states induced by chronic persistent high-dose SCRA use have been reported.

Psychiatric Effects

The use of SCRAs has been associated with psychiatric morbidity. SCRA users are more likely than people who use natural cannabis to experience hallucinations and delusions, and there appears to be a greater risk of psychosis with SCRAs than with natural cannabis (see Case Study, SCRA psychosis). In comparison with psychotic episodes associated with the use of natural cannabis, psychotic episodes associated with SCRAs occur more frequently, are more severe and are linked to greater agitation. Presentations to hospital tend to be characterised by paranoid delusions, ideas of reference and a disorganised, confused mental state. Patients are described as having a flat affect, significant depressive symptoms and in some cases suicidal ideation. Although SCRA-associated psychosis can be transient, some individuals may experience psychosis that persists for weeks following acute intoxication. There is evidence that SCRAs may precipitate psychosis in both vulnerable individuals and otherwise healthy people with no history of psychosis.

Dependence and Withdrawal

SCRAs have greater dependence liability and potential for chronic harms than natural cannabis. Tolerance may develop more quickly for SCRAs than for natural cannabis, and a more severe and prolonged withdrawal syndrome is seen on stopping. Box 13.2 highlights the reported features of SCRA withdrawal.

Management of Adverse Effects

Clinicians should be aware that SCRAs will not be detected by most onsite urine drug screening tests. SCRAs do not give a positive result on urine screening tests for natural cannabis. Laboratory techniques have been developed to detect an increasing number of SCRA compounds, but these are currently not widely available to frontline clinical staff. They will also not detect every newly emerging SCRA. The management of SCRA toxicity is symptomatic and supportive, as no antidotes exist. Very little evidence is available on the

---

Box 13.2 Features of the SCRA withdrawal syndrome

- Coughing
- Headaches
- Anxiety
- Insomnia/sleep disturbance
- Difficulty concentrating
- Anger/irritability
- Restlessness
- Depression
- Drug craving
- Nausea
- Diaphoresis
- Tremor
- Hypertension
- Tachycardia

Case Study SCRA psychosis

Danny is a 43-year-old man previously dependent on heroin who successfully completed detoxification and rehabilitation eight months ago. He has been abstinent from all drugs and alcohol since his rehabilitation and is now living in a recovery-orientated hostel.

A few weeks ago, another resident offered Danny some 'spice' explaining that it was synthetic cannabis that was 'cheap, legal and undetectable' on urine drug screens. He also suggested that 'spice' would help with the insomnia which Danny had been experiencing since stopping drugs. Danny decided to try some and found the drug, which he smoked, 'knocked me out'.

Over the next few weeks, Danny began to use spice more regularly and in larger quantities. He found the drug 'moreish' and that it helped him to forget about everything.

One week ago, Danny was brought to the local accident and emergency unit by the police on a section 136 having been found wandering in the street in a confused and agitated state. At assessment, Danny was observed to be experiencing auditory hallucinations and described persecutory delusions that people in his hostel were plotting to murder him that night. On contacting the hostel, the staff explained that Danny had been smoking 'spice' 'all day long' and now rarely left his room. He was due to see a psychiatrist later that week but had gone missing earlier that day.

Danny was admitted to the acute psychiatric ward as an informal patient having agreed that he needed help. On admission a urine drug screen was negative for all drugs. He was treated with antipsychotics and the symptoms improved over the following week. Danny reported intense cravings for 'spice' as well as excessive sweating, agitation and tremor. After the psychosis resolved, Danny explained that he had run out of the drug the day before admission and attributed his symptoms to withdrawal from 'spice', commenting that they felt 'worse than coming off heroin'.

The antipsychotics were stopped and Danny was discharged to a different hostel which offered more intensive recovery support.

management of the harmful or dependent use of SCRAs and it is suggested that clinicians adopt the evidence-based approaches used for other drugs, particularly natural cannabis. There is no evidence to suggest that a particular approach is linked to successful outcomes for SCRA users. Suggested psychological and social interventions include motivational approaches, relapse prevention and reintegration with non-using social networks. No specific medications are indicated for SCRA withdrawal and no substitute prescribing is currently available.

Depressants

Novel Central Nervous System Depressants

As with traditional depressants, a range of depressant NPSs have been detected with dissociative, hypnotic and sedative properties. Central nervous system (CNS) depressants can decrease the rate of breathing, decrease heart rate and lead to loss of consciousness and even coma or death. Taking large or frequent doses can lead to tolerance, withdrawal and dependence.

Hypnotics: GHB/GBL

Gamma-hydroxybutyrate (GHB) and its pro-drug gamma-butyrolactone (GBL) have a relatively low prevalence of use in the UK, but despite this their health costs can be relatively high compared with other drugs because of their intrinsic toxicity (including their single-dose lethal toxicity), high dependence liability and potentially life-threatening withdrawal syndrome. GHB/GBL is most commonly sold as a clear liquid and diluted in a drink for consumption. Typical recreational doses are usually only a few millilitres of the drug. Other preparations are also available, including powder.

Acute Toxicity and Overdose

GHB/GBL has a steep dose–response curve, whereby even a small increase in dose can cause a very large difference between desired recreational effects and serious toxic effects, such as impaired consciousness and coma. This steep dose–response relationship differentiates GHB/GBL from other drugs. Overdose, with loss of consciousness, is common. This occurs not only as a result of using large concentrations over a short period, but also when GHB/GBL is used in combination with other CNS depressants, including alcohol. The imprecise measurement of GHB/GBL doses taken for recreational use can also result in overdose. The adverse effects of GHB/GBL occur at a variety of doses, indicating the individual response to the drug. There is no available antagonist or antidote.

The use of GHB can lead rapidly to the onset of neurological, cardiovascular and other clinical effects, which may be life-threatening. Signs of acute toxicity can vary from sudden drowsiness to unresponsiveness and profound coma. Patients with acute intoxication typically develop signs of acute toxicity rapidly, but will also improve rapidly, provided they receive appropriate supportive care.

CNS depression typically persists for one to three hours, with patients making a complete recovery within four to eight hours. Coma accounts for a significant proportion of presentations to hospital. Some patients may fluctuate from deep coma to sudden awakening with agitation/aggression. In dependent users, recovery for acute toxicity may coincide with onset of withdrawal symptoms (see the next section).

Dependence, Tolerance and Withdrawal

GHB/GBL has a high dependence liability and is associated with rapid onset of tolerance and subsequent physiological withdrawal syndrome. Dependent users will often use multiple daily doses, with those severely dependent dosing every hour for 24 hours a day. The withdrawal syndrome can be severe, with agitation and delirium. GHB/GBL withdrawal has a rapid onset, which can happen 30 minutes after the last dose. However, more typically, symptoms occur after a few hours or even up to 48 hours after the last dose. GHB/GBL withdrawal typically lasts five to seven days, but can be significantly longer, with symptoms reported up to 21 days. It can be life-threatening and must be treated as a medical emergency if confusion, delirium, hallucinations and/or severe agitation are present. Timely treatment may also reduce the escalation of symptoms.

Withdrawal Symptoms

GHB/GBL withdrawal symptoms include agitation, aggression/combativeness, insomnia, anxiety, confusion, nausea and paranoia, hallucinations (visual and auditory) and depression. Physical symptoms include miosis, vomiting, diarrhoea, abdominal pain, nystagmus, myoclonic jerks, tremor, tachypnoea, dyspnoea, tachycardia and hypertension. Severe withdrawal symptoms can include delirium, seizures (which may become life-threatening), psychosis (mimicking the first rank symptoms seen in schizophrenia) and rhabdomyolysis.

Medically Assisted Detoxification

Dependent users who wish to stop should be strongly encouraged to seek medically assisted detoxification, as self-detoxification from GHB/GBL can be dangerous in dependence and should be avoided. If dependent users want to reduce GHB/GBL use without medical assistance they should do so in very small increments and seek support and monitoring from health professionals. GHB/GBL withdrawal must be considered a medical emergency.

There is some limited evidence that withdrawal symptoms can be treated effectively with a combination of diazepam and baclofen, although the latter is not licensed for GHB/GBL withdrawal.

Benzodiazepines are most typically used for medically assisted withdrawal management using a symptom-led scale to determine the need for treatment (typically a modified CIWA scale). High benzodiazepine doses may be required in severe cases or when treatment is delayed (e.g. in excess of a total daily dose of 100 mg diazepam in divided doses is sometimes required). Baclofen may be started at the same time as diazepam, although some argue that patients should be 'preloaded' a few days before cessation of GHB/GBL.

Planned elective GHB/GBL detoxification is a bio-psychosocial intervention (see Case Study, GHB/GBL withdrawal). As well as the pharmacological component, psychosocial

Case Study GHB/GBL withdrawal

Steven is a 37-year-old gay man attending for help with his use of 'G' (GHB/GBL). He has been using the drug for the last three years and consumes it in a liquid form, which he dilutes in a non-alcoholic beverage. He initially used the drug to moderate the unwanted agitation he experienced when using methamphetamine and to facilitate sexual performance; however, over the last year his use of GHB/GBL has increased dramatically and it is now the only drug he uses.

Steven describes his current use as '1 ml an hour' and uses throughout the day by carrying diluted GHB/GBL in a water bottle wherever he goes. At night, he doubles his dose so he can sleep 'for a few hours' before resuming hourly dosing when he wakes.

When he first used GHB/GBL, Steven enjoyed the relaxing and slightly euphoric effect of the drug, which he described as 'like alcohol but without the hangover'. Now that he is using hourly, he describes the only benefit as preventing the onset of withdrawals. Withdrawal symptoms are described as initially consisting of increased anxiety, intense drug craving and sweating. For Steven, these symptoms begin around 90 minutes after his last dose. If he is unable to consume GHB/GBL, his symptoms develop to include a coarse tremor, intense body pain and confusion. He has been admitted to hospital on two occasions after running out of GHB/GBL and on one of these occasions required intubation and transfer to intensive care as his withdrawals could not be controlled without a general anaesthetic.

Steven now wants to stop using GHB/GBL completely and is requesting a detoxification. The treating team decide that, given the history of severe withdrawals, a medically assisted inpatient detoxification is indicated. They plan to use benzodiazepines as first line and also consider the use of baclofen, although there is only limited evidence to support its use. Aware of the high rates relapse associated with GHB/GBL misuse, the team put in place an intensive preparatory and post-detoxification programme aimed at supporting abstinence.

interventions (PSI) are essential both prior to and following detoxification to enable sustained changes to patterns of drug use. There are no psychological interventions specific to GHB/GBL and those utilised by drug treatment services for other drugs will be most appropriate. Assisted withdrawal is supported by psychological interventions as part of the overall outpatient care plan – for example, motivational interventions, cognitive behavioural therapy, relapse prevention, SMART recovery or other mutual aid, mindfulness, self-help groups, medication education group, family support and involvement and case management review.

Dissociatives: Ketamine and Analogues

Introduction and Brief Pharmacology

Ketamine is a widely available medicine, but its use in a recreational environment gives it a 'novel' context. Ketamine is a predominantly sedative drug, but its complex neurochemical profile reflects its actions as a psychostimulant, dissociative, anaesthetic and analgesic substance, with amnestic properties.

Ketamine is a derivative of phencyclidine (PCP), and both are arylcyclohexylamines. Like PCP, ketamine stimulates the cardiac and respiratory functions, though it is less toxic and shorter acting than PCP. Ketamine shows affinity for mu, delta and sigma opioid receptors, and affects monoamine transporters. It is a non-competitive NMDA receptor antagonist that acts as a dissociative anaesthetic with analgesic and amnestic properties. Ketamine also acts at dopamine D2 and 5-HT2A serotonin receptors. The activation of 5-HT2A receptors is thought to account for the perceptual disorders and hallucinations.

Most ketamine used in the UK for recreational purposes has been manufactured in clandestine laboratories. Illicit ketamine is typically in the form of a powder or fine crystal, but may also be available in pill form. Ketamine powder is typically insufflated (snorted), although it can be injected. Subjective experiences associated with the use of ketamine depend on dose. At low doses, it produces distortion of time and space, visual and auditory hallucinations and mild dissociative effects. It can also have stimulant-type properties. At high doses, it produces more severe dissociation, known by some users as the 'k–hole', where the user experiences feelings of intense detachment and perceptions appear completely divorced from reality. Ketamine effects occur approximately five minutes (but up to 30 minutes) after insufflation and in a matter of seconds or minutes after injection and smoking. The effects are generally short-lived, typically lasting one hour, depending on dose.

Acute Toxicity

There are few severe acute physical health consequences associated with acute ketamine intoxication, with no adverse outcome reported from large overdoses where no other substances are co-ingested. Even in large doses, ketamine is characterised by its ability to cause unconsciousness, amnesia and analgesia, while sparing airway reflexes and maintaining haemodynamic stability. Coughing and swallowing reflexes are maintained with minor suppression of the gag reflex, even when a user is very intoxicated. Nonetheless, ketamine has been associated with acute adverse effects. Ketamine impairs psychomotor performance and clinical features associated with acute intoxication are often related to behaviours resulting from dissociative effects, such as accidents or agitation. Ketamine induces dose-dependent impairments in working and episodic memory, which can have a profound effect on the user's ability to function.

Systemic toxicity with cardiovascular effects can occur as a result of ketamine toxicity, and can be severe. Ketamine stimulates the cardiovascular system, leading to increased heart rate, cardiac output and blood pressure. Risks are increased with co-ingestion of stimulants. Ketamine can cause acute effects, such as agitation or ketamine-related psychotic states. Frequent use of ketamine is typified by increased dissociative symptoms, and can be linked to subtle visual anomalies and depressive symptoms. In contrast, there is increasing evidence that ketamine may be of therapeutic use for the management of treatment-resistant depression, as well as post-traumatic stress disorder.

Chronic and Long-Term Effects

Neurocognitive Effects

Overall, studies have shown that infrequent ketamine users do not appear to experience long-term cognitive impairment. However, frequent and prolonged use of ketamine is associated with neurocognitive impairment. There is evidence in particular of ketamine-induced deficits in working and episodic memory. Frequent ketamine use can impair visual recognition and spatial working memory; the degree of impairment has been correlated with changes in the level of ketamine use. Delusional thinking has also been positively correlated with the amount used by frequent users and has persisted despite abstinence for some people.

Harmful and Dependent Use

Ketamine can be associated with compulsive patterns of behaviour: bingeing, or using without stopping until supplies run out. Frequent ketamine use is associated with tolerance. It is also associated with psychological dependence. Clinical experience suggests that some users show withdrawal symptoms: in cases of sustained and heavy use, the existence of a ketamine withdrawal syndrome must be considered. Small studies have described a number of symptoms associated with ketamine withdrawal, including anxiety, shaking, sweating, palpitations, 'chills', autonomic arousal, lacrimation, restlessness, nightmares, drug hunting, tiredness, low appetite and low mood.

Ketamine-Induced Damage to the Urinary Tract, Kidneys and Gastrointestinal Tract

Ketamine use is associated with damage to the urinary system, which can be severe and in some cases irreversible. Damage can affect the entire urinary tract. Ketamine-induced urinary system damage is associated with severe pain. Users frequently self-medicate for this pain with ketamine, thus perpetuating and exacerbating the urinary tract damage. The urological syndromes associated with ketamine use include dysuria, haematuria, urge incontinence, polyuria and nocturia. These symptoms appear to be related to ulcerative cystitis, obstruction of the upper urinary tract and papillary necrosis. Hepatic dysfunction has also been reported. People with prolonged and heavy use of ketamine have reported intense abdominal pain, referred to by users as 'k-cramps'. Symptoms appear to resolve once the patient stops using ketamine.

Illicit methoxetamine was marketed by drug dealers as a more 'bladder friendly' but similar to ketamine. However, there is emerging evidence suggesting that chronic use of methoxetamine is associated with similar lower urinary tract symptoms as described in chronic ketamine use.

Management of Ketamine Harms

The assessment of harmful and/or dependent ketamine use is similar to assessment of other drug use, with the addition of screening questions on the direct consequences of dissociation (e.g. cognitive impairment, sexual behaviours) and questions on urological symptoms (see Case Study, Ketamine bladder). It is recommended that patients reporting ketamine be specifically assessed for urological symptoms, using a tool such as the International Prostate Symptom Score (I-PSS). Referral to a urology department should be made where appropriate. Treatment interventions for people using ketamine in harmful or dependent ways may include a bio-psychosocial response. This may require joint working between substance misuse treatment services and urology departments. A pain management plan may be required.

Novel Synthetic Opioids

Introduction and Brief Pharmacology

Although synthetic opioids have been misused for a long time, the scale of the problem is increasing. In addition to the diversion of pharmaceutical products, we are currently witnessing the clandestine development and sale of a number of new synthetic opioids, including fentanyl analogues. In recent years, opioids with structures distinct from those used therapeutically have emerged. In Europe, 38 new opioids have been detected on drug markets from 2009 to 2017, including 28 fentanyl derivatives. Fentanyl derivatives currently play a small role in Europe's drug market but pose a serious threat to individual and public health.

Case Study Ketamine bladder

Karen is a 28-year-old woman who has been using around 1 g of ketamine daily for six months since meeting a new partner who is a heavy ketamine user. Prior to this Karen had used a variety of drugs recreationally and without apparent harm. Over the last month, Karen has begun to experience dysuria, polyuria and intermittent haematuria. The dysuria can be so painful that she describes the pain as 'like peeing glass'. She additionally describes a diffuse abdominal pain which varies in intensity but can be so severe that she 'doubles over' in distress. Her partner told her that she is suffering with 'ketamine bladder' and the 'K cramps' and that if she drank more water they would stop. Unfortunately, this made no difference and Karen has now presented to treatment services asking for help.

Over the first few weeks in treatment Karen attempted to reduce her ketamine use, but each time she did so, she found her bladder pain became intolerable leading to a re-escalation in her ketamine use. The anaesthetic effect of the ketamine gave her brief relief, although Karen was aware that it was making the situation worse.

The drug treatment team worked in collaboration with the local urology service and put in place a pain management plan to coincide with a gradual, planned ketamine reduction. Urological investigation showed significant scaring to the inner lining of the bladder which fortunately resolved, along with the symptoms, as the ketamine use decreased.

Karen engaged with the team psychologist and in the course of these sessions decided that she needed to break up with her boyfriend if she was going to stop using ketamine, as he had been clear that he intended to continue his use. Karen initially struggled when abstinent, but was supported in finding a work placement and she also moved back in temporarily with her parents.

Opioid NPSs are typically derivatives of pharmaceutical drugs, such as fentanyl, meperidine and other opioids including AH-7921, MT-45 and U-47700. There are also newly designed fentanyl analogues made by new modifications of the fentanyl chemical structure to avoid legal control, as has been seen with other NPSs. These fentanyls are sometimes known as non-pharmaceutical fentanyls (NPF) and include furanylfentanyl.

The Misuse of Fentanyl and Analogues

Fentanyl is a full agonist at the µ-opioid receptor and is at least 80 times more potent than morphine. When misused it is associated with a significant risk of acute toxicity. Carfentanyl is intended only for veterinary use on large animals, and is not approved for medical use in humans; it is estimated to be about 10,000 times more potent than morphine. Fentanyl has a rapid onset of action, almost immediately following intravenous administration, but its maximal analgesic and respiratory depressant effect may not be noted for several minutes. Following intramuscular administration, the onset of action is from seven to eight minutes and the duration of action is one to two hours. The duration of action of fentanyl when administered intravenously is 30–60 minutes, much shorter than with heroin (four to five hours). This may lead to frequent re-dosing when used recreationally.

Opioid NPS, including fentanyl and its analogues are sold as a powder, tablets or capsules and consumed orally, by inhalation/vaporising, nasal insufflation, sublingually, intravenous injection or rectal administration. In the UK at the current time, fentanyl, fentanyl analogues and other new synthetic opioids are typically mis-sold on the illicit market as heroin or mixed with heroin to increase potency. There are also reports that they are also sold as, or mixed with, other illicit drugs and counterfeit medicines, including alprazolam, MDMA (ecstasy) and crack cocaine [10].

Acute Harms

The number of fentanyl-related overdoses is rising worldwide, with very large numbers of deaths reported in the USA and Canada. In the UK synthetic opioids (including fentanyls) used for non-medical purposes can be described as 'low-use but high-risk' substances. Nonetheless, deaths associated with fentanyl and its analogues, as well as carfentanyl, are increasing. Very often, people who had used fentanyl did not know that they had done so, instead believing they had purchased heroin or another substance. This can result in a user inadvertently consuming a significantly more potent and more unpredictable substance than intended, increasing overdose risk.

Intoxication related to synthetic opioids is associated with miosis, as is the case with most opioids. However, there are exceptions – for example, MT-45 has only a small miotic effect. This may inadvertently reduce clinical suspicion of opioid use. Adverse effects of fentanyl include constipation, nausea, vomiting, itching, cough suppression, nasal burn or nasal drip after insufflation, a bitter taste after oral ingestion, sweating, disorientation, orthostatic (or postural) hypotension and urinary urgency or retention.

Cases of severe fentanyl toxicity are associated with respiratory and central nervous system depression. They are linked to decreased consciousness, apnoea and can lead to deep coma, convulsions and respiratory arrest. Sudden-onset chest wall rigidity may be associated with increased risk of mortality. In comparison to heroin, intoxication with fentanyl and analogues presents with a greater risk of overdose with rapid onset and progression of signs and symptoms. As with other opioids, the combined use of fentanyl with other CNS and respiratory depressants such as alcohol or benzodiazepines is linked to increased toxicity. The longer term use of fentanyls can be associated with dysphoria, anxiety, agitation, depression, paranoia and hallucinations.

Overdose Management

Naloxone is effective in reversing the effects of opioid intoxication, including intoxication related to fentanyl. The UK Medicines Information (UKMi) recommends an intramuscular dose of 400 micrograms is given initially for the reversal of an opioid overdose, with further 400 microgram doses given incrementally every two to three minutes until an effect is noted or the ambulance arrives. The amount of naloxone given in a community overdose situation before an ambulance arrives is unlikely to exceed 2 mg (five 400 microgram doses). However, in cases of fentanyl overdose it seems that more rapid administration and perhaps additional doses of naloxone may be needed in comparison with overdoses of heroin or other opioids. It has therefore been suggested that where there is suspicion that fentanyl is implicated, the importance of calling ambulance or emergency services promptly and transfer to hospital should be emphasised.

Chronic Effects and Dependence

Despite limited evidence, it is assumed that fentanyls, including the novel analogues, have a high potential for harmful use and a high dependence liability. Fentanyls are associated with tolerance and withdrawal symptoms. Reports from users suggest the development of tolerance, withdrawal-like symptoms and physiological dependence are similar to those with other opioids. Characteristic withdrawal symptoms include:

- sweating
- anxiety
- diarrhoea
- bone pain
- abdominal cramps
- 'shivers' or 'goose flesh'

There is little published information on the management of dependence and withdrawal for fentanyl misuse or its analogues. It can be assumed that opioid substitution therapy (OST) may be relevant.

Benzodiazepine NPSs

There is evidence of an emerging market for benzodiazepine NPSs, particularly through internet sales. They are sold as tablets, capsules or blotters in various doses and as pure powders. Benzodiazepines used in the UK without medical supervision appear to belong to a number of categories. In addition to the commonly used benzodiazepines diverted from legitimate sources (e.g. diazepam), benzodiazepines available in other countries but not the UK have been detected on illicit markets, such as Etizolam or Phenazepam. There is also an increase in the use of Alprazolam (Xanax), a drug not available on the UK's National Health Service. As with all illicitly purchased medications, there appear to be high levels of counterfeit products.

In addition, a number of other benzodiazepines, which have not been approved for medicinal use in any country, have been sold on the Internet, generally as 'research chemicals'. Nearly all have been synthesised as potential drug candidates by pharmaceutical companies, but were not subsequently marketed as medication. They include Diclazepam, Flubromazepam, Pyrazolam, Clonazolam, Deschloroetizolam, Flubromazolam, Nifoxipam and Meclonazepam, but it can be assumed that many more will appear.

The evidence of adverse effects of benzodiazepine NPSs is extremely limited, but it should be assumed that harms will be similar to currently available pharmaceutical benzodiazepines and will require similar clinical management. The limited evidence available on the benzodiazepine NPSs suggests that some have a higher potency and/or longer duration of action than traditional benzodiazepines, which in turn may lead to increased sedation and/or amnesia. The high potency can make it difficult for users to accurately measure doses, particularly when consumed as a powder. Tablets can vary greatly in the content of active ingredients, leading to the risk of unintended overdose. There is emerging evidence of severe intoxication following the use of Flubromazolam, resulting in prolonged, severe symptoms including hypotension, rhabdomyolysis and coma. NPS benzodiazepines have a dependence liability that is similar to that of established benzodiazepines. It has been noted however that benzodiazepines such as Alprazolam, with its short elimination half-life and high potency, can cause a more severe withdrawal syndrome and have a higher physical dependence liability than benzodiazepines with longer elimination half-lives.

Hallucinogens

Introduction

The main action mediated by hallucinogen drugs is agonism of the 5HT2A receptor (e.g. LSD, psilocybin), although some hallucinogens work through other mechanisms (e.g. ketamine). Hallucinogen NPSs alter and distort perception to produce intense sensory experiences in any modality, with visual, tactile and auditory perceptual hallucinations most common. There is a wide range of chemicals that produce hallucinosis through agonism of 5HT2A including phenethylamines (e.g. 2-CB), tryptamines (e.g. DMT) and lysergamides (e.g. LSD). Some drugs in these groups also cause other psychoactive effects – for example, stimulant effects. Different drugs have different speeds of onset and length of action. Vaporised DMT has a rapid onset of around one minute and peak psychoactive effect at round five minutes. Bromo-dragonfly drugs can take much longer to cause psychoactive effects, but these can last more than 24 hours. Drugs with slower speeds of onset can result in users re-dosing under the mistaken belief that the drug they have consumed has low potency or purity. Re-dosing before the first dose has taken effect increases the risk of drug intoxication and harm.

Acute Intoxication

Symptoms of hallucinogen NPS intoxication tend to be predominantly psychological rather than physiological. The most common adverse hallucinogen NPS presentation is acute distress, often referred to by the user as a 'bad trip'. Users describe a loss of control, disturbing, frightening perceptions, including synaesthesia, a rapid onset of severe dysphoria with suicidal ideation, marked agitation, paranoia and confusion. Symptoms can rapidly alter, complicating clinical diagnosis. Physical adverse effects include nausea and other gastrointestinal upset, dizziness, headache, tremor, paraesthesia, hypertension and tachycardia.

Traditional hallucinogens such as LSD typically have low systemic toxicity and accidental overdose is rare. In contrast, hallucinogen NPSs can have greater toxicity and a narrower safety ratio. Hallucinogen NPSs also have a broader range of potencies, speed of onset, length of action and subjective effects. There are reports of life-threatening sympathomimetic toxicity associated with NPSs, as well as serotonin syndrome. As a result, potent, long-acting hallucinogen NPSs can cause much greater health harms than traditional hallucinogens, particularly for inexperienced users. The most common adverse hallucinogen NPS presentation is acute distress, often referred to by the user as a 'bad trip'. Users describe a loss of control, disturbing, frightening perceptions, including synaesthesia, a rapid onset of severe dysphoria with suicidal ideation, marked agitation, paranoia and confusion. Symptoms can rapidly alter, complicating clinical diagnosis.

Clinical Management of Acute Adverse Hallucinogen Harms

The large majority of people presenting with acute hallucinogen NPS intoxication can be managed with reassurance, observation and supportive care (e.g. management of airways, if indicated). Rarely, levels of agitation will be such that benzodiazepines are needed for symptomatic control and to keep the patient safe. If benzodiazepines are insufficient then antipsychotics may be used as a second line.

Harms from Repeated Use

Despite the sometimes significant acute psychoactive effects caused by hallucinogens, there is relatively little evidence suggesting long-term harms. Available research does not indicate that hallucinogens cause tolerance, physiological withdrawal symptoms, compulsive use or other criteria of a dependence syndrome. Hallucinogen persisting perception disorder (HPPD) describes a collection of symptoms including perceptual disturbances, usually visual, which can last for months or even years after the ingestion of hallucinogens. Typical visual symptoms include streaks or flashes of light, after-images, visual trails, haloes around the edges of objects, photophobia and intensification of colour. Symptoms generally begin within a few hours of hallucinogen ingestion and often cause significant distress when they fail to resolve. Research is limited and prevalence and aetiology remain unclear. HPPD typically resolves spontaneously; however, anxiety management, particularly techniques supporting the individual to distract themselves from the symptoms coupled with abstinence from all psychoactive drugs is recommended for those with severe symptoms or with symptoms failing to improve after a few weeks (see Case Study, Hallucinogen persisting perception disorder).

Concluding Remarks

Club drugs and novel psychoactive substances pose a challenge for psychiatrists and other frontline clinicians. A large and ever-growing number of substances are available, many of which are purchased through the Internet. Clinical presentations are complicated by consumption of often unknown substances, typically in the context of poly-drug use (including alcohol). Despite an emerging evidence base, our knowledge of the adverse effects of NPS is still limited, particularly the long-term effects. There is also limited evidence relating to treatment of adverse effects

Case Study Hallucinogen persisting perception disorder

Harry is a 20-year-old physics student who presented to clinic three months after his first exposure to any drugs. He reports taking 'a trip' in the form of a pill with friends while on a night out celebrating exam results. Harry describes consuming the tablet and within 30 minutes feeling unwell. He described an intense headache accompanied by 'flickering images, likes clawed hands' in his peripheral vision. His friends had no problems and where enjoying themselves but soon realised that Harry was suffering and so took him home. Harry slept poorly and the next day his symptoms had changed. The headache had gone, but he was now experiencing a number of new symptoms. These included 'visual snow, like an untuned TV', after images where he would see an image persist in his visual field despite looking away from it, and visual trails in the form of 'sparks of light' emitting from his fingertips. He also described patterned surfaces such as wallpaper or curtains as gently moving 'like the sea'. Harry's friends reassured him that the visual experiences would settle down and told him to rest for a few days.

One week later, the visual symptoms were if anything more intense. Harry was now also experiencing pronounced photophobia and had started wearing sunglasses day and night. After two weeks, with no improvement, Harry told his parents what had happened and they arranged for him to see a neurologist. The neurologist found no abnormality on examination but arranged an MRI and CT scan both of which were normal.

Harry was now feeling desperate as the visual symptoms were highly distracting and stopped him from studying. He began to feel increasingly anxious and dropped out of university, returning to live with his parents.

After two months, with no improvement, he approached the clinic for assessment. Prior to his consumption of the pills, there was no previous drug use or previous psychiatric history. Aside from these symptoms, the only other feature was marked anxiety which appeared to intensify his visual symptoms. There was no evidence of depression or psychosis. A diagnosis of hallucinogen persisting perception disorder (HPPD) was made. There are currently no available evidenced-based treatments and the symptoms tend to be self-limiting although they can last months or even years. The clinic commenced cognitive behavioural therapy (CBT) aimed at reducing Harry's anxiety and recommended that he avoid all psychoactive drugs including alcohol.

Over the following three months, Harry completed 12 sessions of CBT and noticed a gradual improvement in his visual symptoms. He avoided all psychoactive substances. Ten months after ingesting the pill his symptoms had completely resolved and he was able to return to university.

This chapter addresses some of these challenges. It provides a simple framework allowing clinicians to build on their existing knowledge and skills relating to traditional illicit drugs. NPSs, like traditional drugs, can be classified into four broad categories based on their psychoactive effect. Clinicians will already be familiar with these categories: predominantly stimulant; predominantly hallucinogen; predominantly depressant; and synthetic cannabinoid receptor agonists. Using clinical presentation as a guide, clinicians can determine the broad group to which an NPS belongs and then make decisions on the most appropriate management of the acute and chronic adverse effects. The chapter describes the specific effects of the most commonly used NPSs within the four categories in more detail. The clinical management of NPSs must take into account the wide differences that can exist between substances within each group and the potential differences such as potency, toxicity and half-life.

References

1 Independent Expert Working Group. *Clinical Guidelines on Drug Misuse and Dependence, Update 2017: Drug Misuse and Dependence – UK Guidelines on Clinical Management.* London: Department of Health; 2017.

2 United Nations Office on Drugs and Crime. *World Drug Report 2018.* United Nations publication, Sales No. E.20.XI.6; 2018.

3 European Monitoring Centre for Drugs and Drug Addiction. *European Drug Report: Trends and Developments.* Lisbon, Portugal: EMCDDA; 2018.

4 Meader N., Mdege N., McCambridge J. The public health evidence-base on novel psychoactive substance use: scoping review with narrative synthesis of selected bodies of evidence. *Journal of Public Health.* 2018; **40** (3): e303–e19.

5 Abdulrahim D., Whiteley C., Moncrieff M., Bowden-Jones O. *Club Drug Use Among Lesbian, Gay, Bisexual and Trans (LGBT) People.* London: Novel Psychoactive Treatment UK Network (NEPTUNE); 2016.

6 Karila L., Billieux J., Benyamina A., Lançon C., Cottencin O. The effects and risks associated to mephedrone and methylone in humans: A review of the preliminary evidences. *Brain Research Bulletin.* 2016; **126**: 61–7.

7 Abdulrahim D., Bowden-Jones O., on behalf of the NEPTUNE group. *Harms of Synthetic Cannabinoid Receptor Agonists (SCRAs) and Their Management.* London: Novel Psychoactive Treatment UK Network (NEPTUNE); 2016.

8 Winstock A., Lynskey M., Borschmann R., Waldron J. Risk of emergency medical treatment following consumption of cannabis or synthetic cannabinoids in a large global sample. *Journal of Psychopharmacology.* 2015; **29** (6): 698–703.

9 Zaurova M., Hoffman R. S., Vlahov D., Manini A. F. Clinical Effects of Synthetic Cannabinoid Receptor Agonists Compared with Marijuana in Emergency Department Patients with Acute Drug Overdose. *Journal of Medical Toxicology.* 2016; **12** (4): 335–40.

10 Abdulrahim D., Bowden-Jones O., on behalf of the NEPTUNE group. *The Misuse of Synthetic Opioids: Harms and Clinical Management of Fentanyl, Fentanyl Analogues and Other Novel Synthetic Opioids: Information for Clinicians.* London: NEPTUNE; 2018.

Addiction Problems in a Family and Social Context

Alex Copello and Ed Day

Conceptual and Service Context

Traditional attempts to help people with problems with alcohol and drugs have been largely focused on the individual user and their characteristics. This stands in contrast with the observation that those close to people with substance use disorders (e.g. close family members or friends) suffer significant and sustained stress that often leads to psychological and physical problems for themselves. Furthermore, in most cases the same people can positively and significantly influence the course and outcome of the alcohol and drug problems of those they are concerned about through their support and encouragement for the user's efforts to change. Therefore focusing exclusively on the individual can provide at best a partial and limited picture of the problem.

The impact of substance use on the family has been explored across a range of studies in different populations across the world with strikingly similar results. Orford and colleagues have described the most prominent elements of the stressful experience of living with a relative who is drinking or taking drugs excessively in multiple studies [1]. These include 'the relationship with a relative becoming disagreeable and sometimes aggressive; conflict over money and possessions; the experience of uncertainty; worry about the relative; and home and family life being threatened.' Good-quality social support for family members is often lacking, and they cope in a variety of ways, including either withdrawing totally and gaining independence or standing up to substance use.

There are at least two very good reasons for considering the families of people with substance use disorders. First, family members experience considerable stress in their own right [2]. Second, family members and other members of an individual's social network are potential co-therapists in helping the individual change their addictive behaviour [3]. Interventions for family members fall into three broad areas [3]:

(1) working with family members to promote the engagement of people with substance use disorders in treatment

(2) the joint involvement of people with substance use disorders and their family and friends in the treatment

(3) responding to the needs of family members and friends in their own right

Alcohol, drug and other addictive behaviours should be seen as occurring in an important social context. Members of this social network can experience negative impacts resulting from the addiction, but also significantly influence its course through the provision of positive support. The present chapter focuses on two forms of help, developed from this perspective and based on evidence and research on family and social networks that draws from different, yet complementary conceptual frameworks.

After a review of what we know about social networks in those with alcohol and drug problems and the impacts of alcohol and drug problems on those families and wider social networks, this chapter describes two interventions, their associated theoretical models and components along with the current evidence base to support their use. The Five Step Intervention [4] aims to help those families affected in their own right through a series of focused counselling sessions or guided self-help. Social behaviour and network therapy [5], on the other hand, aims to help those with the alcohol or drug problem by identifying, developing and enhancing social support for a change in the substance consumption behaviour. Both are structured yet flexible and described in some detail before discussing more broadly the benefits of using a social network focus when working with people with alcohol and drug problems.

What Do We Know about Social Networks?

Social support can be defined as 'resources provided by other people' and has been linked to a wide range of health-related outcomes, including mortality, physical disease and psychological symptoms [6]. Such support appears to protect people from the harmful effects of stress and enhance overall subjective well-being [7], but at the same time it is recognised that social network members may also provide dysfunctional role models, reinforce maladaptive behaviour and provide 'environmental cues' associated with drug or alcohol availability and use [8].

Social networks are 'the set of people with whom an individual is directly involved': that is, those who regularly interact with an individual. The 'personal' network is a subnetwork of closer, personal relationships in the global network, such as family members, friends and other close confidants, and this may be further subdivided into a friendship network, a family network or a work-related network. Various theories have been developed to explain how an individual's social network changes over the life course, but generally speaking the number of informal social contacts increases rapidly in adolescence, followed by a steady reduction back to a few closer relationships as life progresses [9]. Relations with the spouse or close family are more stable throughout the lifespan, but those on the margins of the network are less stable and are influenced by changes in external circumstances.

The general consensus appears to be that the quantity and quality of social relationships in industrialised countries has decreased over the past 50 years [10]. There are a number of possible reasons for this, including greater social mobility, delayed marriage, reduced intergenerational living, increased single residence households and dual-career families. However, qualitative research suggests that people who experience remission of a substance use problem have an increased social connection to others [11], increased reliance on the support of family and friends [12] and increased activities and time spent with non-substance-using social network members [13]. One large epidemiological study reports that personal networks of friends, neighbours and religious groups are first to change in remission, possibly because drug using network members are exchanged for non-users [14].

The Importance of Family and Social Networks for People with Substance Use Disorders

A commonly held perception is that those who have serious alcohol or drug problems tend to be somewhat lonely and isolated from their social networks, yet this is not confirmed by research findings. For example, all participants entering a large trial of the treatment of alcohol problems in the UK [15] were asked about the composition of their social networks in some detail using a validated research tool [16, 17]. The Important People and Activities instrument asks people to nominate up to 12 members of their social network whom they perceive to be important in their lives and with whom they spent most of their time. Secondary analysis of this data revealed that a total of 4,677 important people were named by 740 participants entering routine alcohol treatment in UK services and consenting to participate in UKATT. All participants could name at least one important person, and many could name 12. The mean social network number named across the whole participant sample was 6.5, with a mode of 10. The IPA also looks more closely at the four most important people of all those nominated by each participant. Here, the majority of people named their partner as the most important person, although other family members such as parents, children and siblings were also a frequent choice. Very few participants named their partner as least important person of the four. Other members of close family were predominantly named as second or third most important, and friends were commonly named as third or fourth [18].

A subsequent study of clients in opiate substitution treatment (OST) in the UK National Health Service [8] interviewed 118 participants using a shorter adaptation of the IPA measure, the Important People Drug and Alcohol Interview (IPDA) [19] and identified a total of 820 network members with a mean network size of 6.9 people. Of this group, 378 (46 per cent) were immediate family members; 189 (23 per cent) friends; 97 (12 per cent) extended family members; 51 (6 per cent) treatment professionals or members of self-help groups; 47 (6 per cent) sexual partners; 16 (2 per cent) colleagues from work; and 42 (5 per cent) others. The study revealed that two-thirds of the social network of clients was made up of family members, with the remaining third made up of mostly friends and fewer self-help group members or professionals.

There is also evidence that those who are potentially more complex and isolated also show evidence of connection to their social networks. A study of a homeless population living in hostels in the UK showed that drug and alcohol users have small friendship networks that can often be undermined by arguments, geographical mobility and imprisonment [20]. However, users reported a desire for culturally normative friendships, underpinned by routine and regular contact. Furthermore, the study showed that information and communication technologies are central to the friendships of many homeless drug and alcohol users, keeping them connected to sources of social support for recovery outside homelessness and substance using worlds.

Taken together, the findings from these studies appear to challenge the notion that alcohol and drug users tend to be isolated and cut off from potential sources of social support from others. While the networks of alcohol users tend to include more partners when compared to drug users, family members feature largely for both groups. The average number of social network members across both samples is similar and even those that could be considered more vulnerable and at risk of isolation (e.g. those in the study by Neale et al. [20]) report significant social support networks as well as placing important value on the availability of such networks.

A View from the Social Network Perspective: The Impact of Addiction Problems on the Family Members and Friends of Users

Interesting findings emerge when experiences are viewed from the perspective of the social network. Estimates of prevalence suggest that at least 1.5 million adults in the UK are significantly affected by a relative's drug use, with the associated cost of harm they experience because of this amounting to around £1.8 billion per year [21]. If we considered alcohol use, the figures would be significantly higher. However, the strain on family members is both underestimated and commonly unidentified by health and other services [22]. This strain manifests in a range of psychological and physical symptoms of stress including significant depression and anxiety (e.g. [23]). It has been suggested that the mental health impact of alcohol and drug problems on families constitutes a major but neglected contributor to the global burden of adult ill health [22].

Family members affected in this way tend to suffer in silence, but on some occasions they may approach services for help with symptoms such as anxiety and or depression. However, the underlying cause of stress is often left undiscussed by professional services, and the treatment received is therefore symptom-focused – that is, psychological help for generalised anxiety or depression. Despite this, the evidence suggests that brief specific problem-focused psychosocial interventions can help reduce stress and harms in this family member patient group [24]. There has been a recent increase in studies of the prevalence of being an affected family member of someone with an alcohol problem [25–28]. Studies with large samples confirm the significant extent of the problem and the nature and range of experiences resulting from being close to someone with an alcohol use disorder. On the other hand, it is important to note that suffering in silence also prevents affected family members from having more opportunity to both understand and wherever possible influence the course and outcome of the alcohol and drug problem within the family unit. Being able to help the user's recovery has potential for positive outcomes for the user and for the family as a whole.

It has been argued that one possible barrier to the delivery of help by professionals who come into contact with affected family members is the lack of a clear way of understanding the problem that can guide the person in delivering focused positive help and support. Historically, families have tended to be perceived as part of the problem. More recently, however, understanding the experiences of family members as the manifestation of a wider set of experiences of living with significant stress has led to the development of helpful conceptual models and more focused forms of help.

Conceptual Understanding of the Affected Family Member Experience: The Stress-Strain-Coping-Support Model

Of particular relevance here is the development of the stress-strain-coping-support model of the impacts of alcohol, drug or indeed other non-chemical behaviours with addictive potential such as gambling problems. The model is a simple, non-judgemental way of understanding that has much in common with models that explain the stresses provoked by living with someone with dementia or significant mental health problems. In simple terms, the model assumes that the core experiences of family members faced with these types of problems is fundamentally the same across different substances, family compositions and cultures. As the name suggests, the four key components of the model are 'stress', 'strain', 'coping behaviours' and 'available social support'. The model specifies that the ongoing experience of stress leads to strain, and that this relationship can be influenced by the other two components – that is, the coping behaviours family members adopt towards the user and the amount of social support available to them in relation to this situation. Each component of the SSCS model is described briefly in turn as it is relevant to family members affected by addiction of a close relative.

Stress: Substance use in the family can cause family bonds and relationships to deteriorate, disrupt family life, possibly leading to situations where family members worry about their relatives, where there may be conflict over money and possessions and where there is potential for hostility and aggression [22]. Such situations have the potential to cause stress for the family member regardless of their gender, age, relationship to the user or sociocultural group.

Strain: This stress in turn can lead to substantial strain for the family member. Research across the world suggests that addiction in the family can be stressful enough to put the family members' physical, mental and general health at risk. Family members often report signs of ill health including sleep problems, weight changes and an increase in both psychological symptoms (e.g. anxiety, depression) and physical symptoms (e.g. hypertension, pains, migraine). Furthermore, in addition to the impact on the family members' health, other domains of life can be affected by the stress, such as their work or career, and their friendship networks [1].

Coping: These experiences leave family members faced with the challenging task of trying to understand what is going on and deciding how to deal with the situation. Family members want to find the best way of coping and there is not necessarily any right or wrong answer, although some solutions are considered by family members to be counterproductive. Qualitative interviews and quantitative research with affected family members [29] have suggested that there are three broad methods of coping (although it is worth noting that there are not always distinct boundaries between these and overlap can occur):

(1) Family members often report 'putting up with' their relatives' substance use – for example, giving them money through fear they will commit crime.

(2) Some report 'standing up to it' in an attempt to regain some of the control over family life that has been lost.

(3) Others withdraw from the situation and try to 'gain independence' from the relative by putting distance between them – for example, by leaving or asking them to.

Family members are usually unsure about what to do and struggle to find the best way of coping, and therefore welcome any support, help and advice.

Support: Good social support is an important resource for coping and this plays an important role in the model. When it occurs social support is highly valued, but it has been suggested that this may be rare [29]. Emotional support from people who have been through similar situations themselves is appreciated, as well as the provision of accurate information and practical help. Family members perceive the feeling of 'being backed up' in their way of coping as helpful, as opposed to having support from somebody who criticises their coping methods.

As previously mentioned, affected family members may not seek support as a result of the embarrassment or shame they may feel if others knew about the addiction [1].

Unfortunately this may be reinforced through negative experiences with both personal and professional support systems. Family members have described receiving unsympathetic or unhelpful advice from family and friends [1], as well as feeling that they have received inadequate support or information from professionals, who were often unwilling or unable to talk through various potential coping strategies. Some have even reported feeling blamed by professionals, that the professional was implying that the relative's addiction was the family member's fault. The overall experience of family members suggests that their social networks are often neither helpful nor supportive [1]. There is a need to recognise the multilayered nature of the stress, the complexity of the various coping strategies and the confusion and mixed feelings that may be felt towards the relative [30].

Theory to Practice: The 5-Step Method to Support Affected Family Members in Their Own Right

The stress-strain-coping-support model provided the conceptual basis for the development of the 5-Step Method, which was specifically designed to help family members affected in their own right when they were identified in a range of different service settings (e.g. primary care, generic mental health services). The method recognises that on some occasions the person with the addiction problem may not be ready for (or indeed want) help, yet those people who are close and concerned can be affected to a significant extent by the impact. Furthermore, there is an assumption that direct help for those affected can be beneficial and has the potential to significantly reduce stress and harm.

The method is brief, structured and flexible. The components of the conceptual stress-strain-coping-support model guide interactions between helpers and family members affected, and each of the five steps relates to a part of the model. Table 14.1 illustrates the tasks for each of the steps as well as the component that each task relates to. For a fuller description of the method, see [4].

The elements of the approach are not novel per se; however, the theoretical model allows those delivering the method to structure the discussion and guide the family member within a formulated understanding of the family members' experience. The focus moves from 'hearing the story' – that is, finding out what life has been like and what stressors the family member has experienced – to establishing and addressing the need for information, discussing and exploring coping behaviours and responses along with establishing the availability of specific support related to the experience. Finally, the focus moves to discussing hopes and expectations for the future.

In addition to the specific areas of focus and skills for each step, the process is underpinned by certain key principles. It is important to adopt a non-judgemental style within the interaction with a family member. When faced with these highly complex problems, most family members attempt to respond in ways which they consider will help improve the situation for the user and the family. Attempts to respond are often experienced as difficult dilemmas, which is to be expected given the complexities involved. The 5-Step Method starts from the premise that family members are ordinary people caught up in highly stressful situations and trying to work out ways to respond, as opposed to suffering from deficiencies or causing the addiction problem themselves. With this understanding in mind, the intervention should be delivered in a supportive and non-confrontational manner. Another central principle is that better-informed family members are more able to manage the situation and associated stress. It is important as part of

Table 14.1 Contents of the five steps mapped onto the stress-strain-coping-support model [4]

Contents of 5-Step Method	Component of SSCS model
Step 1: Elicit the family member's story and experiences through active listening and exploring concerns. • Listen, reassure and explore concerns. • Allow family member to describe situation. • Identify relevant stresses. • Identify need for further information. • Communicate realistic optimism. • Identify need for future contacts.	Stress and strain
Step 2: Identify information needs and provide specific targeted information. • Increase knowledge and understanding. • Reduce stress arising from lack of knowledge or misconceptions.	Need for understanding and increased knowledge
Step 3: Identify and explore advantages and disadvantages of coping responses used as perceived by the family member. • Identify current coping responses. • Explore advantages and disadvantages of current coping responses. • Explore alternative coping responses. • Explore advantages and disadvantages of alternative ways of coping.	Coping
Step 4: Discuss and identify current support and ways of enhancing support for the family member. • Draw a social network diagram. • Aim to improve communication within the family. • Aim for a unified and coherent approach. • Explore potential new sources of support.	Social support
Step 5: Discuss further needs for family member, the using relative and or the rest of the family. • Is there a need for further help? • Discuss possible options with family member. • Facilitate contact between family member and other sources of specialist help.	Additional needs

the second step to find out the specific types of information that may help the family member. Finally, it is crucial to accept the idea that each family is unique and as such their problems need to be understood as they apply to the family member and their unique set of circumstances.

The 5-Step Method has become a popular intervention tool for those delivering help to family members affected by substance use disorders. Preliminary effectiveness has been established through a series of research studies in various settings, including primary care and specialist addiction services. This evidence is reviewed in detail elsewhere [24], but research in both primary and secondary care teams has consistently shown a significant decrease in physical and psychological symptoms in family members receiving the 5-Step intervention. The majority of family members interviewed in these studies were able to report one or more positive ways in which the intervention had helped them. A significant number reported feeling relief at being listened to and having the opportunity to talk about what was going on for them, and many were able to be more assertive with their relatives while taking a more open and calmer approach in tackling problems.

Two important challenges for the method include wider implementation as well as further studies testing the method against less structured support and exploring key ingredients.

Social Support for Change in Addictive Behaviours and Social Behaviour and Network Therapy (SBNT)

Bringing the focus back onto those with substance use disorders themselves, there is accumulating evidence that the social environment is an important factor that influences initiation, maintenance and behaviour change [31]. However, in contrast to other chronic diseases such as pulmonary disease or cancer, the problem status (i.e. substance use) of members of the social network is also an important consideration for this group, as are issues such as the stigma of substance use and the role of social norms in guiding behaviour. When the construct of social support was first considered in SUD treatment research it was defined globally and measured using one or two questions in a pre-treatment assessment battery [32]. However, this simplistic approach ignored the fact that support from another person who drinks alcohol heavily may not help the resolution of an alcohol problem, and so its relationship to patient outcome was unpredictable. It was only when social support was differentiated into two distinct constructs (alcohol-specific support and general or global social support) that meaningful associations started to emerge. Whereas general support promotes overall well-being, alcohol-specific support has been directly tied to alcohol use [17, 33].

There is consistent evidence for the role of family support, with both general and abstinence-specific support associated with more abstinent days and less relapse [34–36]. Good family adjustment and functioning is associated with better drinking outcomes [31], whereas negative family behaviours such as withdrawing, avoiding or tolerating drinking are associated with higher levels of drinking [37]. Intimate partner or spousal support is particularly significant, but is generally greater for men than women [31]. The best outcomes occur when support for abstinence comes from all members of the network (family and friends).

Social behaviour and network therapy (SBNT) is an approach that aims to build on this evidence of the influence of social networks by working with people with substance use disorders to identify and develop positive support for their efforts to change their behaviour. A detailed description of this approach is given in the SBNT treatment manual [5], but a brief description of the key components of the intervention is presented here. Originally, SBNT was designed as a flexible, time-limited intervention consisting of eight sessions and based on the principle that social behaviour, social interaction and network support for change can play a central part in the resolution of addiction problems. The approach focuses specifically on developing the clients' natural environment and existing support networks, and where necessary introduce new ones (e.g. self-help groups), in an attempt to develop the conditions to support positive change in substance use during treatment and beyond. As an approach focused on social networks, SBNT also has the potential to help other people affected and concerned by the addiction problem through their involvement in the treatment process. Within SBNT the user is identified as the 'focal person or client' while others involved in treatment sessions are referred to as 'network members'.

Phase 1 of SBNT is to identify the structure of the social network around the focal person, and which members may be supportive of change in their substance use [38]. In practice, SBNT starts by carefully drawing a social network diagram (see Figure 14.1). This allows therapist and focal client to determine how important each network member is to the focal client; how they respond to the presence of the focal client's alcohol or drug problem; and how their help could be enlisted in supporting the focal client's efforts to change. For example, in the case of Frank (Figure 14.1), Sarah, Lee and Sam were all considered as potential early network members as they understood the current situation and could be supportive but non-judgemental. As the work progressed, one of the three childhood

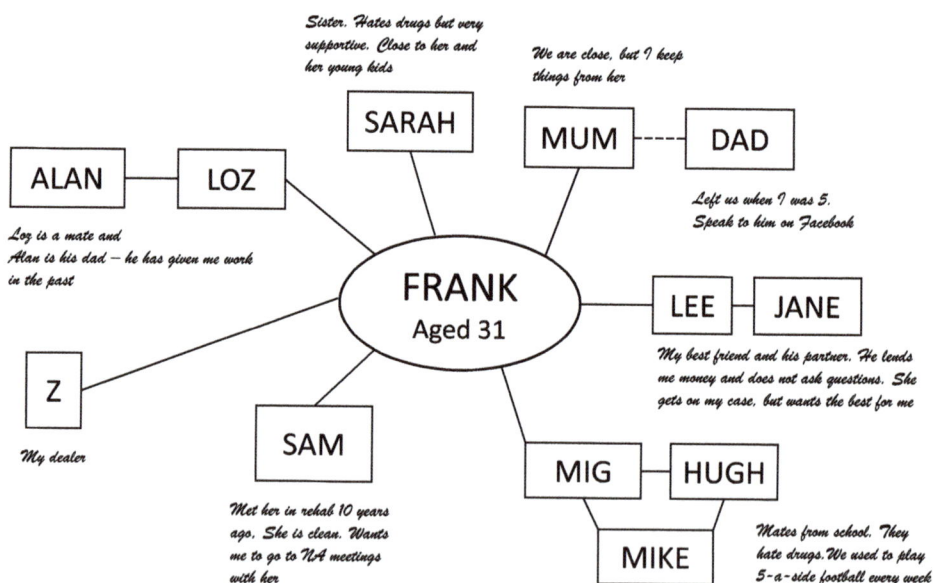

Figure 14.1 A Social Network Diagram constructed with Frank, who has presented for help with heroin and crack cocaine use. This was drawn in response to the request for information: 'Tell me who you have had contact with in the past three months and who has been important to you.'

friends was recruited to increase the opportunity for non-using social activity, and Alan was approached in an attempt to find work.

In practice, the drawing of the social network diagram is an important and powerful therapeutic tool in itself. It enables the focal client and helper to make sense of the focal client's problem in context. In addition to the identification of the focal client's social network through the network diagram, the first session involves two further tasks: conveying the social focus of the intervention approach, and establishing the treatment goal (e.g. abstinence or moderation). Towards the end of session 1 the discussion focuses on who to involve in future sessions. The ideal network member would be readily available to the focal person, agree with their substance use goal (e.g. cutting down, abstinence) and offer positive but boundaried support.

Phase 2 involves building, engaging or mobilising the social network, using a menu of core and elective topics for subsequent sessions. There are four core topics: communication; coping/responding; enhancing social support; and relapse management. In addition, any of four elective topics could be used: basic education on drugs/alcohol; increasing pleasant activities; employment; and minimising support for drug/alcohol use. The broad nature of each topic allows the material to be used when network members are present, but also with the focal person alone in order to engage potential network members or develop networks from scratch. The therapist is encouraged to take an active role, using role play and skill practice within sessions and homework tasks between sessions. The components of SBNT are described in Table 14.2.

Phase 3 focuses on preparing for the future after treatment. The final session is an opportunity to review progress and plan for the network to continue to provide positive support for change. The therapist encourages the focal person and their network members to share responsibility for success.

SBNT was initially developed to help people presenting with alcohol problems and evaluated in the UK Alcohol Treatment Trial [39, 40]. Subsequently SBNT has been adapted and evaluated as a treatment for drug users [41, 42]. The UKATT results showed that SBNT was as effective and cost effective as motivational enhancement therapy (MET), while the evaluation of SBNT with drug users showed that it is feasible and has promise as a treatment for individuals who misuse illicit drugs. Further analysis of UKATT data, using structural equation modelling, showed evidence of a small treatment effect on post-treatment motivation favouring SBNT over MET. Those who received SBNT were more likely than those in the MET group to be actively trying to change their drinking at the end of treatment for three out of five of the treatment outcomes explored [43].

The way of working inherent in SBNT offers different options for those delivering interventions. Considering the social environment can open possibilities for those attempting to change behaviour by tapping into sources of ongoing support from the focal client's natural environment. These sources of support can continue to provide an environment supportive of change in the future and importantly beyond treatment episodes, with potential for sustained maintenance of treatment gains. Support can also be drawn from recovery and self-help groups where this is seen as important for and by the client [9].

Despite the evidence for the important role of families and wider social networks, UK service delivery remains largely focused on the individual substance user, with families and other network members playing a very peripheral role [44]. With very few exceptions, help for those concerned about the user is limited and poorly resourced. One of the most challenging aspects for those delivering interventions like SBNT is the shift in focus from

Table 14.2 Components of Social Behaviour and Network Therapy with brief rationale for their inclusion [38]

Establishing social network	The problem may have alienated some or all potential network members. A first step is to identify who these individuals are and, provided the focal person thinks that they will be supportive, make contact with them, and invite them to take part in supporting the focal person in their efforts to change.
Drinking goal	Members of the network may not agree with the focal person or among themselves about the appropriate change goal. This should be discussed and an agreed goal should be negotiated.
Communication	The focal person and members of their social network may have been communicating ineffectively. Together they may plan and practice improved ways of communicating.
Coping/responding	Network members can explore how they have been coping with/responding to the alcohol/drug problems. There may be ways that they recognise, on reflection, to be counterproductive. They may discuss and practice better ways of coping.
Support	The focal client may not be engaging with network members in a way that is supportive. They could be helped to develop ways of engaging with positive network members more effectively (e.g. by contacting network members at times of relapse risk).
Relapse and support	Network members may have different views about how to respond in the event of relapse. An agreed strategy could be negotiated with network members and with the focal person. The focal person may find it difficult to enlist support from network members when relapse occurs. There is a need to develop a shared understanding of the relapse process and to discuss joint strategies for dealing with lapses. This may include the identification of early signs of impending risk for lapse and possible responses to these.
Alternative activities	The focal person and members of their network may have been undertaking few joint activities which have been pleasant, and hence the focal person has little access to activities that are alternatives to drinking. Together they may be helped to plan such activities and to increase their frequency.
Developing network support	In some cases, it may be difficult for problem drinkers/drug users to identify anyone who might join a positive network for change and it may be necessary to recruit a 'mentor' (e.g. an ex-problem user or a volunteer worker) who can, for a period of time, perform the functions otherwise served by a natural support network.
Social behaviour	Problem alcohol/drug users, at the time of seeking help, often show a lack of skill in social behaviours necessary to make contact with potential network members and engage with them effectively. Skills training can be used to address this deficit. This may involve training in communication skills such as starting conversations, re-establishing contact by telephone with a potential network member, composing a letter to a potential network member or dealing with criticism from a potential network member. The focus of this work is on engaging potential network members as opposed to general social competence.

individual to social in order to incorporate the additional importance of the social environment. However, even conducting the simple task of drawing a network diagram with clients can help to widen the focus of the discussion and provide a more social interpersonal focus. This technique can be taught very simply, and is easily integrated into other ways of working with people with substance use disorders [45].

References

1 Orford J., Velleman R., Copello A., Templeton L., Ibanga A. The experiences of affected family members: A summary of two decades of qualitative research. *Drugs: Education, Prevention and Policy*. 2010; **17** (sup1): 44–62.

2 Orford J., Natera G., Copello A., Atkinson C., Mora J., Velleman R. et al. *Coping with Alcohol and Drug Problems: The Experiences of Family Members in Three Contrasting Cultures*. London: Routledge; 2005; chapter 5, pp 95–117.

3 Copello A., Velleman R., Templeton L. Family interventions in the treatment of alcohol and drug problems. *Drug and Alcohol Review*. 2005; **24** (4): 369–85.

4 Copello A., Templeton L., Orford J., Velleman R. The 5-Step Method: Principles and practice. *Drugs: Education, Prevention, and Policy*. 2010; **17** (s1): 86–99.

5 Copello A., Orford J., Hodgson R., Tober G. *Social Behaviour and Network Therapy for Alcohol Problems*. London: Routledge; 2009.

6 Holt-Lunstad J., Smith T. B., Layton J. B. Social relationships and mortality risk: A meta-analytic review. *PLOS Medicine*. 2010; **7** (7): e1000316.

7 Cohen S., Gottlieb B. H., Underwood L. G. Social Relationships and Health. In: *Social Support Measurement and Intervention* (eds. S. Cohen, L. G. Underwood, B. H. Gottlieb): 3–25. Oxford: Oxford University Press, 2000.

8 Day E., Copello A., Karia M., Roche J., Grewal P., George S. et al. Social Network Support for Individuals Receiving Opiate Substitution Treatment and Its Association with Treatment Progress. *European Addiction Research*. 2013; **19** (4): 211–21.

9 Day E. Building Bridges to Positive Social Identities: The Social Network Diagram and Opiate Substitution Treatment. In: *Addiction, Behavioural Change and Social Identity* (eds. S. A. Buckingham, D. Best). London: Routledge; 2017.

10 Putnam R. D. *Bowling Alone: The Collapse and Revival of American Community*. New York: Simon & Schuster; 2000.

11 McIntosh J., McKeganey N. Addicts' narratives of recovery from drug use: Constructing a non-addict identity. *Social Science and Medicine*. 2000; **50** (10): 1501–10.

12 Granfield R., Cloud W. Social context and 'natural recovery': The role of social capital in the resolution of drug-associated problems. *Substance Use and Misuse*. 2001; **36** (11): 1543–70.

13 Best D., Ghufran S., Day E., Ray R., Loaring J. Breaking the habit: A retrospective analysis of desistance factors among formerly problematic heroin users. *Drug and Alcohol Review*. 2008; **27** (6): 619–24.

14 Mowbray O., Scott J. A. The effect of drug use disorder onset, remission or persistence on an individual's personal social network. *The American Journal on Addictions*. 2015; **24** (5): 427–34.

15 UKATT Research Team. United Kingdom Alcohol Treatment Trial (UKATT): hypothesis, design and methods. *Alcohol and Alcoholism*. 2001; **36** (1): 11–21.

16 Allen J. P., Wilson V. B. *Assessing Alcohol Problems: A Guide for Clinicians and Researchers*. Bethesda, MD: National Institute on Alcohol Abuse and Alcoholism; 2003.

17 Beattie M. C., Longabough R. L. General and alcohol-specific social support following treatment. *Addictive Behaviors*. 1999; **24**: 593–606.

18 Copello A., Walsh K. Families, friends and addiction: Impacts, psychological models and interventions. In: *Addiction Psychology*

and *Treatment* (eds. P. Davis, R. Patton, S. Jackson). Hoboken, NJ: Wiley-Blackwell; 2017.

19 Zywiak W. H., Neighbors C. J., Martin R. A., Johnson J. E., Eaton C. A., Rohsenow D. J. The Important People Drug and Alcohol Interview: Psychometric properties, predictive validity, and implications for treatment. *Journal of Substance Abuse Treatment.* 2009; **36**: 321–30.

20 Neale J., Brown C. 'We are always in some form of contact': Friendships among homeless drug and alcohol users living in hostels. *Health and Social Care in the Community.* 2016; **24** (5): 557–66.

21 Copello A., Templeton L., Powell J. *Adult Family Members and Carers of Dependent Drug Users: Prevalence, Social Cost, Resource Savings and Treatment Responses.* London: UK Drug Policy Commission; 2009.

22 Orford J., Velleman R., Natera G., Templeton L., Copello A. Addiction in the family is a major but neglected contributor to the global burden of adult ill-health. *Social Science and Medicine.* 2013; **78**: 70–7.

23 Ray G. T., Mertens J. R., Weisner C. The excess medical cost and health problems of family members of persons diagnosed with alcohol or drug problems. *Medical Care.* 2007; **45**: 116–22.

24 Copello A., Templeton L., Orford J., Velleman R. The 5-step method: Evidence of gains for affected family members. *Drugs: Education, Prevention, and Policy.* 2010; **17** (s1): 100–12.

25 Berends L., Ferris J., Laslett A. M. A problematic drinker in the family: Variations in the level of negative impact experienced by sex, relationship and living status. *Addiction Research and Theory.* 2012; **20** (4): 300–6.

26 Dussaillant F., Fernandez M. Alcohol's harm to others' well-being and health: A comparison between Chile and Australia. *Alcohol and Alcoholism.* 2015; **50** (3): 346–51.

27 Rognmo K., Torvik F. A., Roysamb E., Tambs K. Alcohol use and spousal mental distress in a population sample: the Nord-Trondelag health study. *BMC Public Health.* 2013; **13** (1): 852.

28 Casswell S., You R. Q., Huckle T. Alcohol's harm to others: Reduced wellbeing and health status for those with heavy drinkers in their lives. *Addiction.* 2011; **106** (6): 1087–94.

29 Orford J., Templeton L., Copello A., Velleman R., Ibanga A. Working with teams and organizations to help them involve family members. *Drugs: Education, Prevention and Policy.* 2010; **17** (sup1): 154–64.

30 Orford J., Copello A., Velleman R., Templeton L. Family members affected by a close relative's addiction: The stress-strain-coping support model. *Drugs: Education, Prevention and Policy.* 2010; **17** (S1): 36–43.

31 McCrady B. S. To have but one true friend: Implications for practice of research on alcohol use disorders and social networks. *Psychology of Addictive Behaviors.* 2004; **18** (2): 113–21.

32 Longabaugh R., Wirtz P. W., Zywiak W. H., O'Malley S. S. Network support as a prognostic indicator of drinking outcomes: The COMBINE study. *Journal of Studies on Alcohol and Drugs.* 2010; **71**: 837–46.

33 Beattie M. C., Longabaugh R. Interpersonal factors and post-treatment drinking and subjective well-being. *Addiction.* 1997; **92** (11): 1507–21.

34 Booth B. M., Russell D. W., Soucek S., Laughlin P. R. Social support and outcome of alcoholism treatment: An exploratory analysis. *The American Journal of Drug and Alcohol Abuse.* 1992; **18** (1): 87–101.

35 Gordon A. J., Zrull M. Social networks and recovery: One year after inpatient treatment. *Journal of Substance Abuse Treatment.* 1991; **8** (3): 143–52.

36 Zywiak W. H., Longabaugh R., Wirtz P. W. Decomposing the relationships between pre-treatment social network characteristics and alcohol treatment outcome. *Journal of Studies on Alcohol.* 2002; **63**: 114–21.

37 McCrady B. S., Hayaki J., Epstein E. E., Hirsch L. S. Testing hypothesized predictors of change in conjoint behavioral alcoholism treatment for men. *Alcoholism: Clinical and Experimental Research*. 2002; **26** (4): 463–70.

38 Copello A., Orford J., Hodgson R., Tober G., Barrett C. Social behaviour and network therapy – basic principles and early experiences. *Addictive Behaviours*. 2002; **27** (3): 345–66.

39 UKATT Research Team. Effectiveness of treatment for alcohol problems: Findings of the randomised UK alcohol treatment trial (UKATT). *BMJ*. 2005; **331** (7516): 541–4.

40 UKATT Research Team. Cost effectiveness of treatment for alcohol problems: Findings of the randomised UK alcohol treatment trial (UKATT). *BMJ*. 2005; **331** (7516): 544–8.

41 Copello A., Williamson E., Orford J., Day E. Implementing and evaluating social behaviour and network therapy in drug treatment practice in the UK: A feasibility study. *Addictive Behaviors*. 2006; **31** (5): 802–10.

42 Day E., Copello A., Seddon J. L., Christie M., Bamber D., Powell C. et al. A pilot feasibility randomised controlled trial of an adjunct brief social network intervention in opiate substitution treatment services. *BMC Psychiatry*. 2018; **18** (1): 8.

43 Cook S., Heather N., McCambridge J. Post-treatment motivation and outcome 9 months later. Findings from structural equation modelling. *Journal of Consulting and Clinical Psychology*. 2014; advance online publication.

44 Copello A., Orford J. Addiction and the family: Is it time for services to take notice of the evidence? *Addiction*. 2002; **97**: 1361–3.

45 Day E. *Routes to Recovery via the Community*. London: Public Health England; 2013.

Addiction Recovery Mutual-Aid Organisations

John F. Kelly, Alexandra Abry and Brandon G. Bergman

Introduction

Alcohol and other drug use disorders and related conditions confer a prodigious burden of disease, disability and premature mortality in middle- and high-income countries globally [1, 2]. The economic costs of these on most societies also often runs into the hundreds of billions annually. In response, most societies implement various public health, social policy and treatment measures to address these endemic problems. While professional treatment implementation efforts are considerable, the prevalence and chronic nature of these conditions and long-term susceptibility to substance use disorder (SUD) recurrence – especially during the first five years of recovery – mean that professional resources alone are typically stretched to cope with demand for long-term recovery monitoring and management strategies that can support and sustain remission over the long term. Perhaps in tacit recognition of these challenges, particularly by sufferers and their families themselves, a number of indigenous, free community-based peer-led resources have emerged and grown substantially in many countries to help initiate and sustain recovery-related changes.

The oldest and most prevalent among these are mutual-help organisations (MHOs; also referred to as mutual-aid or self-help groups), such as Alcoholics Anonymous (AA), Narcotics Anonymous and other 12-step-based entities, as well as newer entities, such as SMART Recovery, LifeRing, Women for Sobriety and Celebrate Recovery [3]. These organisations differ in origin, scope, prevalence, theoretical orientation and behaviour change and maintenance strategies. At the same time, there are many therapeutic elements common to these ostensibly different organisations, which may confer the majority of the therapeutic benefits derived from engagement [4, 5].

Mutual-Help Organisation Theory and Evidence

In this section, we describe five major MHOs that focus on helping individuals with SUD and other addictive disorders: 12-step MHOs; SMART Recovery; LifeRing; Women For Sobriety; and Celebrate Recovery. First, we briefly outline each of these organisation's origin, growth and prevalence. This is followed by a description of their theoretical orientation and purported mobilisers and mechanisms of behaviour change. In the final section under each of these MHOs, we review the research evidence on their effectiveness, cost-effectiveness and evidence for mobilisers and mechanisms of behaviour change. We begin with the oldest, and largest, of these MHOs: AA and other 12-step MHOs.

12-Step Mutual Aid

Origin, Growth and Prevalence

The 1920s and 1930s in the United States saw the rise of The Oxford Group, a religious organisation based on Christian principles wherein many alcoholics sought refuge, despite the fact that the group was not explicitly designed for those seeking recovery from alcoholism [3, 6]. In 1935, while on a business trip to Akron, Ohio, an Oxford Group member by the name of William Griffith Wilson, who had been abstinent from alcohol for several months, found himself at risk of relapse. Another Oxford Group member and former school friend of Wilson's, Edwin ('Ebby') Thatcher, had instilled in him the importance of 'talking to other drunks' in order to stay sober himself. Recognising he was about to begin drinking again, Wilson picked up the hotel lobby telephone and eventually found 'another drunk' through another Oxford Group member. This person happened to be an alcohol-addicted physician who lived in Akron, Dr Robert Holbrook Smith. Smith (known today as 'Dr Bob') reluctantly met with Wilson (known today as 'Bill W.'), but the meeting turned into several hours of conversation in what would later be identified as the first ever Alcoholics Anonymous meeting [6]. In their meeting, both men identified how connecting over their shared experiences and struggles could foster hope, understanding and strength. With the help of the continued daily support of Bill W., Dr Bob managed to stay sober. This included them both continuing to meet with other alcoholics and they soon developed a network of support operating through the Oxford Group meetings. Over time, however, there was increasing discomfort in this fledgling alcohol-recovery support organisation (which was to become AA) surrounding its emphasis on religion, as well as its non-alcohol addiction-specific focus [6]. Therefore, this fledgling group broke away from the Oxford Group to focus explicitly on those who struggled with 'alcoholism' and in 1939 published the so-called Big Book (*Alcoholics Anonymous*), documenting for the first time the initial 12-step recovery programme that the first several dozen cases had followed to achieve recovery [7].

As AA continued to grow rapidly throughout the 1940s and early 1950s, the organisation gained more experience in the application of the 12-step programme and was also gaining experience in how best to run AA groups and organise the now international entity. It formally documented these organisational policies and elaborated its thinking about its 12-step programme in a subsequent text entitled, *Twelve Steps and Twelve Traditions* [6, 8]. These 'traditions' continue to serve as guidelines designed to facilitate optimal group functioning and unity among members. One tradition, for example, includes having only a single membership requirement, which is 'the desire to stop drinking', while another tradition outlines the group's commitment to neither support nor oppose any outside causes (political, religious or otherwise) so as not to detract from the group's main purpose [8]. AA also decided to remain financially self-sufficient (Tradition 7), declining to take or seek outside donations or to have property of any kind. This principle of 'corporate poverty' [8] also limited donations from AA members themselves, with most countries prohibiting members from donating more than US$3,000 per year.

AA's model has since resonated with countless millions of individuals who have sought help and support from AA for nearly a century. Since its inception, the organisation has grown exponentially, spreading across the United States and throughout the world. AA reports that as of 2019 there were more than 125,000 registered groups with over 2.1 million members across 181 countries worldwide [9]. These estimates are likely conservative, however, given that AA does not maintain formal membership lists and relies instead on reports from only those groups that have general service offices [9]. AA's most recent membership survey in the USA (in 2014) characterises its members as consisting of slightly more males (62 per cent), white (89 per cent) and employed or retired (92 per cent) members [10]. AA members report attending an average of two to three meetings per week, with 86 per cent reporting that they have a 'home' group, and 82 per cent reporting they have a 'sponsor' (a mentor, typically with more sober time and recovery experience). Particularly intriguing is that members' lengths of sobriety span a wide range of time, with a somewhat even distribution (27 per cent reporting less than 1 year, 24 per cent 1–5 years, 13 per cent 5–10 years, 14 per cent 10–20 years and 22 per cent more than 20 years) [15]. Overall, members report being sober for nearly 10 years on average [10].

Theoretical Orientation and Purported Mobilisers and Mechanisms of Behaviour Change

In the introduction to the Big Book (*Alcoholics Anonymous*, 1939), Dr Silkworth – an addiction physician at a New York city hospital who treated Bill W. on several occasions, but not a member of AA – posited that individuals with alcohol addiction suffer from something akin to, though not technically, a physiological 'allergy', which triggers uncontrollable alcohol craving and consumption [7]. This so-called allergy is, according to Silkworth, indicative of a set of biological attributes that are unique to individuals with alcohol addiction. This theory lends itself to the idea of 'powerlessness', which is central to the 12-step ideology and refers to the belief that individuals with alcohol addiction have lost control over their alcohol use, and need to find another source of power beyond themselves for help [8]. The need to surrender oneself to a 'higher power' is also fundamental to AA. A higher power can take many forms, ranging from a more formal deity, to an individual's AA sponsor or to the AA organisation itself [7, 8].

The main AA text also posits that certain characterological factors such as 'selfishness' and 'self-centeredness' play a role in the development and maintenance of alcoholism [7]. For example, 'selfishness' and 'self-centeredness' purportedly foster fear and resentment in the individual, leading to continued alcohol use. Other personality flaws, referred to as 'character defects', are outlined in Steps 6 and 7 of the Twelve Steps and Twelve Traditions [8]. These are, according to AA, the result of insatiable, fear-driven urges to satisfy one's instinctual drive for security (both emotional and financial), social status and sexual relationships [7]. When taken together such ideas foster the notion that alcoholics are disturbed by 'unsatisfied demands' that ultimately lead to 'character defects', which includes heavy alcohol use as well as 'spiritual decay'. The ideas expressed in The Big Book [7] and the Twelve Steps and Twelve Traditions [8] suggest that AA views addiction as being caused and maintained by psychological, physical and spiritual factors. These three primary factors are akin to contemporary theories that can be applied to addiction, such as the stress and coping models, self-medication and psychodynamic models, as well as the biological disease model.

Assuming AA does in fact view addiction as having complex, multifaceted and physical roots, it might follow that AA is supportive of the use of medication treatment. However, anecdotal evidence has raised concern that as an organisation AA is not supportive of the use of medication treatment among its members. While some evidence suggests that AA members are generally supportive of the use of relapse prevention medications (e.g. acamprosate, naltrexone, disulfiram) and psychotropic medications (e.g. antidepressants, antipsychotics) [11], there is also evidence that some individuals oppose the use of such medications (e.g. see [12]). However, research on the latter group has found AA participation to be unrelated to individuals' opposition to medication use, which may instead be a perspective more generally held among some individuals in or seeking recovery, rather than one that is unique to AA [3, 12]. Nonetheless, due to the importance of medication treatment for some individuals in recovery, AA published a pamphlet to somewhat clarify its position, stating that is wrong to deny members the right to medication treatment [3].

However, as this quote from the Big Book shows, AA believes spirituality above all to be the solution for members: 'The great fact is just this and nothing less: That we have had deep and effective spiritual experiences which have revolutionized our whole attitude toward life' [7, p. 25]. Originally put forth in 1939, the idea that members achieve recovery through spiritual awakening has prevailed to present [13]. This purported mechanism of change has since garnered empirical attention as part of a larger body of research on the mechanisms of behavioural change in AA which is discussed in more detail below.

Evidence for Effectiveness, Cost-Effectiveness and Mobilisers and Mechanisms of Behaviour Change

Given its growth and success in helping members achieve and maintain sobriety AA and to some extent other 12-step organisations such as Narcotics Anonymous (NA) have garnered significant empirical attention. Hundreds of studies have demonstrated AA's benefits and efficacy in helping individuals attain sobriety and recover from alcohol and other drug problems. These effects have been summarised in various meta-analyses and narrative reviews that cover decades of research (e.g. see [14, 15]). A recent Cochrane review [16] has evaluated the efficacy of AA and professionally delivered treatments that facilitate AA involvement (i.e. Twelve-Step Facilitation [TSF]) compared to other clinical interventions (e.g. cognitive-behavioural therapies [CBT], motivational enhancement therapy [MET]) and other 12-step programme variants (i.e. TSF that varied in style or intensity from the intervention condition) for adults with alcohol use disorder. Researchers examined a total of 27 studies yielding 36 published reports and found that when compared to other clinical interventions or 12-step programme variants, AA/TSF often led to significant and often substantial advantages in continuous abstinence and remission, as well as in percent days abstinent (PDA), though to a lesser degree than aiding continuous abstinence. For other important outcomes including measures of drinking intensity and alcohol-related consequence, AA/TSF produced better outcomes in approximately half of the reports and performed equally as well as other treatments in the other half. Of note, there was only one instance across all studies and all outcomes where TSF/AA performed worse (on PDA) than the comparison treatment, which was in a study of dual-diagnosis participants. However, a meta-analysis of the research on participants who suffer from psychiatric illnesses in addition to alcohol/drug addiction found fairly consistent benefits on par with members without such psychiatric comorbidity [17]. Overall, however, AA/TSF produced lasting changes that were not only as effective as, but in many cases better than, other interventions. Moreover, of the five economic studies included in the review, four found substantial cost saving benefits for AA/TSF relative to other treatments (e.g. CBT). Consequently, AA's free and widespread availability, along with its effectiveness and cost-effectiveness, has been described as the closest thing in public health to a free lunch [18].

In another recent systematic review researchers examined the effectiveness of 12-step MHOs in reducing illicit drug use when compared to a range of psychosocial interventions (e.g. cognitive behavioural training, medication treatment, relapse prevention), and in some cases to no 12-step MHO attendance [19]. Among the seven studies included in the review, there were no differences in primary drug outcomes (e.g. abstinence, reduction in drug use) when comparing 12-step programmes to other psychosocial interventions. The finding that 12-step programmes are equally as effective as various other treatments for drug use is somewhat inconsistent with the largely positive findings from the Cochrane systematic review, and should be interpreted with caution given the small number of studies included in the review coupled with the heterogeneity in comparison conditions across studies. Nonetheless, the overall body of existing evidence on AA/TSF points to 12-step groups as an effective, low-cost and accessible resource for individuals in or seeking recovery.

With the demonstrated efficacy of AA/TSF come questions regarding the mechanisms of behaviour change through which 12-step organisations help to facilitate continued remission from alcohol addiction. As previously mentioned, AA claims that spirituality is the main mechanism through which change occurs and recovery is achieved [7]. However, emerging empirical evidence suggests that this is only true for a minority of those who attend AA with high addiction severity [13]. Thus, rather than helping members through a single primary mechanism, evidence supports the notion that AA helps different people in different ways, suggesting that people may use AA differently to help to cope with various challenges present in their own particular life contexts and stage of recovery [13]. For example, men have been found to derive benefit from AA's ability to help them cope with high-risk social situations without drinking. In contrast, women have been found to derive more benefit from AA's ability to help them to cope with negative affect without drinking, thereby decreasing their risk for relapse [13, 20]. Moreover, older adults (aged 30+ years) benefit from AA through its ability to help them eradicate high-risk/heavy drinkers and adopt abstainers into their social networks, whereas young adults (18–29 years) are more likely to benefit by eradicating heavy drinkers from their social networks but not by adopting abstainers into their networks [13]. This may be due to the fact that the social networks of young people are more likely to contain heavy drinkers, and the low proportion of young people in AA may mean it is more difficult for these younger participants to find new sober friends in AA and thus adopt more abstainers through AA [21].

In addition to fostering spirituality, facilitating adaptive social network changes and increasing abstinence self-efficacy, AA has been shown to work also by decreasing craving and impulsivity [13]. In sum, the mechanisms research so far has explained approximately 50 per cent of the direct effect of AA on increasing abstinence and reducing relapse risk. Studies of moderated multiple mediation (e.g. [20–22]) that detail the relative importance of different mechanisms and how these differ across different individuals show that the benefits that people derive from AA participation differ in nature and magnitude, influenced by degree of addiction severity, gender and age.

As noted, support for AA's model coupled with the increased availability of illicit substances and addiction to other drugs has led to the adaptation of the AA model for those seeking recovery from drugs other than alcohol [3]. To date, the largest of these groups is Narcotics Anonymous (NA), which was founded in 1953. Many other substance-specific 12-step organisations have since emerged, including Marijuana Anonymous (1989), Cocaine Anonymous (1982) and Crystal Meth Anonymous (1994) [3]. In recognition of the overlap between comorbid psychiatric illnesses and substance use, dual-diagnosis MHOs – for example, Dual-Disorders Anonymous (1982), Double-Trouble in Recovery (1993) – have also developed in an effort to concurrently address both sets of challenges [3]. Furthermore, Al-Anon (1951), Alateen (1957) and Nar-Anon (1968) were established using the 12-step model to support family members of addicted love ones. Yet, despite the success of AA and the numerous groups that were established using the 12-steps and 12-traditions model, many non-12-step MHOs emerged as alternatives. Non-12-step MHOs are examined next.

SMART Recovery

Origin, Growth and Prevalence

In describing SMART Recovery it is first necessary to consider its precursor, Rational Recovery (RR). RR emerged in the late 1980s in opposition to AA and many of its defining features [6]. Its founder Jack Trimpey strongly rejected AA's spiritual components and conceptualisation of addiction as a disease, as well as several of its other defining principles. The organisation consequently put forth guiding principles that stood in direct opposition to those of AA. For example, inspired in part by Albert Ellis' rational emotive behavioural therapy, Rational Recovery conceptualised the process of recovery from addiction as one driven by individual self-control, rather than peer support or spiritual experiences. Unlike AA and other MHOs, Trimpey further divided Rational Recovery into two organisations: the Rational Recovery Self-Help Network, which was not for-profit, and Rational Recovery, which was a for-profit organisation intended to provide professional addiction services. In 1994 the Rational Recovery Self-Help Network broke from the Rational Recovery organisation and its founder to become the group, Self-Management and Recovery Training, also known as SMART Recovery.

Leaving behind Rational Recovery's outward opposition to AA but maintaining its cognitive behavioural roots, SMART Recovery draws on evidence-based practices. Its aim is to 'support individuals who have chosen to abstain, or are considering abstinence from, any type of addictive behaviour (substances or activities), by teaching how to change self-defeating thinking, emotions, and actions; and to work towards long-term satisfactions and quality of life' [23]. The organisation has grown both nationally and internationally since splitting from Rational Recovery, with SMART Recovery currently reporting that there are more than 2,700 weekly meetings held across 24 countries, including more than 1,500 meetings in the United States alone [3, 23].

A systematic review of 12 studies on SMART Recovery (eight peer-reviewed studies and four unpublished dissertations) characterised its membership as follows: the mean gender distribution ranged from 39 per cent to 71 per cent male; the mean age of participants ranged from 34 to 51 years; the majority of participants were Caucasian; between 31 per cent and 63 per cent of participants were employed in either part- or full-time positions; and co-occurring mental health problems were found to be common among members [23]. These somewhat broad ranges in demographic characteristics can be attributed to heterogeneity across studies in the systematic review, which included a variety of different sample sizes and sample groups (e.g. dual-diagnosis participants, custodial offenders). Moreover, although SMART Recovery has a secular orientation, the majority of its members report believing in a God or higher power (60.7 per cent) and attending AA in addition to SMART Recovery (85.2 per cent) [3].

Theoretical Orientation and Purported Mobilisers and Mechanisms of Behaviour Change

SMART Recovery views addictions and compulsions as complex maladaptive behaviours that individuals can recover from using self-directed change [3, 6]. It therefore endeavours to equip members with the tools and techniques necessary to create and maintain motivation to abstain from addictive substances and activities; cope with urges to use substances or engage in addictive behaviours; manage thoughts, feelings and behaviours; and achieve a balanced lifestyle. The group further advocates for the 'appropriate use of prescribed medications and psychological treatments' and is committed to evolving with scientific knowledge. SMART Recovery is different from other mutual-help organisations in that, while still capitalising on peer support dynamics, meetings are led by trained facilitators, are didactic (e.g. teaching cognitive behavioural coping skills) and teach self-reliance and self-empowerment. The organisation's reliance on trained facilitators provides elements of standardisation and 'quality control' from group to group, optimising adherence to the SMART model, but the training element may also limit its growth compared to the more laissez faire approach of other MHOs like AA where anybody can start a meeting anywhere in the world as long as it adheres roughly to the 12 traditions [8].

Evidence for Effectiveness, Cost-Effectiveness and Mobilisers and Mechanisms of Behaviour Change

To date, only a very small number of studies have evaluated the effectiveness of SMART Recovery. In their systematic review, Beck and colleagues reported that there was only one randomised controlled trial (RCT) that evaluated the effectiveness of attending SMART Recovery [24]. Specifically, Campbell and colleagues evaluated the effect of SMART Recovery participation on outcomes related to substance use when compared to participation in Overcoming Addictions, a web-based application informed by SMART Recovery, either alone or in combination with SMART Recovery [24]. Researchers found that participants across all three groups improved on drinking-related outcomes (per cent days abstinent, drinks per drinking day and alcohol-related problems) at the three month follow-up. However, between the three and six month follow-up the Overcoming Addictions and Overcoming Addictions + SMART Recovery groups slightly regressed, whereas the SMART Recovery only group continued to improve on substance use outcomes. It is important to note that the meeting rates for the SMART Recovery only and Overcoming Addictions only groups dropped from an average of 3.17 to 1.86 in-person meetings and from 5.85 to 3.02 online meetings, respectively, between the three and six month follow-ups, with 78 per cent of SMART Recovery and 66 per cent of Overcoming Addictions participants attending no meetings between follow-ups. Although the meeting attendance rate for SMART Recovery dropped more sharply than that of Overcoming Addictions and the majority of participants did not attend SMART Recovery meetings between three and six months, the SMART Recovery only group continued to improve on substance-related outcomes, suggesting that SMART Recovery could have positive, enduring effects even with low levels of meeting attendance. Though one could speculate that this continued improvement could be due to the cognitive behavioural skills they have developed, or to the recovery-specific social support derived from face-to-face SMART Recovery meetings – as evidenced in literature examining AA [13, 22] – much more research is needed to examine the efficacy of SMART Recovery and its mechanisms of behaviour change.

Most recently, Zemore and colleagues conducted the first longitudinal study to evaluate substance use and related outcomes among those attending non-12-step MHOs [25]. In this study, researchers surveyed non-12-step (i.e. LifeRing, Women for Sobriety and SMART Recovery) as well as 12-step meeting attendees at baseline, six and twelve months. Although their evidence suggests that SMART Recovery, WFS, LifeRing and 12-step groups are equally as effective, participants who self-identified SMART Recovery as their primary group at baseline had significantly worse substance use outcomes (alcohol abstinence, total abstinence, no alcohol problems) when compared to 12-step members after controlling for covariates. However, this effect was no longer evident once researchers controlled for participants' baseline alcohol goals, which ranged from complete lifetime abstinence to controlled substance use.

Although the aforementioned study represents a positive step towards a better understanding of the effectiveness of SMART Recovery (as well as other non-12-step MHOs), the group has received relatively little empirical attention since its inception overall, despite steady growth. Existing evidence suggests there are benefits associated with SMART Recovery participation. For example, studies characterising members' perceptions suggest they find SMART Recovery's meetings, group experience and cognitive behavioural tools to be helpful to their recovery [5]. Preliminary evidence from a pilot study of SMART Recovery members also suggests that a longer length of affiliation with the group and frequent meeting attendance are associated with increased self-efficacy to refuse substances [26]. In light of these encouraging findings and SMART Recovery's continued growth, there are numerous research opportunities available to assess the efficacy of SMART Recovery in relation to other mutual-help organisations, as well as potential healthcare cost savings associated with the group.

LifeRing

Origin, Growth and Prevalence

James Christopher held the first meeting of SOS – an acronym for both Save Our Selves and Secular Organization for Sobriety – in North Hollywood, California, in 1986 [6]. Initially turning to AA for help with his recovery, Christopher found himself uncomfortable with its emphasis on spirituality and a higher power, as well as its conceptualisation of alcoholism as a disease. SOS thus emerged as an abstinence-based secular organisation that views alcoholism as an illness with psychological, biological and genetic factors. As SOS does not have a clearly defined course of action for its members, individual members are responsible for forging their own paths to sobriety, although they are encouraged to use the experiences of group members who have achieved sobriety as guidance [3]. There has been very little research on SOS membership, with Connors and Dermen conducting the largest survey of SOS members (n = 158) to date [27]. The response rate for this study was particularly low (approximately 15–29 per cent), but provides the only glimpse of SOS membership, which found that SOS members are largely Caucasian, male, well-educated and non-religious [3, 27].

As the consequence of a legal issue over its name, the largest chapter of SOS changed its name to LifeRing Secular Recovery in 1999 and then established itself as its own national organisation in 2001 [6]. A membership survey issued by the LifeRing organisation in 2005 (n = 401) found that members were largely Caucasian and well educated (80 per cent attended some college, 44 per cent had undergraduate degrees or higher) [28]. Of note, 45 per cent of respondents reported being diagnosed with a co-occurring mental illness and approximately one-third of members reported that they attended AA in addition to LifeRing.

Theoretical Orientation and Purported Mobilisers and Mechanisms of Behaviour Change

LifeRing follows a secular recovery model and strongly emphasises the importance of developing an individualised, self-driven path to recovery wherein each member is responsible for strengthening their 'sober self' and weakening their 'addict self' [28]. Empowering the sober self involves three components known as recognition, activation and mastery, which serve to recognise the existence of the sober self and its role in guiding the individual to their current place in life, to live a sober life and to face the challenges recovery poses, and developing one's own Personal Recovery Program (PRP), respectively. Personal Recovery Programs can either develop organically, or be more strategically cultivated with the help of Recovery By Choice, the organisation's workbook that helps members develop their PRP across nine recovery-related domains [3].

Evidence for Effectiveness, Cost-Effectiveness and Mobilisers and Mechanisms of Behaviour Change

Beyond the organisation's 2005 member survey LifeRing has received very little empirical attention since its inception. As previously mentioned, Zemore and colleagues conducted the first longitudinal study to compare non-12-step MHOs (i.e. LifeRing, Women for Sobriety and SMART Recovery) to 12-step MHOs [25]. They found all groups to be equally effective, but that those who affiliated with LifeRing at baseline had significantly lower odds of total abstinence at six and twelve month follow-up. However, this effect was no longer evident once researchers controlled for participants' baseline alcohol goal, which ranged from complete lifetime abstinence to controlled substance use. More research is needed to better understand LifeRing members and the impact of LifeRing on substance use and related outcomes.

Women for Sobriety

Origin, Growth and Prevalence

Born from the belief that women in recovery have needs that differ from their male counterparts, Women for Sobriety (WFS) was established in 1975. Jean Kilpatrick, a woman in recovery, found that AA did not meet her needs and endeavoured to create a space wherein women, free from gender-role expectations and independent from men, could join together to share experiences, shed feelings of guilt and shame and forge individual paths to recovery with the help and support of their peers. WFS is primarily based in the United States, though the organisation also has a small number of groups in England, Canada, New Zealand and Australia (an estimated total of 150–300 groups worldwide) [6]. Its membership base is relatively modest, with estimates suggesting the organisation is comprised of 1,000–2,000 members [8], the majority of whom are Caucasian, middle-class and well-educated [29].

Theoretical Orientation and Purported Mobilisers and Mechanisms of Behaviour Change

As reflected in the group's Thirteen Statements of Acceptance, WFS is largely centred on affirming each individual woman's value and worth, which leads women to increased self-confidence and the belief that they are able to overcome their drinking and other problems.

These statements, which include affirmations such as 'I am a competent woman and have much to give life,' and 'Problems bother me only to the degree I permit them to' were also created with the intention of building up, rather than minimising, the self [6]. Kilpatrick viewed minimalisation of the self as inherent to AA's principles, which she asserted was appropriate for 'arrogant' men, but damaging to female alcoholics who struggled with self-esteem and confidence [8]. The centrality of confidence-building affirmations in WFS is further reflected in the group's meeting structure. At the start of each meeting, each member introduces herself by saying her name, followed by the statement 'and I am a competent woman' [6].

Other defining features of WFS include the organisation's belief that lifetime membership and use of sponsors (as in AA) fosters dependency rather than independence, and therefore neither uses sponsors nor encourages lifetime membership. Related to this notion of independence, WFS encourages members to take credit for their own abstinence and does not embrace anonymity as one of its principles, leaving it up to each individual member to decide whether or not to disclose their status as a person in recovery and a WFS member [6, 30]. Furthermore, WFS is abstinence based and draws on cognitive strategies, positive reinforcement, relaxation techniques and meditation, among other strategies, to help members to change their behaviour and attain sobriety.

Evidence for Effectiveness, Cost-Effectiveness and Mobilisers and Mechanisms of Behaviour Change

WFS has received very little empirical attention. In their study comparing non-12-step groups (i.e. LifeRing, Women for Sobriety and SMART Recovery) to 12-step groups, Zemore et al. found that Women for Sobriety was equally as effective as the other 12-step and non-12-step MHOs among active members [25]. As with other non-12-step groups, much more research is needed on WFS to better understand its ability to engage and retain members, its effectiveness and to identify which factors (other than gender identity) set this group's membership base apart from that of other MHOs.

Celebrate Recovery

Origin, Growth and Prevalence

In contrast to the overtly spiritual emphasis of AA and 12-step MHOs, and the secular emphasis of most of the others mentioned so far (LifeRing, SMART; to a lesser extent WFS, which contains spiritual elements), John Baker established Celebrate Recovery in 1991 at Saddleback Church in California to be overtly religiously oriented. After entering recovery with the support of AA, Baker sought to create a separate group wherein he could openly discuss his Christian values and beliefs [3]. Building upon the 12 steps for those seeking a 'Christ-centered' treatment, he created an additional Eight Recovery Principles that delineate the group's Christian interpretation of the concept of a higher power and that are supported by Christian scripture [3, 31]. Baker outlined his inspiration for Celebrate Recovery – developed through his vision from God – in a letter to his pastor, Rick Warren. Warren provided his blessing for the group, prompting Baker to hold the first Celebrate Recovery meeting, which 43 people attended. The organisation has since grown, with the faith-based MHO reporting that it currently operates more than 14 types of groups across 35,000 churches worldwide, as well as in prisons, recovery houses, universities and rescue missions.

Theoretical Orientation and Purported Mobilisers and Mechanisms of Behaviour Change

Celebrate Recovery meetings follow a similar format to other 12-step meetings and are not only open to those with substance use problems, but also anyone who is having trouble changing a problematic pattern of behaviour [3]. Meetings typically start as one large group and then break into smaller groups based on content and gender. Members are encouraged to have individual mentors, who function much like an AA sponsor, but who place a more explicit emphasis on spiritual growth. Celebrate Recovery members also have 'accountability partners' who are at a similar stage in recovery, who are facing similar challenges and who can provide extra support between meetings and through prayer [3].

For members ready to progress further in evaluating their past and their decisions, Celebrate Recovery has step study groups. The group's 12 steps, based on those of AA, guide members' step work with the addition of biblical comparisons – e.g. '1. We admitted we were powerless over our addictions and compulsive behaviours. That our lives had become unmanageable. I know that nothing good lives in me, that is, in my sinful nature. For I have the desire to do what is good, but I cannot carry it out. (Romans 7:18).' The organisation's Eight Recovery Principles, known also as 'the Beatitudes', are from Christian scripture (e.g. 'Happy are the pure in heart' and 'Happy are those whose greatest desire is to do what God requires') and are also believed to help members pave a way towards 'wholeness' and 'spiritual maturity'. Together, these steps and principles are designed to support members in or seeking recovery.

Evidence for Effectiveness, Cost-Effectiveness and Mobilisers and Mechanisms of Behaviour Change

Formal research on Celebrate Recovery, its membership and its efficacy is lacking. Due to its broader focus on problematic patterns of behaviour (including, but not limited to, substance use), it is possible that the group could attract a larger group of members seeking support than a group focusing only on substance use would. Conversely, the group's broader focus could also act as a deterrent to some who may experience the group as being less cohesive and find less mutual identification among members [3]. Such questions require empirical investigation to answer and could be examined in preliminary research designed to first characterise the Celebrate Recovery membership base.

Discussion and Future Directions

In addiction it is arguably the initial social factors (observational learning, initial offers, support for initial use) that lead to positive expectancies about substance use and initial exposure, which in turn lead to behavioural experience, learning and related psychological changes. With repeated exposure the now well-known physiological changes in the brain that cause addiction occur [32]. In recovery, the same processes occur in the same direction; social changes towards non-substance-using social networks (e.g. those often provided by MHOs) lead to psychological changes ('unlearning' processes of de-conditioning, and new learning processes involved in cognitive restructuring) which in turn lead to abstinence-based physiological re-adaptations and change.

Several lines of research suggest that the abstinence-oriented social support provided by mutual-aid can help to provide assiduous daily monitoring and support (e.g. through an AA sponsor) that can facilitate avoidance of exposure to high-risk conditioned cues, provide immediate social reward and impart new cognitive and behavioural coping skills to mitigate stress-related relapse risk. This is likely to lead to neuroendocrine and neurobiological changes (e.g. accelerated upregulation of dopamine D2 receptor density; decreased stress hormones such as corticotropin releasing factor [CRF]/cortisol, and increased oxytocin) among affected addicted individuals [33].

As noted, although each MHO has its own particular theory about how best to address substance use disorders or other addictive behaviours, there are many commonalities. Group therapy theory holds promise for conceptualising some of the benefits of MHO participation because it espouses social dynamic interpersonal constructs and has many similarities with mutual aid [34]. The group theory therapeutic elements of universality, cohesion, instillation of hope, catharsis, observational learning, imparting of information and altruism are all arguably operating within and across MHOs, which all run similarly in group format and are by nature social interpersonal organisations. In fact, in several studies conducted across different MHOs including 12-step and non-12-step, that have investigated systematically members' responses regarding what they perceive they gain from MHO participation, many such elements emerge as most important, particularly the sense of belonging ('universality') and togetherness ('cohesiveness') and instillation of hope [35].

Research across several treatment approaches suggests that the majority of professional interventions use common processes (i.e. they all contain a therapeutic supportive relationship that mobilises motivation for change, active coping and change self-efficacy [36]). It is also possible that the main benefit of MHOs is that they provide access and exposure to therapeutic components that mobilise the same helpful recovery mechanisms that are mobilised by formal interventions [13], but can do this for free, over the long term, in the communities in which people live [4]. This is the essence of what is called recovery management [37]. While preliminary research exists supporting a range of MHOs, more rigorous research will help to determine whether certain MHOs offer particular advantages over others, and whether certain subgroups of individuals appear better suited to some than others.

References

1 Degenhardt L., Whiteford H., Hall W. D. The Global Burden of Disease projects: What have we learned about illicit drug use and dependence and their contribution to the global burden of disease? *Drug and Alcohol Review*. 2014;33 (1):4–12.

2 Rehm J., Mathers C., Popova S., Thavorncharoensap M., Teerawattananon Y., Patra J. Global burden of disease and injury and economic cost attributable to alcohol use and alcohol-use disorders. *The Lancet*. 2009; 373 (9682): 2223–33.

3 Kelly J. F., White W. L. Broadening the base of addiction mutual-help organizations. *Journal of Groups in Addiction and Recovery*. 2012; 7 (2–4): 82–101.

4 Kelly J. F., Magill M., Stout R. L. How do people recover from alcohol dependence? A systematic review on mechanisms of behaviour change in Alcoholics Anonymous. *Addiction Research and Theory*. 2009; 17 (3): 236–59.

5 Kelly P. J., Raftery D., Deane F. P., Baker A. L., Hunt D., Shakeshaft A. From both sides: Participant and facilitator perceptions of SMART Recovery groups. *Drug and Alcohol Review*. 2017; 36 (3): 325–32.

6 Humphreys K. *Circles of Recovery: Self-Help Organizations for Addiction*. Cambridge: Cambridge University Press; 2004.

7 Alcoholics Anonymous. *Alcoholics Anonymous: The Story of How Thousands of Men and Women Have Recovered from Alcoholism*. 4th ed. New York: Alcoholics Anonymous World Services; 2001.

8   Alcoholics Anonymous. *Twelve Steps and Twelve Traditions*. New York: Alcoholics Anonymous World Services; 1952.

9   Alcoholics Anonymous. *Estimates of AA Groups and Members as of January 1, 2019*. New York: Alcoholics Anonymous General Service Office; 2019.

10 Alcoholics Anonymous. *Alcoholics Anonymous: 2014 Membership Survey*. New York: AA World Services; 2014.

11 Rychtarik R. G., Connors G. J., Dermen K. H., Stasiewicz P. R. Alcoholics Anonymous and the use of medications to prevent relapse: an anonymous survey of member attitudes. *Journal of Studies on Alcohol*. 2000; **61** (1): 134–8.

12 Tonigan J. S., Kelly J. F. Beliefs about AA and the use of medications: A comparison of three groups of AA-exposed alcohol dependent persons. *Alcoholism Treatment Quarterly*. 2004; **22** (2): 67–78.

13 Kelly J. F. Is Alcoholics Anonymous religious, spiritual, neither? Findings from 25 years of mechanisms of behavior change research. *Addiction*. 2017; **112** (6): 929–36.

14 Emrick C. D., Tonigan J. S., Montgomery H. A., Little L. Alcoholics Anonymous: What is currently known? In: *Research on Alcoholics Anonymous: Opportunities and Alternatives* (eds. B. S. McCrady, W. R. Miller). New Brunswick: Rutgers Center of Alcohol Studies; 1993; pp 41–76.

15 Tonigan J. S., Toscova R., Miller W. R. Meta-analysis of the literature on Alcoholics Anonymous: Sample and study characteristics moderate findings. *Journal of Studies on Alcohol*. 1996; **57**: 65–72.

16 Kelly J. F., Humphreys K., Ferri M. Alcoholics Anonymous and other 12-step programs for alcohol use disorder. *Cochrane Database of Systematic Reviews*. 2020 (3).

17. Tonigan J. S., Pearson M. R., Magill M., Hagler K. J. AA attendance and abstinence for dually diagnosed patients: A meta-analytic review. *Addiction*. 2018; **113** (11): 1970–81.

18 Kelly J. F. Are societies paying unnecessarily for an otherwise free lunch? Final musings on the research on Alcoholics Anonymous and its mechanisms of behavior change. *Addiction*. 2017; **112** (6): 943–5.

19 Bog M., Filges T., Brannstrom L., Jorgensen A.-M., Fredriksson M. K. 12-step programs for reducing illicit drug-use: A systematic review. *Campbell Systematic Reviews*. 2017; **13** (2).

20 Kelly J. F., Hoeppner B. A biaxial formulation of the recovery construct. *Addiction Research and Theory*. 2015; **23**(1): 5–9.

21 Hoeppner B. B., Hoeppner S. S., Kelly J. F. Do young people benefit from AA as much, and in the same ways, as adult aged 30+? A moderated multiple mediation analysis. *Drug and Alcohol Dependence*. 2014; **143**: 181–8.

22 Kelly J. F., Hoeppner B., Stout R. L., Pagano M. Determining the relative importance of the mechanisms of behavior change within Alcoholics Anonymous: A multiple mediator analysis. *Addiction*. 2012; **107** (2): 289–99.

23 Beck A. K., Forbes E., Baker A. L., Kelly P. J., Deane F. P., Shakeshaft A. et al. Systematic review of SMART recovery: Outcomes, process variables, and implications for research. *Psychology of Addictive Behaviors*. 2017; **31** (1): 1–20.

24 Campbell W., Hester R. K., Lenberg K. L., Delaney H. D. Overcoming addictions, a web-based application, and SMART recovery, an online and in-person mutual help group for problem drinkers, part 2: Six-month outcomes of a randomized controlled trial and qualitative feedback from participants. *Journal of Medical Internet Research*. 2016; **18** (10): e262-e.

25 Zemore S. E., Lui C., Mericle A., Hemberg J., Kaskutas L. A. A longitudinal study of the comparative efficacy of Women for Sobriety, LifeRing, SMART Recovery, and 12-step groups for those with AUD. *Journal of Substance Abuse Treatment*. 2018; **88** (1): 18–26.

26 O'Sullivan D., Watts J. R., Xiao Y., Bates-Maves J. Refusal self-efficacy among

SMART recovery members by affiliation length and meeting frequency. *Journal of Addictions and Offender Counseling.* 2016; **37**: 87–101.

27 Connors G. J., Dermen K. H. Characteristics of Participants in Secular Organizations for Sobriety (SOS). *American Journal of Drug and Alcohol Abuse.* 1996; **22** (2): 281–95.

28 Nicolaus M. *Empowering Your Sober Self: The LifeRing Approach to Addiction Recovery.* Oakland, CA: LifeRing Press; 2014.

29 Fenner R. M., Gifford M. H. Women for sobriety: 35 years of challenges, changes, and continuity. *Journal of Groups in Addiction and Recovery.* 2012 ;7 (2–4): 142–70.

30 Kaskutas L. A. A road less traveled: Choosing the 'Women for Sobriety' program. *Journal of Drug Issues.* 1996; **26** (1): 77–94.

31 Brown A. E., Tonigan J. S., Pavlik V. N., Kosten T. R., Volk R. J. Spirituality and confidence to resist substance use among celebrate recovery participants. *Journal of Religion and Health.* 2013; **52** (1): 107–13.

32 Volkow N. D., Koob G. F., McLellan A. T. Neurobiologic advances from the brain disease model of addiction. *New England Journal of Medicine.* 2016; **374** (4): 363–71.

33 Hostinar C. E., Sullivan R. M., Gunnar M.R. Psychobiological mechanisms underlying the social buffering of the hypothalamic-pituitary-adrenocortical axis: A review of animal models and human studies across development. *Psychological Bulletin.* 2014; **140** (1): 256–82.

34 Yalom I. D., Leszcz M. *The Theory and Practice of Group Psychotherapy,* 5th ed. New York: Basic Books; 2005.

35 Kelly J. F., Greene M. C., Bergman B. G. Recovery benefits of the 'therapeutic alliance' among 12-step mutual-help organization attendees and their sponsors. *Drug and Alcohol Dependence.* 2016; **162**: 64–71.

36 Longabaugh R., Donovan D. M., Karno M. P., McCrady B. S., Morgenstern J., Tonigan J. S. Active ingredients: How and why evidence-based alcohol behavioral treatment interventions work. *Alcoholism: Clinical and Experimental Research.* 2005; **29** (2): 235–47.

37 Kelly J. F., White W. L. *Addiction Recovery Management.* New York: Springer; 2011.

Index

For EU product safety concerns, contact us at Calle de José Abascal, 56–1°,
28003 Madrid, Spain or eugpsr@cambridge.org.

www.ingramcontent.com/pod-product-compliance
Ingram Content Group UK Ltd.
Pitfield, Milton Keynes, MK11 3LW, UK
UKHW040951090126
466816UK00019B/360